FIT FOR AMERICA

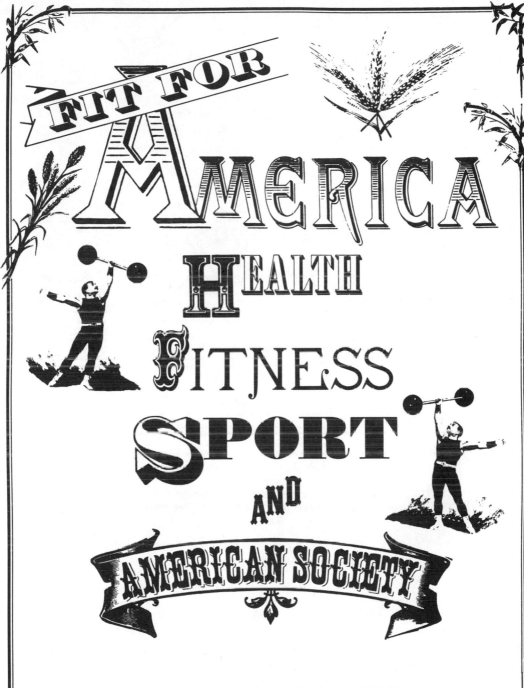

FIT FOR AMERICA

HEALTH FITNESS SPORT

AND

AMERICAN SOCIETY

HARVEY GREEN

THE JOHNS HOPKINS UNIVERSITY PRESS
Baltimore and London

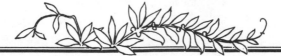

Johns Hopkins Paperbacks edition, 1988, published by arrangement
with Pantheon Books, a division of Random House, Inc.

The Johns Hopkins University Press, 701 West 40th Street
Baltimore, Maryland 21211
The Johns Hopkins Press Ltd., London

Library of Congress Cataloging-in-Publication Data

Green, Harvey, 1946–
Fit for America.

Reprint. Originally published: New York : Pantheon Books, 1986.
Includes index.
1. Physical fitness—United States—History.   2. Health attitudes—United
States—History.   I. Title. [GV510.U5G74   1988]   613.7′0973   88-45393
ISBN 0-8018-3642-5 (pbk.)

*Research for this book was made possible in part by a grant from the
National Endowment for the Humanities, a federal agency.*

Book design by Amy C. Titcomb

In Memory of Warren Susman
Mentor, Scholar, Inspiration

1.8

· CONTENTS ·

Contents

· PREFACE ·

We often think of the world in metaphor, with our bodies as the touch-stone. We speak, read, and write of the "body politic" or a "corpus of data." Such images may be the easiest to comprehend because they are so close to us.

With an understandable bias to the present, most of us think that the ideal of "good health" and the ways people try to achieve it have been a constant throughout modern history. The differences between the past and present seem only a matter of degree. The advances of medical and biological sciences have lengthened our lives, and thus our expectations are greater than our forebears'. Yet it is not true that our vision of health and our notions of the ideal body size and shape are the same as those of a century and a half ago. Similarly, we of the last quarter of the twentieth century did not invent aerobics, weight-lifting, exercise machines, "health" foods, or the variety of other ways we employ to attain the bodily state we desire. But if there has been continuity between the 1830s and the 1980s, there has also been change. Americans of the last century became interested in health, fitness, and sports for different reasons and with different hopes for themselves and for the human race than we have today. Those of the thirty years before the advent of the Civil War had ideas and concerns different from the individuals of the three decades that followed the conflict. Americans of the turn of the century and the 1920s and 1930s had theories, thoughts, and plans of action different from and in addition to those of the early nineteenth century.

This study investigates those ideas, realities, and the solutions offered to problems of health and fitness as they changed over a century. It is primarily an analysis of the American middle class—that group above the level of subsistence but below the realm of great wealth, who participated in a market economy and bought many if not most of their goods and services. The range of sources investigated includes trade materials such as catalogs of goods and advertising; diaries, letters, and journals; artifactual materials; professional texts such as medical books and athletic instructional manuals; and advice books and household guides. No one of these sources is adequate by itself. Trade catalogs do not tell the researcher that people bought items (although a series of references over time would be a strong indication of such behavior). Diaries, letters, and journals are by definition individualistic, and perhaps a product of people eccentric because they kept or saved them. Artifacts are mute, and some may survive because they were not used, while the most commonly used pieces were "used up" and discarded. Professional texts, instruction manuals, and advice books tell us what people were supposed to do, but leave open the question whether people really did those things. Taken together, however, these sources might provide an image that is valid and from which conclusions can be drawn.

The themes of regeneration and renewal run continuously through this book, as does the idea of individual responsibility for one's social position. The latter is, as James C. Whorton has demonstrated, a corollary to the widely held idea that nature (an expression or metaphor of God's work and will) is essentially good, and human maladies or complaints are a result of people's inability to live within that system without being victimized by their own passions.

The constancy of complaint and urging for our fellow citizens to better themselves physically arose from essentially different sources between 1830 and 1860, 1860 and 1890, and 1890 and 1940. In the three decades before the Civil War, the millennial spirit of religious enthusiasm and a concern for the fate of the republic after the death of the great leaders of the eighteenth century provided the impetus to reform human beings and their society. After the war, the new maladies of the growing urban and village middle class, off the farm and working away from home, as well as new

technologies and new theories about disease, stimulated a renewed drive for
health. By the 1890s, a profound sense of cultural pessimism had set in
among many of the nation's middle class, as well as its elites, and they turned
to new activities and new foods and developed a new standard of the human
body. Sport, the "strenuous life," breakfast cereals and other health foods,
body-building, and the ideas of innovators such as John H. and William K.
Kellogg, Charles W. Post, Bernarr Macfadden, and Dudley Sargent altered
the way Americans responded to their own bodies and their culture.

The subject of health and fitness had received scant attention until recent
years. Ronald Numbers's *Prophetess of Health: A Study of Ellen G. White*,
Stephen Nissenbaum's *Sex, Diet, and Debility in Jacksonian America: Sylvester Graham and Health Reform*, and Paul Starr's *The Social Transformation of American Medicine* are valuable studies. James C. Whorton's *Crusaders for Fitness: The History of American Health Reformers* has been both
an inspiration and an invaluable source of information. Donald J. Mrozek's
Sport and American Mentality, 1880–1910 treats the rise of sport in a
sophisticated analytical framework. These books are essential to any student
of American culture. It is my hope that this study, by looking at some
different sources and analyzing some different questions, will enlarge our
understanding of this complex phenomenon of which we continue to be a
part.

· ACKNOWLEDGMENTS ·

Many people have aided in the preparation of this book. The board of trustees of the Strong Museum have for many years encouraged research and writing that investigate American cultural life between 1820 and 1940. Bill Alderson, director of the museum, has also been a consistent advocate of this and other works in the humanities. Without their enthusiastic support, this project could not have come to pass.

Research for this book was funded in part by a grant from the National Endowment for the Humanities, and I am very grateful to the Endowment staff, particularly Andrea Anderson, for their support and aid. Several libraries were extremely useful in the course of my research, and I was fortunate to have the help and enthusiasm of some very fine librarians. Mary Huth and Karl Kabelac of the University of Rochester Library's Division of Rare Books and Manuscripts kept a watchful eye out for materials that might be useful from the time they knew of the project, and were always available when I needed them. Spencer Crew, Lorene Mayo, and John Sleckner of the Collection of Business Americana, Archives Division, National Museum of American History, Smithsonian Institution, gave me access to the incredibly rich collection for which they care, and their colleagues Michael Harris of the Division of Medical Sciences, Ellen Hughes of the Division of

Community Life, and Gary Kulik of the Department of Social and Cultural History were enthusiastic and accessible during my trips to Washington. Albert Kuhfeld and Elizabeth Ihrig of the Bakken Library in Minneapolis, Minnesota, helped guide me through the complicated history of electricity and electrotherapy in the nineteenth and early twentieth centuries, and Nick Westbrook of the Minnesota Historical Society pointed me in the direction of that organization's rich resources on the immigrant experience with sport in the upper Midwest. The staff at the Houghton Library of Harvard College helped me find Horace Fletcher's papers, and directed me to other collections in their vast and well-organized holdings.

I am especially indebted to Elaine Challacombe and Kathy Lazar of the Strong Museum Library. Throughout the long gestation period of this project, they went out of their way to find important sources for me, and in the process began to build a major collection of research materials on nineteenth- and early-twentieth-century American culture. No book of this sort is ever possible without great librarians, and my institution is blessed with a staff of them.

The National Endowment for the Humanities provided funds for a colloquium of scholars that convened in May 1984 for the purpose of analyzing and criticizing the plan for this book and the exhibition that will accompany it. Neil Harris brought his immensely broad knowledge of American popular culture and material culture to bear on the project, and provided helpful commentary throughout the long writing process. Dr. Edward Atwater, who holds an advanced degree in the history of medicine as well as an M.D., helped me place the series of often "irregular" medical practices within the broader framework of American and Western medical history. Michael Harris, who is both a pharmacist and a first-rate curator at the National Museum of American History, not only was of immeasurable aid in the analysis of the direction of this project, but also was instrumental in the location of key artifacts that altered the direction of my analysis. Throughout the year, Donald Mrozek gave me the benefit of his creative genius and the example of his evidently boundless energy. Don suggested possible speakers for a symposium, worked over my plans and outlines, and graciously helped in innumerable ways. His own works have been an inspiration and an example of clear thinking. I hope I have been able to utilize all these talents in the best way.

Mary Lynn Stevens Heininger helped me with some of the research, especially on Bernarr Macfadden, and also read and commented on the manuscript in her usual perceptive manner. She is a trusted partner and a good friend. Rita Kuder, Wanda Lodico, Janet Otis, and Mary Hall, all volunteers at the Strong Museum, pored over periodicals and other primary sources to locate relevant materials. They have been clever, creative, and dogged in their labors.

Many of the Strong Museum's curatorial staff have made this project better than it ordinarily might have been. Chief among those is Patricia M. Tice. She not only researched and acquired many critically important artifactual materials for the book and exhibit, she spent a number of hours reading the manuscript and analyzing it with her own considerable skills in the English language. The project is far better for her efforts. Deborah A. Smith came to the museum late in this effort, but has been instrumental in locating, researching, and cataloging a superb collection of photographic and other paper materials. Mary-Ellen Earl Perry paid particular attention to the clothing and fine arts that constitute the artifactual evidence used in this book, and Blair and Margaret Whitton provided encouragement and enthusiasm, as well as the relevant artifacts of childhood for the project. Gretchen Fuller graciously helped with word processing whenever she could.

Melissa A. Morgan coordinated the complicated operation of getting approximately two hundred artifacts photographed for this book. She was prompt, organized, and helpful, especially when what seemed like a good idea on paper made a substandard photograph. The Strong Museum is fortunate to employ two extraordinarily fine photographers. Tom Weber and Michael Radtke photographed and printed all the images of the artifacts and illustrations in the Strong collections, and their work is not only technically superb, but exemplary of the way an image can interpret the visual world.

Kathryn Grover, director of publications at the museum, deserves special recognition for her efforts in transforming this manuscript into a book. We worked together feverishly—nights, weekends, and holidays, in addition to the "regular time" we could get to work on the project—and her contribution as editor and conscience are inestimable. Judy White was somehow able to read my handwriting and enter the manuscript into a word processor. As well as handling the mechanical parts of the job, she was ever vigilant for those areas where I was unclear, and encouraging about those where I had succeeded. Without Kathryn and Judy I would have not finished the book.

Wendy Wolf of Pantheon Books, a first-rate editor, not only carefully worked over the manuscript but supported and pushed me from our earliest discussion of the project in 1981. All historians should be as fortunate as I have been in my dealings with editors and publishers. Kathryn's only drawback is that she roots for the Red Sox while Wendy and I favor the Yankees.

Susan Williams, to whom I am lucky enough to be married, gave me encouragement and counsel throughout the project. As a curator at the Strong Museum, she also helped find, research, and analyze artifacts related to the book and exhibition. Even as she was working on her own book on Victorian dining, she was always looking out for research materials essential to my work. Often I would find research cards on my desk with quotations and citations that proved to be critical, and it was she who had found them. She understood when I disappeared every night and weekend to write during the long haul of 1984.

Other family members helped, with their support and their forbearance. My parents, Herman and Bess Green, have been important for their constant support of my career choice and their genuine interest in the work. My mother- and father-in-law, Helen and George Williams, similarly have supported and tolerated the historians' sometimes odd hours.

Friends and colleagues help not only the substantive but also the emotional element of a book. William B. Waits, Mark Connelly, and Bill McGrath were there when they were needed. I am also indebted to good friends Linda and Michael Kirschen, Sam and Mimi Tilton, Peg and Andy Hemenway, and the numerous faithful and talented baseball players who made my summers bearable as I tried to write.

My greatest debt, however, is to Warren I. Susman, who died suddenly in April 1985. He was my mentor at Rutgers, and more than any other individual helped me to learn to think about history and becoming a historian as a process of understanding and explication. His sense of scholarship as a complex and humane process that must be broadly conceived and his unquestioned brilliance as a thinker have been both inspiration and challenge. He died before he could read this manuscript, and it is much the poorer for it. In both his intensity for teaching and his commitment to cultural history, I have an example for a lifetime.

Harvey Green
Rochester, N. Y.

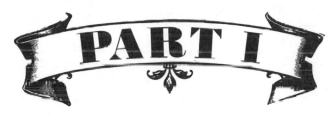

PART I

MILLENNIAL DREAMS AND PHYSICAL REALITIES, 1830–1860

CHAPTER ONE

HEALTH, MEDICINE, AND SOCIETY

The struggle of men and women of great heart against prejudice, superstition, and vice has inspired authors and readers
for centuries. In "The Young Doctor," a short story in the
July 1841 issue of *Godey's Lady's Book*, Timothy Shay Arthur
(1809–1885) utilized this theme to address a controversy that
erupted in the United States in the 1830s and that persists to this
day: the nature of proper medical treatment, the role of physicians
in American society, and the definition of good health. The dramatic tension in the story centers around the sickness of "Mrs.
Absalom," a crotchety lady with no use for one of her attending
physicians, young James Barclay. She scoffed at the young man's
recent medical training and his reliance on new theories of treatment, which she thought "as good as nothing." She considered
"mustard plasters and foot-baths, with perhaps a little rhubarb"
useless.[1]

She preferred Doctor Bailey, her trusted physician of many years
who had just taken Barclay on as a partner. Unlike Barclay, an
"eclectic" physician, Bailey was a product of the "heroic" school

of medical practice. Followers of Benjamin Rush, heroic physicians favored decisive intervention in the course of a sickness. Most often this meant bleeding and the ingestion of calomel, a tasteless white powdered form of mercuric chloride, which was thought to promote recovery by relieving the pressures wrought by the "morbid excitement" of disease. Mrs. Absalom

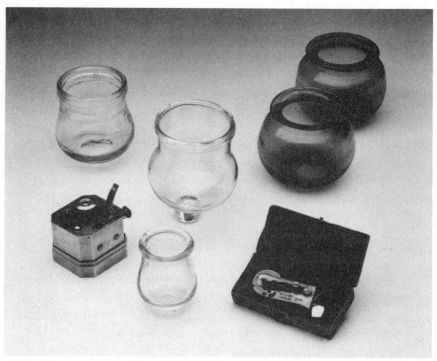

Scarificators contained multiple blades that, when pressed on the skin, created numerous wounds, to which heated glass cups were usually then applied. As the cups cooled, the pressure within them dropped, and blood flowed through the wounds and into them, allegedly relieving the congestion within. Leeches were also used to bleed patients, and Americans commonly kept them readily at hand to treat minor problems at home. Clockwise, from lower left: scarificator, probably European, brass, steel, 1800–1850; bleeding cups, American, free-blown and blown-molded glass, ca. 1850–1900; leech bowls, American, free-blown glass, ca. 1820–50; lancet, Wiegand & Snowden, Philadelphia, Pa., brass, steel, leather, 1823–55.

argued with her husband, who admitted his respect for the seasoned veteran: "Well, I like Dr. Bailey, too, I must confess. . . . But I know I would like him much better if an imaginary *click* of his lancet did not sound in my ears, accompanied by visions of his calomel bottle, whenever I think of him or see him." But Mrs. Absalom's confidence in Bailey's methods was steadfast. History was on her side. "Not less than forty or fifty times . . . [had] her arm, just above the inside of the elbows," been lanced.[2]

Bailey bled Mrs. Absalom several times, but each procedure provided only brief relief, followed by more intense pain. Only when she was weakened to near death did she submit to Barclay, who prescribed a foot bath in a hot solution of mustard powder and a mustard plaster. The treatment worked, validating the claims of "eclectic" medicine even for Mrs. Absalom.

Mid-nineteenth-century readers would have recognized the author's blunt biblical reference in his choice of the patient's name. Absalom was King David's favorite son, but he was killed for rebelling against his father. Mrs. Absalom nearly died; she was saved only when she became too weak to rebel against Barclay's ministrations. Arthur was careful to point out that Barclay was a trained physician—he had three years of intensive study—and

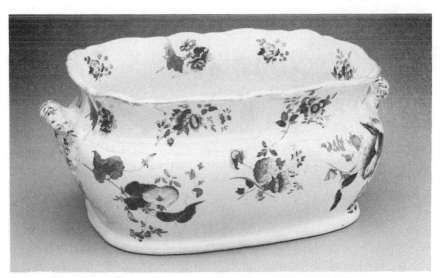

Footbaths were commonly used to relieve the symptoms of internal sicknesses. Footbath, William Adams & Sons, Staffordshire, Eng. Transfer-printed and enameled earthenware, ca. 1830.

was therefore a legitimate authority figure, whom patients ignored at their peril.

Barclay's position was a mediating one—between the "heroic" physicians and their radical opponents, the "botanics," or "Thomsonians." Followers of Samuel Thomson (1769–1843), Thomsonians maintained that diseases resulted from a "clogging of the system," which was best alleviated by purgation and sweating. Unlike heroic physicians, Thomsonians insisted that only distillates of native vegetable flora were appropriate treatments. They rejected bloodletting and treatment with mineral compounds, such as calomel, and favored medical education through empirical observation rather than through formal medical schools.[3]

Thomsonianism was extremely popular in the United States. Thomson obtained a patent for his system in 1813, and for the next twenty-five years he sold the rights to it to thousands of primarily rural Americans. By 1840

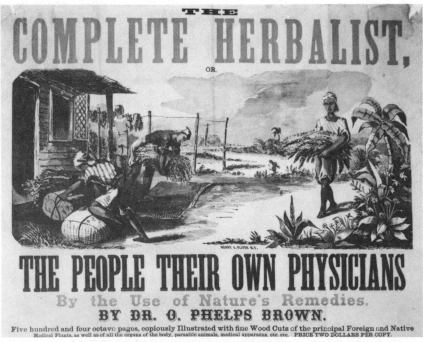

Like most self-help books, The Complete Herbalist *attacked physicians and commented on moral as well as physical aspects of living. Broadside, Henry A. Oliver, New York, N.Y., ca. 1855.*

he claimed to have sold the rights to his secrets to more than one hundred thousand families. His two books, *Thomsonian Materia Medica* (1825) and *A New Guide to Health* (1822), were the essential texts for the faithful, and a multitude of local Thomsonian medical societies were formed. Like adherents to the other political religious and social movements of the early nineteenth century, Thomsonians attended conventions (the first was held in Columbus, Ohio, in 1832), published periodicals (the *Thomsonian Recorder*, for example, was first published in 1835), and established schools (the Botanica-Medical College, for example, was founded in Columbus in 1840).[4]

The fact that botanic physicians were trained in a college was itself a change from Thomson's original purist antipathy to formal medical education, and it shows how his ideology of medical treatment had been incorporated into American medical practice. Some physicians were selective in their subscription to Thomsonianism. In 1829 New Yorker Wooster Beach broke from Thomson, formed a "Reformed Botanic Practice," and established a medical school in Worthington, Ohio. He included basic traditional medical and physiological training in his curriculum and was part of a group of physicians who called themselves "eclectics." In 1836 they published their own magazine, the *Eclectic Medical Journal.* Young James Barclay, then, was probably an "eclectic," combining botanic medicines with his formal training and his professional association with Bailey, a more traditional "heroic" physician.[5]

Thomsonianism, in its purest form, had by the 1850s become too extreme for both physician and patient. Thomson's unrelenting rejection of both nonvegetable substances and formal scientific education irritated many of his fellow critics of the American medical establishment. William Alcott, for example, asserted in an 1838 article that their almost religious devotion to Thomson's methods was as problematical as "regular" physicians' reliance on the lancet and calomel bottle.[6] Moreover, some patients discovered that Thomson's recommended treatments could be as great a shock to the system as those he condemned: note his reputed prescription of "spicy and emetic botanicals, steam baths, and enemas laced with cayenne pepper."[7]

Two other major groups ministered to the health of the nation. Homeopathic medicine originated in Germany in about 1800. "The true method of cure," wrote its most well-known advocate, Samuel Hahnemann (1755–1843), "is founded on the principle of *similia similibus curantur . . .* it is

7

necessary in each case to choose a medicine that will excite an affection similar to that for which it is employed."[8] Homeopaths theorized that disease was as much mental as physical and that the artificially induced weaker symptoms replaced the patient's original discomfort, thus allowing the body to overcome them. They also thought that extremely weak solutions were more dynamic in their effects on the body than concentrated solutions and that proper diagnosis was possible only by a detailed report by the patient to the doctor. The emphasis on personal interaction and easy-to-endure dosages made the treatment extremely popular, in spite of the "regulars'" opposition to it.

Dr. William Wesselhoeft established the first homeopathic medical school, the Allentown Academy in Bath, Pennsylvania, in 1835, and the method's popularity soared in the United States, owing in part to its apparent success during the great cholera epidemic of 1832. A particularly vicious and fast-acting disease, cholera was characterized by acute stomach and

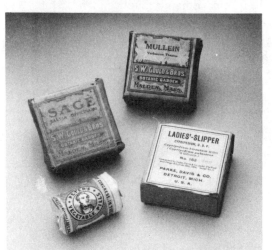 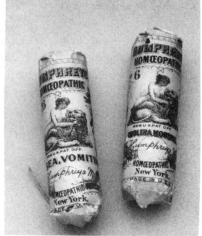

Left: Botanic medicines consisting of dried herbs and other flora. S. W. Gould and Bros., Malden, Mass.; and Parke, Davis & Co., Detroit, Mich.; ca. 1850–80.

Right: These packages of homeopathic medicines illustrate the religious symbolism of the "peaceable kingdom," an image common in the era of great religious revivals. Dried herbs from Humphrey's Homeopathic Medicine Co., New York, N.Y., ca. 1855.

intestinal pain, rapid dehydration due to diarrhea, and death. The terrifyingly rapid course and spread of this contagion made survival a powerful argument for any medical treatment. It was an especially opportune moment for the homeopath's methods, since the personal relationship of physician and patient was undoubtedly welcome in the midst of the terror of epidemic. Homeopathy flourished in the antebellum era and declined by the 1890s, but it never completely disappeared from the pantheon of medical theories.

The entire medical profession—heroic, homeopathic, or botanic—encountered an unending hostility to its methods and its claims for professional authority from 1830 until at least the 1860s. Calvin Owen, a farmer and cabinetmaker from the little town of Penfield, New York, typified this attitude. On March 30, 1853, Owen, then fifty-five years old, related in his diary the story of one Calvin Clark, who "was taken sick with fever." As was the custom, Clark was not allowed to drink any cold water to relieve the fever, but "while he was burning up with a raging fever he . . . sliped of the bed and creept to a pail of water in the room, and took two harty draughts by puting his face into the pail, but not being satisfied yet, he undertook to tip the pail, and in his weakness to hold it, it tiped over and fell from a bench and dashed on him, and in the fall roused up the watchers," who had fallen asleep; they summoned a physician who "without hesitation declared that he must die in a few hours." Clark was then allowed to drink more water, since the physician thought "any further doctoring was useless." By the next day Clark was on the way to recovery, a result that led Owen to surmise that

> most, if not all of the remedies now used by Alopathic doctors will
> be abandoned, or will be rejected by the people, for instance such
> as arsenic, Mercury and Calomel in all its preparations, antimony,
> sulphates, and nearly the whole class of *drugs.* And also the indis-
> criminate use of the *Lancet.* This *Butchering* System of Medical
> Treatment has too long been tolerated.[9]

"It does seem to me," Owen concluded, "that there would not be so much pain and suffering by the human family; if there were no doctors in the world."[10]

Twenty years earlier, the voluble and charismatic vegetarian reformer Sylvester Graham had expressed nearly the same sentiment. "It were better for mankind," wrote Graham, "if not a particle of medicine existed on the face of the earth." He argued that a physician's task was to "teach the laws of life, . . . [learn] the nature and causes of disease," and "when sickness occurs . . . remove these, and help nature restore the system." In 1843 Charles Grandison Finney, one of the most important religious revival ministers in pre–Civil War America, similarly condemned "almost the whole class of physicians, who instead of trying to prevent disease . . . go about and give this pill to one man and another to another man, without knowing whether it will kill or cure."[11]

Lay health reformers captured the public's attention because their attacks were part of a broader social and intellectual analysis and critique of American culture. Much of the reformers' activity was grounded in contemporary religious convictions about the imminence (or remoteness) of the Second Coming of Christ and the possibility that human behavior might or might not influence the timetable. It was an attitude new in nineteenth-century America and contrasted starkly with the ideas of Original Sin and election, which were fundamental to the faith of seventeenth- and eighteenth-century settlers in the New World. According to the Puritans, all were tainted from birth with the stain of Original Sin, and God arbitrarily chose a few "elect" to be saved, thereby demonstrating His mercy.

By the 1820s, however, ministers and the faithful (whose numbers increased dramatically after a series of revivals swept through the country) demonstrated slightly greater optimisim about insuring salvation. Rejecting both Original Sin and arbitrary salvation, many argued instead that the human race could improve itself and that Christ's reappearance would occur only after human civilization had evolved to that state of perfection that would then endure for a millennium, or one thousand years. Millennialism offered both a peril and a hope. The awesome responsibility for arriving at the state of grace and perfection rested squarely upon human shoulders— but the task was comprehensible and, therefore, possible.

Good health—the avoidance of disease, debility, and "premature" death —thus took on extraordinary importance. Physical degeneration was a spiritual as well as medical or physiological problem. Adherents to Sylvester Graham's vegetarian creed argued "that the millennium, the near approach of which is by many so confidently predicted, can never reasonably be expected to arrive until those laws which God has implanted in the *physical*

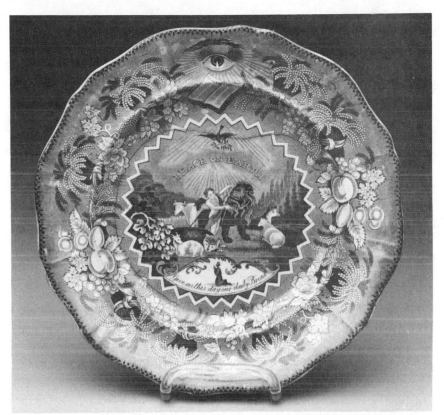

Depicted on this common tableware piece is the prophecy of Isaiah, when the lion shall lie down with the lamb. This promise of peace was the hope of the Second Coming, and the plate gives visual testament to the equation of abundance (fruits and sheaves of wheat on the border) and piety (in the center). Dinner plate, "Millennium," Ralph Stevenson and Sons, Staffordshire, Eng. Transfer-printed earthenware, 1832–35.

nature of man, are, equally with his moral laws, universally known and obeyed."[12] Reformers combined and sometimes confused morality and health, arguing that to be "regenerate" was certainly to be free from disease. They indirectly assumed that strength and longevity would increase as the race advanced to a more perfect overall condition. By regenerating, or renovating, the spiritual and physical state of the citizenry, they thought, the polity could survive the threats of the growing sectional and slavery controversies, become rejuvenated, and the millennium might come.

The belief in access to bodily and spiritual salvation coincided with a broader cultural challenge to traditional institutions—governmental, economic, and religious—and traditional social and class organization that characterized Andrew Jackson's America. President Jackson attacked eastern bankers, in particular the Bank of the United States, and decentralized their financial power. The percentage of free white men who could vote increased dramatically during his administration, shattering the domination of government by the propertied classes. Jacksonian Democrats were hostile to elites in general, whether they were bankers, lawyers, or doctors, who allegedly drained both blood and money from the unsuspecting and trusting patient. By confusing and trying to impress patients with his knowledge of the secrets of medicine, the physician did not consolidate his authority, but instead revealed himself to be the charlatan that Jacksonian Americans such as Calvin Owen thought he was. Laws licensing physicians were repealed in all but three states by 1845, thereby allowing the general populace to treat themselves. Physicians' own actions also helped undo their claims to authority. As the rapid expansion westward made work for more practitioners, they organized new medical schools, often requiring only sixteen weeks of training, some even without formal entrance requirements.

The coterie of health reformers—dietary faddists, water-cure specialists, animal magnetizers and electromagnetizers, and physical educators—shared in varying degrees an opposition to the established medical profession and held to the common conviction that American culture (ultimately world culture) needed their ministrations because the nation was declining. Set against the millennial hopes of the 1830s and 1840s, this idea of a fall from a nobler age galvanized their efforts at reform.

In September 1829 the *Journal of Health*, a monthly magazine intended for the general public as well as the medical profession, was first published in Philadelphia. Editors John Bell and D. M. Condie proposed that the magazine consider the "properties of the air, its several states of heat, coldness, dryness, moisture and electricity"; the effects of food and drink; exercise; clothing ("a cause of disease, when under the direction of absurd fashions"); and "bathing and [its] functions, and the use of mineral waters." It was almost immediately influential among practitioners in health-related fields. In 1830 Edward Hitchcock, professor of chemistry and natural history at Amherst College and the first professor of physical education in the

United States, called the *Journal* "a work conducted by some of the ablest physicians in our country."[13]

The *Journal* lasted only four years, despite impressive endorsements. Bell and Condie had made one tactical error: They misjudged just how hostile most Americans still were to formally trained physicians.

> The *Journal of Health* will on all occasions be found in opposition to empiricism; whether it be in the form of nursery gossip, mendacious reports of nostrum makers and venders [sic] or on recommendations of even scientifically compounded prescriptions, without the special directions of a physician—the only competent judge in the individual case of disease under his care.[14]

The *Journal* warned its readers in clear language of the dangers of the "misapplication of medical maxims, and the consequent misuse of medicinal substances." The physician would eventually be summoned, but only after the disease was "beyond the reach of art" and mistreated "by means of remedies which the parents and nurse had gathered from the 'Family Oracle' or 'Domestic Medicine' or the like."[15]

Lay health reformers saw themselves as interpreters of science rather than medical professionals, and thus considered nature superior to "art" or "artifice," prevention preferable to cure, industrial development hazardous, the economic costs of illness too high, and physical circumstances and condition linked directly to individual morality. As individuals, many of the most important health reformers—William Alcott, Sylvester Graham, James C. Jackson, Orson Fowler, and Mary Gove—experienced (or at least said they experienced) a typical life course of abusing their bodies, suffering debility, finally discovering hygiene, then advocating reform, and ultimately subscribing thoroughly to the belief in the efficacy of the healthful life. Central to their ideas—whatever their particular passion—was the conviction that they were not exceptional in their need for regeneration. All around them they saw signs of debility and decline that could be corrected.

The notion that the human form was decaying was ancient; even the earliest Christians believed that, since Adam's fall, the earthly body had lost any claim to perfection. More immediate to the early-nineteenth-century experience was eighteenth-century English poet John Dryden's lament that the English peoples were "a pampered race of men" who had "dwindled" from "long-lived fathers."[16] Edward Hitchcock implied that Americans of 1830 had declined from their healthy forefathers and mothers, when he asserted that a "weakened society" and religion could not be "successfully met and countered by the puny arm and shrinking sensibility of dyspepsy. It needs the resolution, the assured faith, and energetic action of our Pilgrim Fathers."[17] By 1850 degeneracy was so widespread that one of the century's most popular advisors, Catharine Beecher, complained:

> Multitudes abuse their bodies because they do not know the mis-chiefs they are perpetrating. Perhaps as many more go on in courses that they know to be injurious because these matters are never urged on their attention and conscience as matters of *duty*. All the strong motives of religion and the eternal world are brought to bear, from the Pulpit and at the Sunday-school, to enforce certain duties that are no more important to the best interests of man than those "laws of health" which are so widely disregarded.[18]

Beecher further argued, "if the American people were a strong, hardy, unexcitable race, like the German laborers that come among us . . . rules for the selection of diet would be of less importance."[19]

Critical to the reformers' ideology was the conviction that the land—the physical space that was America, and, by extension, the earth—was perfect, and thus achieving perfection was possible if Americans would seize the opportunity. In his popular *Young Man's Guide* (1835), William Alcott warned his readers, "It is for you to decide whether this *greatest* of free nations shall, at the same time, be the *best.*"[20]

Alcott also equated the health of the polity and the health of the individual. The complex relationship between a perfect and balanced nature, religious piety, material abundance, and political virtue was well known in the early nineteenth century. In 1798 political theorist David Tappan commented that "virtue is the soul of republican freedom" but warned that "luxury tends to extinguish both sound morality and piety." It was an awesome and exhilarating challenge, as Alexander Hamilton had pointed out: "It seems to have been reserved for the people of this country, by their conduct and example, to decide the important question, whether societies of men are really capable or not of establishing good government from reflection and choice."[21] By the beginning of his administration in 1817, James Monroe thought he had an answer to Hamilton's query: "The United

States have flourished beyond example. Their citizens individually have been happy and the nation prosperous. . . . Blessed, too, with a fertile soil, our produce has always been very abundant, leaving, even in years the least favorable, a surplus for the wants of our fellow-men in other countries. Such is our peculiar felicity."[22]

The political orations, Fourth of July speeches and sermons, and newspaper editorials of the first half-century after the Declaration of Independence were filled with such invocations to American greatness. Writing on the fiftieth anniversary of the Declaration, Edward Everett asserted, "It is in this way that we are to fulfill our destiny in the world. The greatest engine of moral power, which human nature knows is an organized, prosperous state."[23] But as Everett was writing, two of the last surviving leaders of the generation that made the Revolution lay dying: both Thomas Jefferson and John Adams died on July 4, 1826. It was now the task of their children and their children's children to shape and mold the characters of future generations, and thus continue the American experiment.

Not everyone was optimistic. Minister Timothy Flint, also writing in 1826, was troubled by the very abundance Monroe and Everett found so comforting. "Increasing wealth," he wrote, "rolls the tide of fashionable vice over the land. Who that reflects must tremble for the consequences."[24] He was joined by Lyman Beecher, probably the best-known minister of his day, who wrote in 1829:

> All which is done to stimulate agriculture, commerce, and the arts is, therefore, without some self-preserving moral power but providing fuel for the fire which is destined to consume us. The greater the prosperity the shorter its duration, and the more tremendous our downfall, unless the moral power of the Gospel shall be exerted to arrest those causes which have destroyed other nations.[25]

> Indeed, our Republic is becoming too prosperous, too powerful, two extended, too numerous, to be governed by any power without the blessed influence of the Gospel.[26]

Amherst College professor Edward Hitchcock agreed: "No nation becomes rich and prosperous, without becoming also luxurious and debilitated," and pointed out how "luxurious, enervated, dyspeptic Rome, sunk an easy prey before the brawny arm of the Goth and Vandal." In 1844 cabinetmaker

Calvin Owen similarly summoned ancient history to attack luxury and ambition: "I would appeal to History, particularly of Greece and Rome, to show that human virtue were no where unaccompanied by those noxious seeds of ambition, which have been the ruin of all former republics. In this country, the sovereign power is being corrupted by the love of wealth and personal grandeur; and tocsin [an alarm bell] *may* not be sounded, until! *alas!* the knell of liberty shall be tolled."[27]

By 1833 even the traditionally optimistic Fourth of July oration had a tone of worry. Edward G. Prescott asserted in Boston that "our country presents a situation hitherto unparalleled among men. We are suffering, not like the nations of Europe from a debt which bows us to the earth under our vain efforts to discharge it, but from a state of prosperity which is perhaps even worse."[28] The connection between material abundance and decline was stated more directly by Boston clergyman Andrew Bigelow in 1836:

> It is with nations as with individuals, that prosperity . . . is the parent of vice. . . . In the long festival of peace which has smiled upon us, the very sunshine of our fortunes has hatched out a pernicious brood of evils. The political atmosphere is becoming charged with noxious miasmata, which threaten grievous distempers to society. . . . We see luxury, the bane of all republics, spreading its infection and eating as a gangrene into the vitals of the state."[29]

The metaphorical link between individual health and the vitality of the nation was close indeed. The very abundance of land and economy that so intoxicated political orators could, and indeed would, be the undoing of the great governmental experiment. For both governments and individuals, the solution lay in altering the practices and minds of individual Americans.

Economic abundance was not the only threat to the survival of the republic. As Prescott was fretting over "the state of prosperity" in the summer of 1833, southern states, especially South Carolina, were asserting their right to nullify a federal law they found onerous. The "nullification" crisis was severe enough that physician Charles Caldwell began his *Thoughts on Physical Education* (1834) with the pessimistic conclusion that "The embittered strife of parties . . . and the growing discontents of geographical sections, seriously threaten the repose of the country, not to say the integrity of the Union." The immediate issue was a tariff—"the tariff of abominations," as South Carolina Senator John C. Calhoun called it—but the greater question was whether the nation would endure. Caldwell thought the country's only hope was to improve the mental, physical, and moral character of the people through education. "On the redeeming influence of such improvement alone," he wrote, "can the American people safely and confidently rely, for the attainment of that degree of national prosperity, greatness, and glory, and that amount of individual happiness, which is placed within their reach."[30]

For ministers such as Lyman Beecher, religion was the critical element in this process of changing American behavior. Some ministers even welcomed the economic trials that the Panic of 1837 visited upon the people, because, as Baltimore's Reverend George W. Burnap said at the time, "the cause of religion will ultimately be promoted by the present commotions in the commercial world." The perception that there were grave inequities, injustices, and other imbalances that threatened the establishment of a moral society provoked a spate of reforms directed at social and individual improvement. In addition to the religious revivals that occurred between 1820 and 1860, a mixture of local and national organizations was formed to improve the conditions of incarcerated criminals, ameliorate treatment of the insane, moderate the use of alcohol, abolish slavery, improve the schooling of children, end war, and secure rights and the vote for women.[31]

Nearly all of these movements generated organized opposition. Antiabolitionist mobs attacked demonstrators and proponents of abolition; crusaders for women's rights encountered hostility in the press and in government, and pro-saloon and pro-liquor forces fought the "cold water armies" that sought to prohibit alcohol consumption. Splinter religious sects were spawned that even the revivalist camp found disturbing. Most of these groups tended to preach a doctrine of premillennialism—that is, that the Second Coming was both imminent and would come without warning. For them, there would be no gradual evolution toward a better, more moral society, but a sudden, terrible presence, and then, for the chosen, a millennium to bask in the glory and light of Christ's presence.

One of the most extreme and most popular of these groups were the followers of Reverend William Miller, who had calculated the end of the world to be April 23, 1843. The Millerites attracted attention in newspapers

17

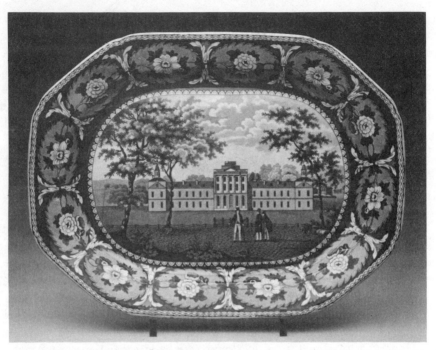

Large urban hospitals—here depicted as a bucolic environment—were a source of pride for Americans, and the regular Georgian style of the building marks it as a product of Enlightenment ideas of order and rationality. Platter, "Hospital at Philadelphia," W. Ridgway, Cobridge, Eng. Transfer-printed earthenware, 1830–55.

and in general day-to-day conversation. Theodosia Dunham, a teacher who moved from Philadelphia to Camden County, North Carolina, heard of the Millerites from her friend Kate in February 1843.

> Miller has been preaching in Philadelphia and thousands of persons went to hear him and many are fully convinced that the world is really coming to an end on 23 of April next. . . . *I would not be in the least surprised if something dreadful should happen,* for the *people are getting so bad* I do not know what *will* become of us.[32]

The Millerites allegedly gathered together on a hill in upstate New York to await the end, having abandoned their worldly possessions. When Christ did not appear, Miller announced an error in his calculations; he reexamined the Scriptures and announced that the new Judgment Day was to be in 1844. Dunham's friend Kate commented that "the 23 of April and all the set days are past, I believe, and the world is continuing on its unvarying way."[33] Once again, a now-diminished flock waited. When the day and night passed without incident, the Millerites declined precipitously into a tiny and dedicated sect that advocated that judgment would be forestalled until sufficient preaching and conversion had occurred.

The emotional nature of revival meetings, whether in churches or in tents in the countryside, caused some to question the healthiness of conversion. In 1834 Charles Caldwell linked religious enthusiasms to insanity and proclaimed that "the inordinate sum of insanity, which prevails in the United States, is too plain to be held in doubt." He posited that "madness is the result of cerebral excitement, rendered deleterious by the excess in quantity. . . . Nor can any cerebral irritant be more noxious, either in kind or degree, than the cankered and fierce religious and political passions which are constantly goading the American brain." In *Phrenology Known by Its Fruits* (1836), a book whose title suggests an attack on a different fad of the nineteenth century, pro-revival physician David M. Reese took on the antievangelical arguments of Doctor A. Brigham, who linked night revival meetings and the emotional "excesses" of the conversion experience to "nervous and hysterical diseases, apoplexy, palsy, consumption and death." Reese suggested Brigham should instead attack the "multiplied and multiplying parties, soirees, quilting, levees, and converzationes [*sic*] of the ladies, and the secular, political and festive assemblages of the other sex . . . the theatres, circuses, concerts, museums, or other public places of amusement . . . [which] are thronged even on the Sabbath."[34]

Reese and Brigham were not simply squabbling over minor points of religious orthodoxy. They were arguing about issues of significance for bodily health as well as religion and social reform. Brigham maintained that the brain was the origin of both debility and health; Reese favored the idea that the heart was the seat of affections and, to some extent, of afflictions. But whatever their differences, they agreed that, in Reese's words, "the country is rampant with intemperance, dyspepsia, puerperal [postpartum] fever, repelled eruptions, insolation [sunstrokes], onanism, ill health, intermittent fever, liver complaint, amenorrhoea [cessation of menstruation], meonorrhagia [excessive menstruation], leucorrhea [vaginal discharge], epilepsy, paralysis, inflammation of the bowels, licentiousness, and excessive *bodily*

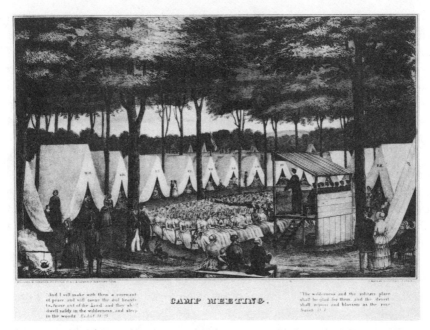

CAMP MEETING.

Outdoor revival or "camp" meetings were a vital part of the religious revivals that swept through the United States before the Civil War. "Camp Meeting," D. Needham, Buffalo, N.Y., lithograph, ca. 1855.

exertion." Moreover, as Reese asserted, "no other disease is probably increasing faster in our country than insanity! . . . It already prevails here to a greater extent than in any other country."[35]

The incidence of insanity was not the only area in which the United States was found to compare unfavorably with other nations. In 1829 the *Journal of Health* implied that Europeans, for decades characterized as decadent in relation with the New World, were somehow more adept at caring for their young. The magazine found that in Paris and London in 1818 and 1827, respectively, nearly one-sixth of all deaths were children less than one year old. In Philadelphia, "during a period of twenty years ending January 1, 1827, the proportion of deaths of children under a year old, to the whole numbers, is rather more than a fifth."[36] The samples are statistically unsophisticated to a twentieth-century analyst and the comparison flawed because the sample populations are similar neither in time of accumulation, nor duration. But the important point for the *Journal* was that there was a fearful problem of infant mortality that mothers had to solve. Surely the republic was in danger.

Women were criticized in 1830 for their allegedly sedentary habits, many of which were part of the fashionable activities of the era. Housework was thought to bolster health, and in 1830 "females in the middling classes" were considered more robust than their more fashionable wealthy sisters, who were "apt to confound occupation or industry, with exercise," the *Journal of Health* observed. "It is this error, we are persuaded, which has fixed many a female to her piano, her needlework, her books or drawing . . . together with the fashionable manufacture of scrap-books, scrap and tables, and other toys . . . [which] can never supply the place of even in-door exercise."[37]

Concern for working-class men was also manifest in 1830. In a remarkably prescient article on January 13, 1830, the *Journal of Health* enumerated the occupational hazards of certain trades. Gilders, the publishers found, were subject to "giddiness, asthma, partial palsy, and a death-like paleness of visage" that resulted from inhaling mercury vapor, "since it is by the aid of this metal that the process of gilding is performed. . . . Ulcers in the mouth, salivation, universal languor, and trembling . . . an especial intolerance of sound . . . [and] an insufferable stammering" were also ill effects of exposure to mercury. Miners of the metal's ores similarly suffered from "convulsions, tremors, palsy, and vertigo." The author went on to detail the specific ailments and hazards endemic to pottery glazers, glassmakers, stonecutters, masons, blacksmiths, locksmiths, gunners, founders, and "Plasterers and Makers of Lime . . . [who] are affected with laborious breathing, have a wan pallid visage, and digest badly," a result of the gases they inhaled and the generally damp environs of their work.[38]

In addition to the direct threats of occupational hazards and sedentary habits, health reformers identified still another, more complex and perhaps more insidious force undermining individual and national health in the mid-nineteenth century: stress. Twentieth-century Americans tend to think of emotional stress as a product of the age in which they live, but recognition of the impact of worry and care upon mental stability and physical well-being dates back to well before the Civil War. In 1830 Edward Hitchcock maintained that "nervous maladies [are] already a formidable national evil." These "maladies" included a variety of mental conditions—timidity, memory loss, inability to concentrate, jealousy, irritability, hopelessness—as well as physical problems—indigestion, headache, and other internal discomforts —and were linked, according to Hitchcock, to excesses of study, of political fervors, of religious enthusiasm, of food, and of drink. He warned that "the leaven is spreading wider and wider; and by its fermentation, is secretly heaving up the foundations of society. The ravages of these complaints," he cautioned, "will always go hand in hand with luxury, intemperance, and excess of every kind."[39]

Charles Caldwell agreed with Hitchcock in an assessment published in 1834, though he identified more specific causes of "mental commotion" in America: "Party politics, party religion, and the love of wealth. . . . a more ardently money-loving and keenly money-seeking people than the Americans does not exist." He attributed the inordinate amount of "harassing and giddy excitement" in the United States to the lack of long-established lines of hereditary wealth and to a political system which encouraged individuals to seek the power and "standing" that could be achieved through money.[40]

Catharine Beecher built upon the analyses of Hitchcock, Caldwell, and her father, Lyman Beecher, to develop her own critique of American society. She placed more emphasis on women and their place in the problems and solutions of the nation, and in particular on the effects of their ambition for wealth and status. But her analysis took a different approach from those of her predecessors: she identified stress as a problem for socially aspiring rural people who had succeeded in the marketplace economy that had begun to dominate the northeastern United States in the 1830s:

> In our country towns and among the industrial classes it will be found that the taxation of care and labor on the brain of women is even worse and greater than it is in the same class of our cities. The wives of rich farmers often are ambitious to carry out plans of labor and wealth with their husbands, while at the same time, their daughters must be sent to boarding-school, and all the habits and tasks of city life must in consequence be mingled with other cares.[41]

Beecher's allowance that city life and its "habits and tasks" exacted a price on the health of Americans suggests that she thought her audience familiar with many of her contemporaries' indictment of cities.

Beecher's assertions were part of a critique of American society that found it wanting when compared with that of the sturdy American colonials and Revolutionaries. "Our great-grand-parents," wrote the editors of *The Young People's Mirror and American Family Visitor* in 1849, "lived to a great age, and never thought of complaining or lying down to die, til they reached the meridian of life. They were stout, strong, and worked like beavers, and never spent the midnight hours in dancing." Beecher similarly admired her ancestors' superior health and activity. "Their physical strength, and their power of labor and endurance, were altogether beyond anything witnessed in the present generation."[42]

Like Beecher, the *Young People's Mirror* was especially hard on American women. The magazine shrieked: "How have their daughters degenerated!" Beecher was more nostalgic than shrill:

In former days, when women spun and wove, and made butter and cheese, their daughters were their intelligent and well-trained assistants; and in the style of dress and all the details of life were simple, and easy, and comfortable. These days have passed away.

Like those ministers and laymen who fretted over the imminent demise of a republic too undisciplined not to be seduced into luxury and laziness by the abundance of the American land, Beecher saw a fearful decline from the "Golden Age" of American family life, labor, and political virtue—the seventeenth and eighteenth centuries—a degeneration that left its mark on the mental and physical features of the populace.[43]

The class distinctions Beecher described were also products of the new era of industrialization and urbanization. "In the palmy days of our early Republic, all classes rose with the sun, and all the hours of labor, even for the highest, were by daylight. And their social gatherings were ordinarily ended when the nine o'clock bell gave warning that all well-ordered families should retire to rest." The Industrial Revolution and the rise of a class of people with substantial amounts of leisure time did not indicate to Beecher that an aristocracy like that of Europe would soon occupy American soil, but she wondered, "Why should not the American people set an example to the Old World of customs conformed at once to the laws of health, the laws of God, and the spirit of their own boasted institutions?"[44]

Like her father Lyman, Catharine Beecher identified much of the health of the nation with that of the individual. But unlike him, she believed that the people's physical and mental condition, and ultimately the fate of their soul, could be altered by human action. Although she wished to believe "all men are equal in rights and privileges, and that no aristocracy can flourish here," Beecher was forced to concede that "another class [of American women] . . . live to be waited on and amused [and] are as great sufferers for want of some worthy object in life, or from excesses in seeking amusement." The result was a "brain and nervous system exhausted by too much care and too much mental excitement in their daily duties."[45]

This conclusion was descended from medical theories accepted for more than a century. "This system [of medicine]," Benjamin Rush wrote in 1809, "admits of only a single disease, consisting of different forms of morbid excitement, induced by irritants acting upon a previous debility."[46] The way to relieve tension and pressure and reestablish the body's equilibrium was through "depletion," or bleeding and purging the circulatory and digestive system—hence the lancet and calomel.

Physicians before Rush had begun to classify diseases by symptoms in order to deduce cures, and nearly all had agreed in some measure about the general nature of disease. Fredrick Hoffmann (1692–1742) and William Cullen (1712–1790) thought disease was a result of external forces disrupting the equilibrium of the body's "nervous tone." John Brown (1735–1788) presaged much of the medical debate of the nineteenth century with his elaboration of the theory of two competing states of the body: *sthenia,* or tension, and *asthenia,* or ease. Rush and other physicians refined these ideas, offered lists of diseases, and, in some cases, recommended various compounds to be administered for each sickness. Similarly organized but more amateurish popular publications were also available.

The course of a typical serious disease—with its terrifying and sudden relapses and often severe treatment—of the pre–Civil War era in part explains the power of self-help medical guides. In 1837 Elijah Inman, aged fifty, entered an unidentified physician's care on May 28, complaining of "chills, pain in the head and side, difficulty of breathing, and cough from which there was little or no expectoration." He had "been the subject of pectoral disease since he had [had] the measles 25 years [before]" and had most recently taken a dose of calomel, "which purged him frequently for three days." Even though Inman's pains had subsided somewhat, the physician found his "tongue very dry and much coated with . . . fur . . . [his] countenance pallid, [with] moderate emaciation." His prescription was somewhat eclectic—a "breast plaster, antimonial mixture, [and] Flax seed for tea."

Two days later, on May 30, Inman's physician concluded that the "Blister [raised by the plaster had] drawn [the] cough loose." Inman continued to take an "antimonial mixture," and by June 2 his pains were gone completely, but he experienced "some lightness in breathing, [and his] bowels [were] very open." By June 10, however, the patient had taken a turn for the worse. "Nervous symptoms [were] more apparent," the physician noted. "When spoken to, [the patient was] confused [and] has not been out of bed [for] . . . two days . . . emaciation greater, Pulse Smaller, skin somewhat soft. Muscular tremor now and then." The physician then prescribed carbonic ammonia, camphor, and opium to be administered every three hours. The doctor's next visit, three days later, found Inman suffering from "tremors of the hands and arms" and an inability to control the passing of his bowels. He prescribed a "little arra Root [arrowroot] seasoned with Cassian," as well as an enema "to be repeated every 2nd or 3rd hour or immediately after every loose stool." Plasters were applied to Inman's legs and feet.

Two weeks later, Inman could eat, and his countenance [seemed] somewhat brightened up." But he was "still insensible," and complained of his legs "where the Blister was." He slept and ate still better two days later and was given "calomel and opium" pills, "one every 3 hours," supplemented later was an "Enemata," wine and "Calf's Jelley," a gelatinous liquid prepared by boiling calves' meat and bones.

Over the next two weeks, the patient's happy progress was interrupted, as his doctor found him weak and with blood and mucus in his stool—for physicians of the early nineteenth century, an indication that the crisis point of the disease had been reached. If the patient survived this alarming—but, physicians thought, inevitable—period of greatest danger and most violent reaction, there was thought to be a considerable chance of full recovery.

A month after beginning treatment, Inman seemed improved, though he complained of "great tenderness of the sacrum [lower pelvic vertebrae] and hips." Prescribed for the tender areas were a "charcoal and yeast cataplasm, renewing them every 4th hour . . . [and] half a pint of wine daily and more if sinking [were] greater."

Apparently the first "crisis," when Inman passed a quart of blood, was not the turning point in his illness after all. The doctor visited on July 5 and found his patient's "debility very great." He "had a severe shivering fit [and his] pulse scarcely perceptible." The doctor prescribed "doses of spirits in addition to the wine" every four hours as well as camphor and opium.

The spirits were credited with having revived Inman by July 10. The prescription was continued and supplemented with "acid nitric lotion" to wash "the sacrum and hips [which were] sloughing very deeply." Inman's condition evidently improved between July 16 and July 30, since the doctor characterized the discharges from the "sloughs" and "sinuses in the direction of the gluteal muscle" as "healthy." He prescribed a continuation of "the nitric acid wash, wine & c. as before [and] . . . the calf Jelley highly seasoned."

Inman's improvement was again forestalled when, on August 5, the doctor reported that he felt "very much oppressed" by his inability to move his bowels for the past eighteen hours. His cough lingered, his "sores filled up," and he was given "calomel—to take the powder, and if it [did] not operate in 4 hours, [to] take some oil" (probably castor oil). Nine days later the prescription had an unintended effect: Inman "was taken with very severe purging and much debility and sinking . . . about a pint of pure Blood passed at one discharge" of his bowels, which appeared "as if their whole contents were continually pouring out." The prescription that was then written was the most extensive yet: "Gum Arabic for drink, Isinglass to be Boiled in milk and seasoned oil of cinnamon, Calf Jelley, Enema after every loose Stool, [continuing] the wine with Quinine and Zinc."

Later the doctor reported, "After using the medicines, [the] purging ceased." Inman ate "a little veal, the first he [had] taken in a solid state." He began vomiting and was ordered to take "Soda Powders with 10 drops of Zn [zinc] opii [opium] every two hours." Inman recovered throughout late August and September, troubled only occasionally by diarrhea, and, on October 4, 1837, the physician termed him "cured."[47]

The physician's use of both vegetable (mustard) and mineral preparations (zinc and calomel, among others) demonstrates that he was not a follower of botanic, or Thomsonian, medical theory, and the lack of any reference to bleeding or cupping suggests that he may have moved away from that particular "heroic" treatment. But as "eclectic" as he may have been, the doctor's overarching theories of the human constitution and the nature of human affliction seemed to have been those of Rush and his contemporaries. Calomel was used to purge the system, which it most certainly did. And the passage of blood with the stools may have been viewed as a form of "bleeding." Moreover, the use of plasters, which raised painful blisters from which "fetid" and presumably infected fluids drained, indicated a persistence of the belief that such treatments drew off the infection and conducted it out of the body, either through natural or man-made orifices. In any case, bleeding, blistering, and other forms of purgation continued as important forms of relief and treatment throughout the nineteenth and early twentieth centuries. Theodosia Dunham, the emigrant Camden County, North Carolina, schoolteacher, evidently endured much of this form of treatment in 1842. "You cannot imagine," her friend Julia wrote, "how sorry I was to hear of your sickness, how much you must have suffered Leeching, Cupping, Bleeding, and Blistering and then to crown the rest dieting and darkness."[48]

Elijah Inman's serious disease and dramatic recovery came about after he had endeavored to treat himself (with calomel), and perhaps only after twenty-five years of living with his cough. He was acting as many other Americans were, and as he was advised to by a significant number of his most respected fellow citizens—ministers, laymen, and nonmedical scientists. The primary vehicle used by these lay health advisors was the self-help book. By 1830 most Americans in the northern states could read, and after the invention of the steam printing press in 1835, general stores all over the country were supplied with an assortment of inexpensive volumes that advised readers on deportment, marriage, education, and health.

One of the most prolific and popular of the self-help writers was William Alcott. Born in 1798 in Wolcott, Connecticut, his poor health led to his initial interest in the healer's art, but he rapidly came to distrust physicians. He moved to Boston in about 1830, where he worked as an editor of the *Annals of Education* and *Juvenile Rambler.* He moved on to the editorship of S. G. Goodrich's immensely popular *Peter Parley's Magazine* in 1832 but not before he had finished *The House I Live In,* a guidebook for young adults that offered a simplified general anatomy lesson as well as recommendations for proper cleanliness, exercise, and diet. By 1839 the book was in its seventh edition, and Alcott had become a leader in the rapidly formed and powerful lay health movement. He wrote nearly a hundred self-help guides, including *The Young Wife* (1837), *The Young Husband* (1837, in its twelfth edition by 1851), *The Young Housekeeper* (1838), *Vegetable Diet* (1838), and *Lectures on Life and Health: or, The Laws and Means of Physical Culture* (1853). *The Young Mother* (1836), a manual for raising children, was perhaps his most successful book: by 1855, nineteen years after it was first published, it was in its twentieth edition.

Although Alcott rejected the "everyone their own doctor" approach to medicine, he did believe that laymen and women must serve as their own hygienists. In distinguishing between medicine and hygiene, Alcott was perhaps more sophisticated intellectually than were many of his more extreme contemporaries, such as the whole-wheat flour vegetarian Sylvester Graham. He believed that trained physicians possessed skills necessary for social welfare, abilities not immediately available to anyone who wanted to practice the healer's art. He also believed that patients should negotiate an annual contract with physicians, deducting from a set stipend a minimal cost for each day ill; should the patient remain healthy all year, Alcott reasoned, the doctor ought to get the full stipend.[49]

Like others of his time—revivalist minister Charles Grandison Finney, in particular—Alcott envisioned a truly Christian society as a sort of hygienic millennium, in which all the citizens would have as perfect bodies as possible. Like nearly all commentators on the American scene since the seventeenth century, Alcott assumed that the land space of America was itself perfect in its order and composition, thus placing the responsibility for health with the individual.

This individual moral responsibility for physical salvation and perfectionism was a secular counterpart to the religious responsibilities that ministers everywhere were proclaiming for their flocks. And just as ministers assumed that they should maintain their position as mediators, helpers, and translators of the word of God, reformers of Alcott's persuasion retained respect for physicians and their training. Thus medicine in the pre–Civil War era was more than a simple war between drug-toting doctors armed with lancets, leeches, and calomel, on the one hand, and "botanics," homeopaths, and hygienic laymen and women, on the other. The *Journal of Health,* the *Boston Medical and Surgical Journal,* and other periodicals that shared their bias for professional physicians agreed with lay reformers in their critique of gluttony; the intemperate use of "ardent spirits," "patent" medicines, and "quack" drugs; the alleged lassitude of the wealthy; and popular sensational literature ("too stimulating of the passions"). Like the reformers, they supported exercise, fresh air, sunshine, and balanced or moderate diet.[50] By the 1840s, physicians began to alter their own views, perhaps because of the success of people they considered quacks—Thomsonians, nostrum vendors, homeopaths, and ultimately the "discoverers" of the "water-cure." Thus physicians of all but the most diehard "heroic" persuasion commonly combined purgation and medicinal-herbal treatments.

Hygienists, doctors, ministers, lay critics with no particular training in the physical sciences, politicians, and political thinkers all shared the view that the United States was a nation with the makings of an exemplary democratic government, a land rich in resources and potential, and a people capable of achieving perfectibility in anticipation of the millennium. They also agreed, however, that the American people did not as a group approach the state of perfection and grace necessary for Christ's Second Coming. In fact, by the 1830s there was near-universal agreement that the nation had degenerated from the great men and women of the colonial and Revolutionary era. What was to be done? Some preached prevention—changes in diet, dress reform, and physical education. Others advocated cures using water or electricity. Their theories would influence perceptions and manifestations of both problems and solutions for the next hundred years.

CHAPTER·TWO

SPICES AND THE SOCIAL ORDER

"We may safely take it for granted, after long observation," wrote a contributor to the *Southern Review* in 1829, "that almost every man, woman, and child in this country, habitually eats and drinks twice as much every day ... as is necessary." A quarter of a century later, Catharine Beecher warned that the results of such unrestrained behavior were severe.

> Physicians and physiologists maintain that there is more sickness and death caused by excess in the *quantity* taken than by the violation of any other law of health. The reason of this is that men have so abused nature that *appetite* has ceased to be a guide to most persons as to the amount of food needed. Mankind collects a great variety of foods to tempt the palate, and then eat one thing after another till they feel full, and can eat no more. In this way the stomach receives far more than is required to nourish the body, and thus the nervous powers, together with the lungs, kidneys, bowels, skin, and lymphatics, are overtaxed to throw out of the system this excess.[1]

Critics also condemned American cooks' methods. "Frying," wrote Edward Hitchcock in 1830, "is the worst of all the simple modes of cookery. . . . Of all common articles of food, those that are saturated with butter or fat, while at a boiling heat, are the most pernicious." The author of *New Hydropathic Cook-Book* (1853), Russell Trall, was a physician who regarded water as the greatest healing and health-preserving agent available to men and women. "Nutrition," wrote Trall, "is the replenishment of the tissue, not the accumulation of fat. . . . The latter is a disease, and a fattened animal, be it a hog or an alderman, is a diseased animal. . . . Fat men, fat women, fat children, and fat pigs, are not examples of excessive nutrition so much as of deficient excretion." Trall was doing battle with a formidable foe here; for generations solid animal fats were thought healthy fare, providing energy, nutrition and, equally important, flavoring to the cookery of both the poor and the wealthy. Moreover, an ample girth had for centuries been equated with wealth, since to be fat was a visible sign of excess, and therefore success. Since few people knew of or were diagnosed as having died of heart failure, no equation had been made between slimness, health, and longevity.[2]

The pace of American life was also a problem for the health-conscious. "Students and men of business," wrote Beecher, "rush to their noontide meal with brains throbbing with excitement and the circulation all disarranged. And the laboring classes do the same in reference to their excited muscular system. Both should allow half an hour of quiet to mind and body before setting the stomach to its labors." Not only did people rush to their meals; they also rushed through them. "Food is thrust into [the stomach] half masticated, and one bolus follows another before the needful process for each can be effected," Beecher observed. "Americans took half of the ideal minimum of thirty minutes for the noontime feeding, and then rushed back to the job: "The brain, nerves, and muscles are all set to work again —thus drawing off the blood needed by the stomach to perform its digestive process."[3] Beecher's arguments and advice were based on the commonly held assumption that all bodily and mental functions required "vital energy," or "nerve force," and that the body's reserve of this force was limited. The system was endangered when the body's equilibrium was disturbed, a condition that occurred when immoderate behavior, such as overeating, diverted energy to one bodily function, thereby overstimulating that one area or system. Ultimately such activity would debilitate anyone.

Training for the great gorging began at an early age, Beecher noted, much to her horror, from the molasses on hot cakes to the popular candies—all "sources of debilitation, disease, and death to the young." Parents were urged to select "unmixed and simple food," and not to yield to children's passions for sweets. Americans had to understand that "the chief attractions to social gatherings" among "the lower states of society" were *eating and drinking*. But just in proportion as man becomes elevated, this lowest species of enjoyment gives place to higher and more refined pleasure."[4] Overeating, then, was a working-class vice. Beecher craftily appealed to the aspirations of all classes in a society in which certainly the illusion, and in some cases the reality, of social and economic advancement were present. Clever enough to realize that her own Calvinist Protestant support for moderation would be rejected as prejudiced hostility to the hedonism of the hefty meal, she marked that enthusiasm with the stigma of social ineptitude. Part of the success ethic of Jacksonian America was that social advancement—indeed, simply maintaining one's station—involved more than money. Class consciousness and social desire were the keys to reform.

American cooks did not silence critics if they only abandoned frying and fatty foods and ate more slowly. The citizenry had also developed a dangerous taste for "condiments"—spices and sauces that heightened and sometimes transformed the flavors of foods and stimulated the appetite to an unnatural degree.[5] Common offenders included mustard and the hot red peppers that were native to the United States, as well as imported black pepper.

Condiments were also thought to inhibit the effects of chewing, salivation, and according to Trall, the involuntary actions of the tongue. Salt was a particularly onerous compound to Trall. "Common salt is in no sense dietical. It is entirely a foreign irritant, and its free employment renders the blood putrescent, the solids dry and rigid, the muscles inflexible, and the glands obstructed. The notion that it is essential to life and health is positively disproved by the experience of the millions of Japanese, who have never known its dietic use."[6] How Trall knew of the "millions of Japanese" in 1853, before Matthew Perry sailed into Tokyo Bay to "open" the Japanese Empire is not clear, and his information was not, in any case, accurate.

There was also a history of support for condiments with which reformers had to contend. In 1830 Edward Hitchcock identified five types of condiments in his *Dyspepsy Forestalled*: fats, sweets, acids, salt, and spices. He condemned only fats. He thought sugar and honey were "among the most nutritious of all substances" and the "acid condiments . . . undoubtedly serviceable with some kinds of food." He reserved his greatest praise for salt, and applauded spices' helpful stimulation of the digestive powers.[7] Tradition, folk beliefs in the efficacy of certain compounds to ward off disease, and the fact that many of the ingredients used in cooking were probably too decayed to be enjoyed without spices convinced most Americans that they ought to use "condiments" liberally.

Reformers attacked Hitchcock's position and criticized condiments for being "inflammatory in nature, and stimulating to the nervous system. . . . Articles preserved in salt, sugar, or vinegar, are neither as easily digested, nor as healthful as those in the natural state."[8] The "natural state" did not necessarily mean uncooked, either for meat or for vegetables. Nearly every cookbook and household manual urged broiling, boiling, or roasting all foods. Meat was seldom efficiently refrigerated, and it putrified quickly. And many linked the spread of cholera in 1832 to eating unboiled vegetables. Most health advisors—except the few vegetarians—suggested lean meats, and many argued that animal organs, especially kidneys and liver, were "wholly unfit for food," since they were part of the animals' excretory systems. Meat of herbivores was thought to be the least harmful and that of pigs, the most commonly eaten meat in pre–Civil War America, the most dangerous to health because of the slops they were fed. Slaughterhouses were criticized for improper and incomplete bleeding, since "the more bloody any kind of animal food is, the more unclean and putrescent."[9]

If American taste buds had been corrupted, how could people find their way to the clean and "natural" state of culinary and digestive grace? Beecher pointed to the way children responded to their initial experience with "condiments" and to the strong flavors of organ meats. Their sense of taste, she said, was "acute" because they were innocent and thus closer to meeting the requirements of a pure and Christian life. "The simple and natural taste of childhood," she wrote, "can be restored by drinking nothing but water, and a perfectly simple and healthful diet." By regarding children as exemplary of human potential, Beecher revealed the dramatic change in American ideology that had occurred in the early nineteenth century. By 1850 children were not considered fonts of sin and wickedness but rather as pure, simple, and uncorrupted examples of what humans could be. Human society

33

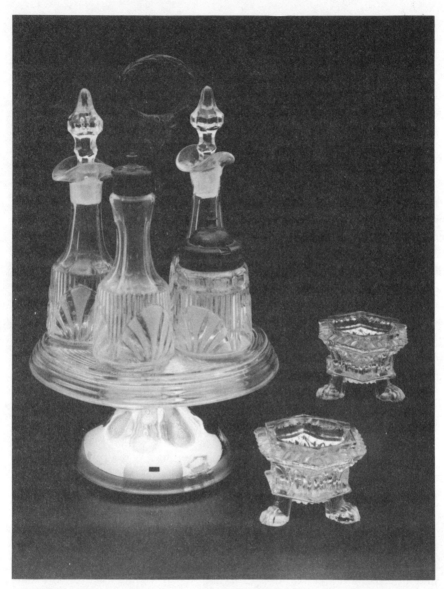

The presence of caster sets and salt cellars in American homes suggests that reformers convinced few Americans that condiments such as vinegar or pepper led to dyspepsia and even drunkenness. From left: caster set, Boston Silver Glass Co., probably Boston, Mass., silvered and pressed glass, ca. 1865; salt cellars, American, pressed glass, ca. 1830–60.

—even their parents—corrupted them. Children's behavior was proof not only of the accuracy of reformers' beliefs but of the culpability of adult society.[10]

Failure to account for age and, accordingly, for digestive capability could lead both children and "excitable" adults to trouble. Trall advocated a meatless diet of milk, bread, fruit, and vegetables for sensitive young stomachs. "Cool, slow, and phlegmatic" adults, he continued, could safely eat more stimulating food, but persons "full of habit and excitable temperament" should stop at bread, fruit, and vegetables. This warning was especially powerful for parents concerned about their own and their children's futures in the mobile society of pre-Civil War America. "Many young children," wrote Beecher, "would be saved from early death by attention to these rules."[11] In an age when young couples were increasingly leaving the close-knit kinship networks of family and community to move to rapidly growing cities, such inexpensive popular advice books as Beecher's or Alcott's volumes provided the support that was left behind. Such scare tactics were remarkably effective in their own time, especially when infant mortality was common and mothers, aunts, and grandmothers were not present to comfort and counsel the young mothers.

These would-be reformers and experts on the diet and debility of Americans had powerful enemies, or so they thought, in the popular authors and literati of the nation. Trall castigated most cookbooks as collections of recipes that "mix and mingle the greatest possible amount of seasonings, saltings, spicings, and greasings into a single dish. . . . No wonder the patrons and admirers of such cook-books are full of dyspepsia, and constipation, and hemorrhoids, and biliousness of every degree, and nervousness of every kind." He saved special vitriol for an estimable foe, Sarah Josepha Hale, editor of *Godey's Lady's Book* and author in 1852 of the *New Book of Cookery.* Trall heaped condemnation on her recipe for pork head "cheese," a luncheon or supper dish "highly seasoned with pepper, cayenne, and salt [to be] eaten with vinegar and mustard."[12]

For "natural" physiologists, and to a lesser extent for physicians, "stimulation" was troublesome for both the "excitable" person and for the culture as a whole. The fluidity of American society that so enthralled most Americans, surprised such foreign travelers as de Tocqueville and Mrs. Trollope, and lured immigrants from Europe was also a destabilizing force. Even as Beecher applauded a society with no aristocracy, she worried about controlling the masses of people—especially the Irish and German immigrants escaping famine and political unrest. As historian Karen Halttunen has shown, the growing urban centers were viewed both as places of opportunity and pits of deception and insincerity—full of "confidence men and painted women" who waited for the noble and naive rural bumpkin to fall into their clutches.[13]

Reformers connected bad eating habits and social disorder precisely because they viewed the world, the human body, and any efforts at reforming or reshaping them as part of one organic whole. Morality and health as well as physical strength and mental stability were all linked, in the end, to both the nation's future and the fate of each Americans' soul at Judgment. The fear that the "passions" would become uncontrollable and find their expression in crime, in overt sexuality, or even in revolt against the government was ever present in America in the antebellum era. Clerical and lay writers warned that cities could become "volcanoes," ready to erupt in violence. The "passions" of unregenerate men and women and, for conservative ministers, even of those whose religious conversion was borne of the emotional embrace of grace, were an obstruction to the establishment of the good society.[14]

One of the most obvious indications of the citizenry's distance from the state of perfection was its immoderate use of alcohol. The consumption of "ardent" spirits was, by current standards, considerable. Historian William J. Rorabaugh has estimated that in 1830, 5.2 gallons of ninety-proof spirits and 15 gallons of twenty-proof cider—and no beer—were drunk per person per year (as compared with 2.5 gallons of spirits and 25.7 gallons of ten-proof beer—and no cider—per capita annually in 1970).[15] Americans did not indulge merely to get drunk. Many thought alcohol aided digestion, made them stronger, cleared their thinking, and prevented disease. Traditionally trained physicians regularly administered spirits and wine to the infirm, and it was a popular folk remedy in America. Edward Hitchcock systematically attacked each of these contentions in 1830 in his *Dyspepsy Forestalled.* He maintained that it offered at best temporary digestive relief, and as for being an inhibitor of the spread of disease, alcohol's "only value . . . appears to consist, in inspiring confidence in those who employ [it]; and this is a state of mind, more favorable than that of fear, for repelling contagion." He admitted that alcohol did "rouse into action that which already exists in the constitution," but that this was a short-term gain that ultimately resulted

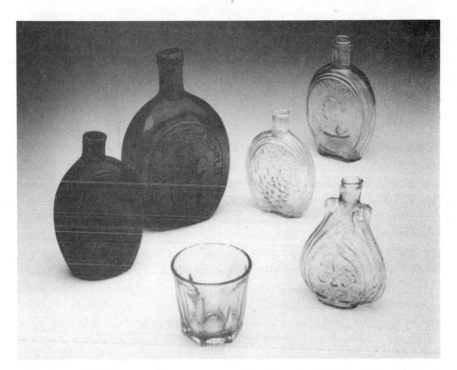

Flasks and bottles—millions were produced—often depicted American popular heroes, mottoes, and other images symbolizing national pride. Whiskey flasks and bottles, American, pressed and blown three-mold glass; whiskey glass, American, pressed glass, ca. 1830–60.

in exhaustion. Alcohol, he concluded, confused "all the mental operations . . . thus entailing upon ourselves the whole hateful train of nervous maladies."[16]

Many critics did not include wines and "malt liquors" in their condemnation of "ardent spirits." The great danger for wine drinkers was the possibility of drinking adulterated goods.

> Wines that have been treated with preparations of lead, in order to destroy their acidity, have, in general, a sweetish taste succeeded by an astringent metal one. Spoiled tart white wines are changed into red, by the aid of sumach, logwood, and various berries: chalk, lime, or magnesia, are employed to take up the excess of acid, and

lead to render them sweeter. . . . The leaves of plants, more or less poisonous, are used to impart an artificial flavour. When these diabolical cordials have attained a proper colour and clearness, they are combined with cider and real wines, according to the conscience or interest of the brewer.[17]

Unlike wines, "malt liquors" (beers and ales) were drunk only occasionally in the United States before the Civil War. The taste for beer and ale as well as brewing technology were brought to the United States by German immigrants who fled the economic and political dislocations of the revolutions of 1848, and the beverages were not a significant part of mainstream culture until the 1870s. Early-nineteenth-century commentators viewed brewery products as invigorating. "Malt liquors, when of good quality, and drunk in moderation, constitute, for many persons, an innocent and wholesome beverage," wrote a contributor to the *Journal of Health* in 1830.[18]

The significant qualifier in the health experts' support of malted beverages and wines was moderation. Intemperate drinking of wine or beers led to drunkenness, which in turn led to numerous evils, including death and insanity. As Beecher commented in 1856, "The abuse of the stomach, brain, and nerves by stimulating drinks, has become so terrible in this nation that the whole country is roused to put an end to *one kind, i.e.,* the *alcoholic* articles." The prohibition of alcohol consumption did not become the law of the land until nearly three-quarters of a century after Beecher's optimistic comment, but counties and states (Maine in 1831, for example) succeeded in "going dry" in the ferment of reform enthusiasm that characterized the era.[19]

The near-universal agreement of physicians and reformers about the ill effects of whiskey has often obscured the significant differences of opinion within that community. R. T. Trall condemned Beecher's recipes in her *Domestic Receipt Book* (1843) because "the wine and brandy she recommends in her cakes, and pies, and pudding sauces are better calculated to make men drunkards, than to make them wise in choosing." Trall's words reveal the hyperbole of the true believer: he was, after all, one of the grand masters of the "cold water army" that favored utter prohibition, rather than mere temperance. The danger was twofold. Those poor souls already addicted to alcohol might be led by their weakness to a lethal overindulgence in brandied cakes, thereby dying from sheer gluttony. For the remainder of the people, Trall and other health reformers saw such recipes as the begin-

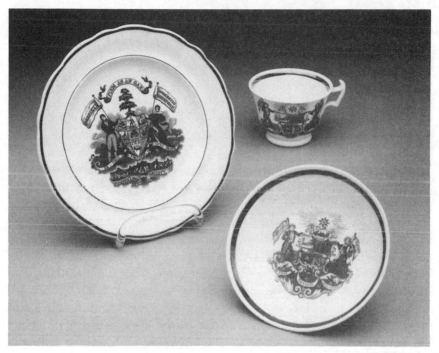

Imported English tablewares such as these were an everyday assertion of a commitment to temperance. Plate, tea cup, and saucer, all transfer-printed bone china, Staffordshire, Eng., ca. 1845.

·ning of a potentially catastrophic pattern of indulgence. Mild and even sweetened liquor-cakes would secretly whet the young and unsuspecting's appetite for drink. The victim (usually male) would then begin to experiment with bolder, less disguised forms of alcohol until he was swept into the vortex of drunkenness, debility, and death. Much like critics a century later who saw inevitable connections between marijuana and heroin, nineteenth-century analysts of the human condition linked the first tastes of drink with the horrible consequences that beset a few extremists. The optimism of some reformers about the perfectability of men and women was counterbalanced and sometimes overmatched by the pessimism of those who saw eventual mass destruction in the amber glow of the glass of spirits, or in the darkened distillates of another of their enemies—the patent medicine salesman.[20]

"The most certain means by which the predisposed, even when guilty of no intemperance, may invite the attack of their lurking enemy," wrote the *Journal of Health* in 1830, "is a plentiful use of pectoral balsams, balms of life, lung restorers, cough lozenges, or indeed any of the list of 'certain cures' in the newspapers." Indeed, many patent medicine "cures" were themselves addictive because they contained alcohol and, occasionally, opium. Laudanum, an extremely popular mixture of the the two drugs, was consistently criticized from 1830 until 1906, when controls were placed on the sale of it.[21]

Health reformers of nearly every cast found themselves in agreement with physicians in their concern about the effects of vastly popular commercially produced medicines, termed "patent" or "quack" remedies. In 1829 the *Journal of Health* attacked the "numerous vegetable syrups made and sold in [Philadelphia], under the title of Panacea." After soundly criticizing "the pompous annunciations of the venders of nostrums" for refusing to list the ingredients of their concoctions (but volunteering what is not contained in them), the journal cited the case of Swaim's Panacea, one of the most popular patent medicines of the late 1820s and early 1830s. Swaim's was found to be laced with mercury, in spite of the manufacturer's claims to the contrary. Twenty-five years later, in 1856, the problem was still with Americans.

> Most of the popular quack medicines, advertised as cures for almost every disease, contain either calomel or quinine, or strong metallic or other poisons, that stimulate the brain or drain the blood [away]. . . . Tonics tend to destroy tone, cathartics tend to produce constipation, emetics tend to debilitate stomach, liver, and bowels, which such medicines are mercury, arsenic, antimony, iodine, and the like are insidious poisons. . . . It is the wise and skillful physician alone who can use these dangerous agents properly.

William Alcott's dissatisfaction with popular pharmaceutics is evident in the title of his autobiography: *Forty Years in the Wilderness of Pills and Powders.*[22]

Concern for and criticism of Americans' choices in liquid refreshment or "cures" did not stop with whiskey and nostrums. One writer in the *Journal of Health* complained in 1829 that "the largest class of strong waters still remains unnoticed, viz., the infusion of Imperial, and Hyson, and Gunpowder; or the decoction of the Arabian berry as, by a paraphrase, coffee is sometimes called." Edward Hitchcock countered the arguments "of nine tenths of the nervous ladies and gentlemen in the land," who claimed that their tea was a *"cure* for their headache" by asserting that "it is most commonly, the cause of it." Tracing what seemed to him an inevitable course of temporary calming followed by increased exhaustion and eventually a greater and greater need for the stimulant, he proclaimed, "How exactly does this course resemble that of the drunkard!"[23]

Tea and coffee were important parts of the day of nearly every American living above the level of bare subsistence. Hitchcock estimated in 1830 that Americans annually consumed one pound of tea and two pounds of coffee *per capita.* In the United States drinking tea—usually but not always a late-afternoon ritual—was an important and enduring carryover from English life. Even some normally uncompromising critics recognized the joys of the tea table and in so doing elicited condemnation from their peers. Hitchcock berated those "advocates of total abstinence from spirit, who would feel exceedingly guilty to offer alcohol to their friends, [who] are often found most devotedly attached to two or three cups of the strongest infusion of Imperial, or Gunpowder, or Young Hyson." Both Hitchcock and the *Journal of Health* cautioned "the feeble, the nervous, the dyspeptic, the hypochondriacal, the gouty," and others prone to weakness to avoid the drink if possible.[24] Coffee, usually drunk at breakfast, and chocolate were similarly characterized as too stimulating, and Americans were urged to forgo them. The battle still rages today.

Although modern medical scientists classify alcoholic beverages as depressants, early-nineteenth-century observers thought them stimulants because they caused loss of motor control, decline in behavioral inhibitions, and a seeming increase in energy. "Alcohol and opium, tea and coffee," Catharine Beecher wrote in 1856, "simply stimulate the brain and nervous system. . . . This stimulus is always followed by a reaction of debility, which is proportioned to the degree of previous stimulation."[25]

For Americans of the pre–Civil War era, "stimulation" was a particularly vexing problem because it made control—of individuals and of the future of society—problematical. The three decades before the war were characterized by rapid economic growth and equally precipitous calamity—the Panics of 1837 and 1857, for example—growing urban congestion, and, at least in the eyes of many established Americans, increasing crime. Prisons of great scale were built all over the Northeast; free land and open spaces, the prison's opposite, were the source of unbounded optimism for some, but a source of discomfort for others. How could the traditional controlling and beneficent forces of community and church, as well as an enduring sense of place, survive in a country in which people seemed to be constantly in motion? Society could never evolve into the type of moral Christian community that would presage the Second Coming if "the tea and coffee stimulants that are undermining the constitution of women and children" and the "alcoholic drinks and tobacco" that caused men to be "debilitated" continued to be as popular as they were.[26]

Health advocates saw in the swirling trail of smoke from a pipe or cigarette an approaching calamity as great as the one they feared from alcohol.

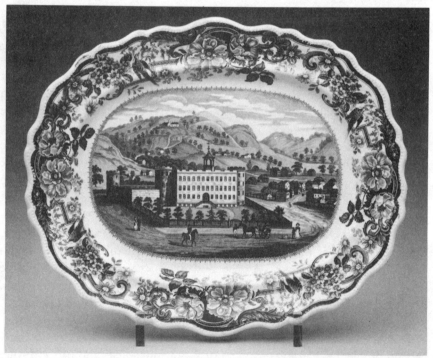

The medieval form of the prison building was a dynamic counterpoint to the gently rolling domesticated hillsides that surrounded it and served as both comfort to the outsider and warning to those tempted by crime. Platter, "Penitentiary in Allegheny," J. and R. Clews, Cobridge, Eng., transfer-printed earthenware, ca. 1835.

The *Journal of Health,* in 1829, termed tobacco "an absolute poison," and linked "the almost constant thirst occasioned by smoking and chewing . . . to the intemperate use of ardent spirits." Edward Hitchcock thought it brought on "the very evils it was intended to remove." American men smoked in spite of such attacks, and evidently thought that "tobacco, in some of its forms, is serviceable for headaches, weak eyes, the preservation of teeth, purifying the breath, [and] cold and watery stomachs."[27] Catharine Beecher was especially unbending in her hatred of smokers and chewers.

> In this nation no one can travel without being constantly made to feel what a selfish as well as disgusting and ungallant habit is induced by the use of tobacco. The majority of ladies are offended by the effluvium of that weed, and disgusted by the marks on the mouth and face, while the puddles of tobacco juice that infest our public conveyances, the breath of smokers, and the wads of squirting chewers, not only defile the dress but keep a sensitive stomach in constant excitement and agitation.[28]

Smoking after dinner or in the library was an activity for men only. Chewing the plug or loose chaw was often banished to the workrooms in the house, or to the barn in the country, and was tolerated only in saloons and clubs in the villages and towns. These were places into which women did not ordinarily venture. Thus inhaling snuff, chewing tobacco, and smoking were immensely popular pastimes for men, not only for the sense of male camaraderie that smoking engendered but also because they thought it healthful.

Like the *Journal of Health,* Beecher was convinced that "this weed is rank poison . . . draining the nervous fountain of thousands of pale and delicate young men" because its effect was "to exhaust the nervous system, to destroy the tone of the stomach, to create a thirst for intoxicating drinks, to irritate the temper, stupefy the sensibilities, defile the house, and offend the neat and refined. . . . It is probable," she continued, "that tobacco destroys more than alcohol, because so many more use it, and so many are led to opium and alcohol by its influence. And yet the clergyman, the church elder, the father of the family, indulge in a useless and dangerous practice, merely to gratify a morbid appetite."[29]

Like other commentators who opposed the use of "the weed," Beecher linked smoking and chewing to the development of other vices that seemed deeply rooted in American behavior. "The use of tobacco," she warned, "lessens the sensibility of taste, and awakens an unnatural longing for stimulus." Beecher's language betrays not only an ambivalence about human nature and potential but also the author's own roots in mainstream nineteenth-century Protestant religion. The yen for condiments, wine, and liquor existed *a priori* in human beings, yet it was "unnatural," a word choice that contradicted the implicit presence connoted by the "awakening" of evil traits. Somewhat like the concept of Original Sin, Beecher viewed the slumbering beast "longing for stimulus" as part of all men and women. Yet like the mainstream of Protestant theologians, Americans seemed unable to accept completely either the determinism of Original Sin or the individual freedom of perfectionism. Hence the seeming contradiction: men, women, and even children in the wrong environment might still avoid their potential roles as implementers of the new society, possessed, as it were, by a latent tendency to do the wrong thing.

Both men and women appeared tangled in a constantly enlarging trap of overstimulation, excitement, decline, and a consequently magnified need for stimulation. "Men are debilitated by alcoholic drinks and tobacco," Beecher wrote, and "women are almost as much injured in the health and comfort by their use of tea and coffee. Multitudes of wives and mothers become feeble, irritable, and miserable from the daily exhaustion caused by these narcotic stimulants. They feel the loss of their tea and coffee almost as much as the inebriate misses his daily libations." The gender distinction enumerated in this critique is obviously simplistic: men drank tea and coffee as well, and presumably suffered from withdrawal when their supply of caffeine was halted. Perhaps the distinction was made for effect—to indict women for their seemingly harmless activities as well as men for their more socially accepted ill habits. Men and women were "so ignorant of physiology as often to imagine that the little strength they have is the gift of the baneful cups which yield only poison. They drink and feel better because a new stimulus is applied to the brain and nerves, to be followed by a new, secret, but certain drain on their nervous fountain."[30]

The new urbanizing world of opportunity was fraught with peril. Fortunes could be lost as rapidly as made. Complexity and conspiracy, reality and illusion, truth and "confidence games" dominated the politics, economics, social relationships, and literature of Jacksonian America. Most obviously a theme in such little-read works as Melville's *The Confidence-Man:*

His Masquerade (1857), it is also present in the serialized popular fiction that appeared in such women's magazines as *Godey's, Peterson's, Demorest's,* and *Graham's.* Who could be trusted in the urban world of vice and fashion, where sincerity and sin coexisted side by side, and often in similar guise?

Even seemingly healthy food could not be trusted. "Frauds and adulteration are more generally perpetrated in articles of food, drink, and medicine, probably, than in relation to all articles of commerce put together," wrote Russell Trall in his *Hydropathic Cook-Book* (1853). Concern about the adulteration of foodstuffs is evident at least as early as the 1830s, when commercial bakers were roundly criticized for artificially stimulating the doughs they baked. In *A Treatise on Bread and Bread-Making* (1837), Sylvester Graham pointed out that public bakers freely experimented with chemicals, especially ammonia.[31] Working-class people, especially those living in the growing cities, were prime customers for commercial bakeries, since many did not have a sufficiently large kitchen stove or the time to bake. Many middle-class Americans, by contrast, still made their bread at home in wood burning stoves until the 1880s or 1890s.

Graham was the early nineteenth century's most famous advocate of whole-grain flours for baked goods. In his *Lectures on the Science of Human Life* (1839), he recalled nostalgically the previous two centuries, invoking the memory of "those blessed days of New England's prosperity and happiness when our good mothers used to make the family bread." For Graham, bread-making was a sacred responsibility, important "in relation to all the bodily and intellectual and moral interests of . . . husbands and children . . . and . . . to the domestic and social and civil welfare of mankind . . . for time and eternity."[32] Like some of the patent medicine hucksters of his era, Graham asserted that the failing health of Americans could be halted and improved by vegetarianism generally and by "Graham" bread and flour specifically. He found great fault with the common practice of using flour from which the bran had been removed, recommending whole-grain flour, "which contains all the natural properties of the grain."[33]

But even "Graham flour" was subject to the dastardly practices of adulteration. Trall enumerated the types of contaminants that unscrupulous purveyors of flour and baked goods used to alter flours and finished products.

The wheat-meal or Graham flour in market, is not infrequently an admixture of "shorts" or "middlings," with old, stale, soured, or damaged fine flour; and fine flour is sometimes—more especially in European markets—adulterated with *whiting, ground stones, bone dust,* and *plaster of Paris.* [34]

Readers and consumers were comforted somewhat by Trall's assurance that the harmful impurities with which these confidence men had betrayed the innocent buyer could be identified by simple tests with sweet-oil or vinegar[35] at home. Trall divided "all breads . . . into *domestic* bread and *baker's* bread," finding "the principle [*sic*] difference" to be "in the greater degree of fermentation to which the latter is subjected, and the alkaline matters which are generally employed by bakers to neutralize the acid created by excessive fermentation." He assured his readers that "the best bread that ever was or ever will be made is unquestionably that of coarse-ground, unbolted meal, mixed with pure water, and baked in any convenient way."[36]

Sylvester Graham was Jacksonian America's most famous and unrelenting advocate of a vegetarian diet. Vegetarianism had been analyzed and discussed for decades before 1830. English physician George Cheyne rejected meat eating in the early eighteenth century and popularized the idea (if not the practice) with his *Essay on Health and Long Life.* In 1815 another English physician, William Lambe, updated Cheyne's work and proposed the meatless diet as a cure for tuberculosis. And Percy Shelley's *A Vindication of Natural Diet* (1813) was reprinted throughout the nineteenth century, as late as 1884.[37]

The debate about vegetarianism intensified in the broader context of reform and criticism that swept the nation during the thirty years before the Civil War. In 1829 the *Journal of Health* defended a primarily vegetarian diet, characteristically comparing American eating habits with those of apparently healthier (and poorer) cultures. Asian and Irish nationals were cited as examples of healthy peoples, and "the Lazzaroni of Naples, with forms so active and finely proportioned, [eat] coarse bread and potatoes . . . [and] a glass of iced water slightly acidilated." Throughout the period, popular magazines and books contrasted the allegedly superior health and strength of nearly vegetarian peasant cultures (none of which had yet emigrated to the United States) with the less healthy meat and fat eaters of the far North (Eskimos and Laplanders) and with the mixed diets of northern

Europeans.[38] In 1856, Beecher continued this trend, suggesting a connection between working with one's hands, poverty, a vegetarian diet, and good health.

> The working people in Ireland live on potatoes. The peasantry of Lancashire and Cheshire, who are the handsomest race in England, live chiefly on potatoes and butter-milk. The bright and hardy Arabs live almost entirely on vegetable food. The brave and vigorous Spartans never ate meat. Most of the hardiest soldiers in Northern Europe seldom taste of meat. . . . Except in America, it is rare that the strongest laborers eat any meat.[39]

The romantic celebration of the peasantry—with their strong backs, long lives, and (assumedly) happy lot—is a variant of the Edenic myth, a "state of nature" in which men and women lived innocently, peacefully, and healthily with one another and among the flora and fauna. This implicit critique of urbanized middle-class and wealthy living remains on safe ground: The working classes are portrayed as beneficiaries of their lot, which was not a vale of tears but an insurance of health. For the wealthy this myth implied that they need only adopt a proper diet to maintain their health and need not worry about the material well-being of the working class. In addition, Beecher juxtaposed the life of the hardy peasant with that of the soldier, presaging the militaristic and strength-related concerns and urgings of the end of the nineteenth century.

Unlike Graham, Beecher did not argue for a strictly vegetarian diet. She allowed that when people "from any cause, need to be not only nourished but *stimulated* by food, then animal food is the best."[40] For most Americans, however, stimulation was unnecessary and potentially dangerous. Physicians were for the most part opposed to vegetarianism in the early nineteenth century because they were convinced that vegetable foods were more difficult to digest than meats, fowl, or fish, and that meats were essential to strength and vitality because they were most like human flesh. Even vegetarianism's most strident opponents warned against eating too much meat, however, since it might lead to "plethora" and excess of blood.

The radical vegetarians—Trall, fellow water-curist Joel Shew, and others —argued that "internal putrefaction" resulted whenever meat was consumed.

Man, in taking his nutrition indirectly by the eating of animals, must of necessity get the original nutriment more or less deteriorated from the unhealthy condition and accidents of the animal he feeds upon, the impurities, putrescent matters, and excretions always mingled in the blood, the flesh, and the viscera of animal substances.[41]

Trall posited a link between blood that had been rendered impure by decayed meats or stimulants. In this sense he was repeating an idea expressed in the 1830s by Graham, who was convinced that disease originated in the disruption of the "vital spirit" caused by stomach disorders, which in turn affected the nervous system.

While vegetarianism was hardly common before (or after) 1830, it was widely discussed in the context of the debates about temperance, criminal reform, abolitionism, and the rights of women. Sylvester Graham stood at the center of the debate, at least in the 1830s and 1840s. Born in 1794, Graham was the seventeenth child of a family that lost its father within two years of his birth. His mother soon afterward became "deranged," and Graham himself was afflicted with tuberculosis in 1810. He recovered, only to suffer a nervous breakdown in 1823, the year he enrolled at Amherst College. In 1828 he entered the ministry, leaving the cloth two years later to participate in the temperance crusade as a general agent for the Pennsylvania Temperance Society in Philadelphia. There he read about anatomy, physiology, and dietetics, research he synthesized into an overall "Science of Human Life." He lectured at Philadelphia's Franklin Institute, and although he was a popular speaker, he remained a minor public figure until 1832, when the cholera epidemic catapulted him to prominence. Cholera attacked the gastrointestinal tract, and Graham posited that overstimulation of the digestive tract by the liquor, spices, and fats that Americans loved to consume had weakened them. When several patients survived after adopting Graham's dietary regimen, he became an important national presence.

Graham argued that the stomach and nerves were intimately connected, and that the origin of all diseases could be traced to that connection. He urged those afflicted with mild cholera to keep clean, avoid damp air, and partake of "Indian meal gruel, or rice-water, or coarse, unboiled wheat-meal gruel, or wheat-bran tea . . . in moderate quantities." He reasoned that because everyone exposed to the contagion was not afflicted with it, personal

48

differences and habits must account for whether or not one succumbed to cholera. He found few if any of those who escaped the epidemic to be unhealthy or in any way intemperate, and circuitously concluded that because they escaped disease they were healthy.[42]

While in New York, Graham founded a boarding house to be run strictly on the principles set forth in his works. The daily routine indicated both Graham's strict Protestant upbringing and his bent for protomilitary arrangements. "The morning bell," he wrote in 1837, "is rung precisely at five o'clock as one hour at least is necessary for bathing and exercise before breakfast."[43] In winter, he generously allowed his boarders to rise at six. The lights were extinguished and the doors closed at ten P.M. A second Grahamite boarding house, established in Boston in 1837, attracted many of the area's political and social radicals, including abolitionists William Lloyd Garrison and Arthur Tappan. The Boston institution was run by David Cambell, a Garrisonian delegate to the New York Anti-Slavery Convention of 1833, which was instrumental in the formation of the American Anti-Slavery Society.

Graham's Boston activities provoked criticism from a broad popular base, including newspapermen, physicians, and bakers (whom he attacked for using chemical additives, superfine and even adulterated flour, and other shortcuts to enhance their "pecuniary interest" at the expense of public health).[44] In 1838, the *Boston Courier* asked "what can surpass that which finds long life in starvation, sees 'moral reform' in bran and cabbage . . . and promises to revolutionize the world with johnny-cake and boiled beans . . . ? Reader, if you wish to preserve your health . . . *eat your victuals and go about your business.*" The *Boston Medical and Surgical Journal* asserted that "a greater humbug or a more disgusting writer never lived."[45]

Professional medical journals also engaged in the debate; the 1836 volume of the *Boston Medical and Surgical Journal* is full of charges and counter-charges about the validity and safety of Graham's brand of vegetarianism. Accusations that Grahamism led to insanity provoked equally vehement denials and counterattacks from Graham, who linked dyspepsia and over-stimulation to a meat-laden diet.

In the conglomeration of reform movements active in Boston in the 1830s, the rancor about Graham's views stemmed in part from his extremist position and his stern conviction that diet, debility, and sexuality were inextricably linked. Graham was convinced that masturbation was a great evil. This belief did not separate him from other critics and advisors of this time. (Henry Ward Beecher, William Alcott, and Timothy Shay Arthur—all prolific authors of advice for the young, old, and in-between—cautioned against the "solitary vice.") But Graham was almost obsessive about the "problem," and his continual connection of diet to morality, and specifically to masturbation, led to his rapid isolation even in liberal Boston circles.[46]

Graham moved from the hot controversies of Boston to the small-town atmosphere of Northampton, Massachusetts, in late 1837. His fame was such that even his adversaries in the *Boston Medical and Surgical Journal* had paid him a grudging compliment in 1836. "No man can travel by stage or steamboat, or go into any part of our country," the magazine asserted, "and begin to advocate a vegetable diet . . . without being immediately asked —'What. Are you a Grahamite?' " But if he was a famous man, Graham was not necessarily an effective one. Once in Northampton, he bombarded the local papers with letters, which were usually so full of self-importance that he became a caricature. In a long, intense letter of 1844 to Alexander Wheelock Thayer, editor of the *Northampton Courier,* Graham attacked not the evils he saw in flesh-eating, but a more general symbol of decay he saw around him. Using an image of pent-up power familiar to Americans of the pre–Civil War era, Graham saw himself as "constituted with a living volcano of philanthropy instinctive and unquenchable. . . . I pour out upon you, my dear friend, the lava of my molten and surging sensibilities, because the fires within me are deeply stirred, and will have out. Fires, not of indignation, but of that sympathy which tastes of death for every man."[47]

What evil had caused this growing pressure in Graham's moral sensibility? "Was ever the human world more rife with human folly and delusion than at present? Did ever human passion more powerfully overwhelm and subvert human reason than at this day?" he asked Thayer. "We boast of the light and refinement, of the civilization and religion, of the intelligence and moral excellence and true piety of our age," he asserted. "And without doubt all these qualities do exist in individuals of the human kind, more largely than ever before." But this concession to religious perfectionism was hardly optimistic, for Graham was convinced that "in equal measure to our increase in intelligence, we have, as an age, refined in wickedness."[48]

As part of his overarching cultural concern, Graham singled out "the obscure and filthy plays of Shakespear [sic]" and claimed that actors "mark for omission all the more shockingly lewd and grossly obscene portions . . . yet when they are reading their expurgated parts in public, they know that every male as well as every female present, has his book before him."

Graham alluded to the "tableaux" presented in theatres, asserting that "it is popular to contemplate with unvailed [*sic*] face and hot-blooded admiration, a nude Venus—not in the marble statue, but living, breathing, acting flesh and blood, in the person of a dancing harlot." He found even stronger words of condemnation for "refined" women, "perfectly modest and chaste," who "throng the public spectacle in so dense a crowd, that her heart sympathetically responds in its strong pulsations to the heart of the *Satyrus* against whose bosom she is necessarily yet willingly pressed."[49]

Strict Freudian analysts would find much evidence with which to build a case for Graham's apparently repressed sexuality and his hostility to women and might link both to the early childhood loss of his father and the fact that he witnessed his mother's madness. Graham regarded women as beings not only incapable of understanding what men could do but also more likely to engage in harmful behavior. Women had "elements in her character somewhat of nature and largely of education—felt rather than understood by herself, which are susceptible to being excited into ruling and ruinous activity; and all the more dangerous because recondite to her own understanding." Women, more than men, were active participants in the increasingly false world of manners, a behavior pattern that unbeknownst to them endangered their souls, and indeed the whole republic.[50]

Graham thus raised the specter that haunted more perceptive analysts of American culture in the era preceding the War between the States: How could an innocent or even a worldly and worthy person strike through the mask, as Melville asked in *Moby Dick* (1851), or see through the surface of the pond, as Thoreau had tried to do? And what would be seen? Graham argued that people could know who they were and who those around them were by what they ate and drank; hence they could control their "baser" passions. Because he linked diet and nutrition not only to physical well-being but to moral and spiritual life, Graham was certain that he could solve the riddle of appearance and reality.

Graham died in 1851. Looking back over fifty years, James Bradley Thayer, Alexander's son, recalled his isolating eccentricities and arrogance with a sympathetic, if critical vision:

He was a strange person, very well known in Northampton with a most inordinate sense of his own merits and powers, and very eccentric. I remember seeing him as he grew infirm, seated in a wheelbarrow, and clothed in a long dressing gown of bedticking, wheeled through the streets to the post office by a man-servant. He is forgotten now, but he used to be quoted as saying that strangers would visit Northampton after he was dead to see the home where he had lived. That never happened, I fear.[51]

The Graham version of vegetarianism never attracted a widespread popular following in pre–Civil War America, but its practitioners and advocates attracted attention in reform groups and colleges and helped define the nature of "health" during an era of widespread concern for the future of the republic and, ultimately, of the whole human race. Grahamism—bran bread, water, and vegetables—was popular among many of the radical communities that sought to reform the United States by separating themselves from the great mass of the population. Members of some of the Shaker communities, Brook Farm, Fruitlands, and many of the "phalanxes" established on the model of socialist Charles Fourier (1772–1837) embraced Grahamism for a time. Certain welfare institutions, such as the Albany Orphan Asylum, also tried the Graham combination of discipline and diet in the 1830s, arousing great controversy in the periodical press.[52]

David Cambell, of the Boston Graham boarding house, took his philosophy westward to Oberlin in 1839, where he became "Steward to the Collegiate Institute." He quickly abolished the elective meat table at the college's dining facility, which provoked great protest even at the nation's most radical reformist institution of higher learning. The outcry against Cambell's rigid interpretation was so great that he was forced to resign in 1841. "Graham clubs" were established at other colleges in the late 1830s, and most, like the one at Wesleyan University, were relatively small (eight to ten members) and short-lived.

Grahamites' hard-line approach to reform also helped undo one of the most active health-related groups of the early 1830s: the American Physiological Society. The organization had consistently increased its membership in the mid-1830s, but it declined rapidly until it disappeared in 1840. In addition to its bias for Grahamism, it failed to maintain its membership because it neglected dress reform, temperance, physical education, school reform, abolitionism, and women's rights. Its narrowness isolated the Society at just the time when American culture was vibrant with a sort of nervous energy to act. Graham's periodical, the *Graham Journal of Health and Longevity,* had at one point a circulation of more than fifteen hundred, but nearly six hundred of those subscribers were delinquent. The journal disappeared in 1839.

Vegetarianism did not, however, die with Grahamism in the 1840s. In fact, the renaissance of the antimeat crusade in 1850 can best be explained as a result of Graham's disappearance from the scene. The American Vegetarian Society was founded in 1850, and at the annual meeting of the Society in 1853, three hundred and fifty members, including such important public figures as Lucy Stone, Amelia Bloomer, Susan B. Anthony, and Horace Greeley, engaged in spirited debate. First fueled by the enthusiasms of the women's rights crusade, this form of vegetarianism was broader-based than Grahamism had been and was supported by the growing activism of women and men who linked the future of the nation to the strength of the home. As the home increasingly came to be defined as that realm separate from and in opposition to the commercial world, women began to assert the connection between their role as nurturers of their families and the moral future of the race and republic. Diet, for which they had primary responsibility, was therefore an appropriate "power base" for both male health reformers and women's rights advocates. Like other reform activities, the vegetarian enthusiasm waned and was swept into the background as the crisis over slavery deepened. By 1855 the annual meeting of the Society was sparsely attended.

Vegetarianism in antebellum America encountered resistance not only because it challenged long-practiced food preferences and the opinions of medical theorists but also because it was a form of prevention rather than therapy—a relatively passive and pessimistic view that constantly risked identification with the social and cultural extremism that had become problematical for mainstream Americans. Moreover, it was in competition with other forms of physical and mental improvement that, though occasionally extremist, still offered people the satisfaction of engaging in some sort of positive action that seemed at least superficially to alter their condition in a more noticeable manner. Rather than simply not eating flesh, men and women might directly improve their lot by using new instruments, new knowledge, or new activities—water, magnetism and electricity, architecture, and calisthenics.

53

THE SPRINGS (AND SHOCKS) OF LIFE

Readied by nearly continuous religious revivals that preached that human and social perfectibility was possible, Americans were quick to seize two routes toward that goal introduced in the three decades before the Civil War. Both the water cure and early versions of "animal magnetism" and electrotherapeutics were promoted as panaceas for human ills, and both were relatively painless in comparison with the blistering, bleeding, and purgation of heroic medicine. Moreover, both forms of treatment suggested positive action, rather than the preventive negativism of vegetarianism—an appealing prospect in a nation that was aggressively expanding in the commercial, political, and geographical sectors. Western civilization did not discover water as a healing agent in the nineteenth century, but only the truly informed knew a form of water therapy was practiced by the Romans. Of course, electrotherapy was new in the nineteenth century. The presumed novelty of both cures was in itself appealing, and helped anchor these forms of treatment in the American therapeutics for decades.

The *thermae* of ancient Rome were integral parts of the city's architecture; taking the baths was a common part of everyday life. Hippocrates had recommended bathing as a therapeutic device, as had Agathinus, whose *On Hot and Cold Baths* was written in the first century A.D. and Galen, whose treatises on medicine were published about a century later. Medieval Europeans of both sexes bathed nude together in the public baths that could be found in most of the continent's cities and towns. These establishments generally included steam rooms, tubs, large pools, and beds for resting. Public baths were systematically closed by the sixteenth century because of the fear of contracting syphilis and other venereal diseases or of helping spread epidemics. Moreover, Catholic and Protestant clergymen campaigned against the corrupt moral behavior and shameless nudity baths promoted. Accusation became reality by the seventeenth century; public baths in Western Europe often were transformed into brothels. In Eastern Europe, the Islamic world, and the Far East, communal bathing endured.[1]

Private bathing, which had none of the associations of disease and licentiousness, virtually disappeared between 1400 and 1700. External bathing was rediscovered in the late seventeenth century, but primarily as a means of treating disease. Fears of massive epidemics receded, and some physiologists asserted connections between both internal disruption and epidermal manifestations and between clean skin and health, though the latter was not much believed until after 1850. In *Some Thoughts Concerning Education* (1693), John Locke recommended foot baths to invigorate and protect infants. Locke's advocacy of such treatment was based on a popular physiological notion that the feet were the sensitive external "pole" of many diseases and disruptions from within; hence, by invigorating the external sensitive portion of the body, debility could be avoided. This theory remained current until the middle of the nineteenth century.

Sir John Fleyer's popular *Enquiry into the Right Use of Baths* (1697) recommended both warm and cold baths to calm and invigorate the body and avoid or ease disease. His theory turned on the assumption that cold water would conduct the disruptive energies of disease out from the skin. By the time Reverend John Wesley's *Primitive Physick* was published in 1747, the clergyman's advocacy of drinking great quantities of water and a regimen of hot and (especially) cold baths had both caught on. Wesley's work remained popular for decades afterward.[2]

The idea that drinking cold water might aid in the treatment of gout and "stone"—a general term used to describe a variety of internal pains—was advocated by Dutch physician Herman van der Heyden in 1644. John

Hancocke's *Febrifugium magnum* (published in about 1720) and John Smith's more popular *Curiosities of Common Water* (1723) both advocated drinking larger quantities of water to relieve fever. Similar publications by other European physicians appeared at about the same time.[3]

In 1830 Edward Hitchcock cited Fleyer and called water "the most promotive of health, strength, longevity, and serenity of mind."[4] The first volume of the *Journal of Health* referred to both John Hancocke and Fleyer in its advocacy of a "Watery Regimen," which the journal's editors maintained, gave "serenity to the mind, and healthful feelings to the body." Their concern in the essay, however, was with "the advantages of water drinking, as detailed by Sir John Floyer [*sic*]." Bell and Condie's list of diseases that drinking large amounts of water was reputed to cure included apoplexy, blindness, gout, convulsions, and madness. Hot water was also recommended over peppermint and laudanum for, respectively, "cramps and pain . . . [and] wakefulness."[5]

Hitchcock considered warm baths a "preservative of health, a restorative of health, and a luxury." The *Journal of Health* agreed and endeavored to combat the "erroneous opinion, that the warm bath is enfeebling, and renders the person using it, more liable to take cold." The authors referred to the ancient Roman traditions of using the warm bath "to renovate vigour exhausted by exertion" and were careful to point out that "during the decline of the Roman empire . . . luxurious indulgences of all kinds were carried to excess." This was an important point for readers of 1829, whose magazines, newspapers, and books taught them that all previous experiments in republican government and all great empires had declined and fallen. For a nation increasingly concerned with its own place in history and the importance of avoiding the seemingly inevitable pattern of rise and fall, this statement was an essential qualifier for any positive reference to the ancient world. Roman bathers had in fact violated the nineteenth-century Christian's vision of propriety: They bathed "four, five, and even eight times a day" in water of "very high heat," a "violent stimulus" that led to "the ready occurrence of debility and disease." Americans who would be healthy —and implicitly, help break the pattern of decline and fall—were admonished to bathe at most once a day in water 88 to 98 degrees Fahrenheit.[6]

Fear of warm baths apparently originated in the popular idea that a warmed torso would "take cold as it cooled" and succumb to any of the diseases classified under the rubric of a "cold." Advocates of the warm bath agreed that "over-heating and fatigue, after violent exercise" was radically different from the feeling enjoyed after the warm bath. "In the former case, the skin is cold and weakened by excessive perspiration. . . . In the second, the heat of the system is prevented from escaping, and has a tendency to accumulate." The authors' argument was further buttressed by their reference to "the Russians, who rush out from a vapour [steam] bath, and jump into the nearest stream of water, or roll themselves in the snow." The implication was that these exotics were a hale and hearty lot perhaps superior to Americans.[7]

The key not just to this argument but to the whole of the external water cure movement is embedded in the early-nineteenth-century theory of the relationship elaborated thus in the *Journal of Health:*

> A very superficial knowledge of the close sympathy between the skin on one side and the stomach and lungs on the other will explain to us how serviceable bathing must be to the latter organs by preserving the former in its proper healthy office—cleansing it of all impurities, keeping it soft and its pores open, so as to allow egress to what, if retained, would cause eruptions on the skin itself, and much internal distress and irregularity of most of the functions of the animal economy.[8]

"There is no portion of the body," wrote Beecher in 1856, "so intimately connected with the stomach and the liver as the *skin.* . . . The lining of the stomach and intestines is in fact only a continuation of the outer skin." Thus she explained why physicians examined a patient's tongue to determine the nature of an illness, and why cleansing the skin was *"one mode of securing a healthy stomach."*[9]

In spite of the urgings of reformers, Americans evidently were not fond of warm baths. In 1834 Doctor Charles Caldwell, in his *Thoughts on Physical Education,* maintained that, "During weeks and months, water touches no parts of many [adults], save their hands and faces." Twenty-two years later Catharine Beecher asserted that "probably more than one half the American people never wash *the whole body* from one end of the year to the other; the face, neck, arms, and feet, being the only portions enjoying this privilege. Even a large part of those who occasionally wash the whole skin, do it only once a week, or perhaps once a month."[10] Bathing in warm water was difficult: it meant firing up the stove and therefore carrying both wood and water to the kitchen. Care of the "face, neck, arms, and feet" was more common not only because it was easier but because American clothing of the era usually had removable collars and cuffs, which were washed and ironed more often than the rest of the garment. Still, by the standards of the later twentieth century, body aroma must have been over-powering.

Nearly all advocates of bathing recommended that everyone who could should use cold water. The first issue of the *Journal of Health* advised, "A habitual use of the cold bath, when no circumstances are present to forbid its employment, while it contributes to the health of the system generally, is an effectual means of removing that delicacy of constitution which renders an exposure to cold alike disagreeable and prejudicial." Hitchcock and —twenty-five years later, in 1856—Catharine Beecher agreed. Physiologists theorized that when cold was applied, "the capillaries contract and send their blood inwards, reporting to the brain the need of the part. Instantly there is a return of a greater supply than before."[11]

By linking cold water bathing and the treatment of disease, water-curists gained popularity in the United States in the 1840s, they followed the intellectual lead of Vincent Priessnitz, a Silesian peasant who, in agony after crushing his ribs in a farming accident, applied cold water bandages to the injury and found relief. By 1829 he had begun to treat with some success the injuries of others in his hometown, Graefenberg, using methods less painful than those used by physicians of the area. Between 1830 and 1842 he treated more than seventy-five hundred patients who journeyed to his facility in Graefenberg and earned more than a quarter of a million dollars. He was still prosperous and preaching when he died in 1851.[12]

Priessnitz's basic technique involved a complicated system of wrapping the patient's nude body with wet bandages, wet and dry sheets, and blankets. For more extreme cases, patients were bathed in very cold (43° –50°F.) water. The most serious cases were treated with the *Wannenbad*, a plunge bath calculated to "bring out" by shock the patient's deeply disturbed condition. Other treatment forms Priessnitz introduced included the douche bath, in which the patient remained still under a column of falling water, and the drop bath, in which the afflicted endured a steady stream of water droplets on a particular area.

Water-based treatments had already been popularized by "steam-doctors" who advocated "blistering," a technique that was based on the theory that blisters on the skin could draw the blood away from a nearby internal inflammation or affliction—inflammation of the lungs thus was relieved by

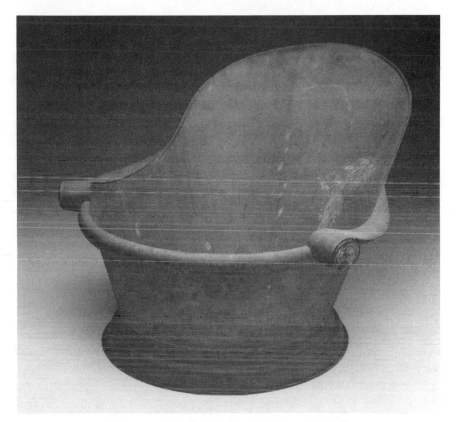

By soaking the lower part of the torso in a sitz bath, hydropathists argued, "female complaints" might be alleviated, as well as various forms of "clogging of the system." Sitz bath, American, tin, ca. 1850.

a blister on the chest. The hydropathists' cold water treatment was, by contrast, still uncomfortable but certainly less painful than the steam treatments.[13]

Hydropathy also meant less serious ailments could be treated at home, and the water-curists' attacks on "regular" physicians were consistent with many Americans' low opinion of doctors. Calvin Owen, the Penfield, New York, cabinetmaker and foe of liquor, slavery, and big banks, had been a believer in the water cure since the early 1840s. A friend's fever had been cured by some "harty draughts" of cold water and an accidental bath in it, despite the physician's disbelief, so when his wife was "attacked with symptoms of *Fever* . . . [and] pains in the head and back" on January 26, 1854, Owen noted that he had not "cal'd any Doctor, but I am treating her Hydropathically, which I believe is the better mode." Within four days, she was "up and about the house again, and . . . seemingly recovered from her sickness." He seems to have used a combination of drinking large amounts and periodic baths. That summer he was himself troubled by a "bad feeling in the region of the heart," a condition he treated by "sleeping in a wet girdle or bandage."[14]

Those Americans who could afford it, or were too ill to be treated at home, or who were unfamiliar with the treatment's methods took themselves to one of the country's many water-cure establishments. The most influential of the institutional practitioners in the United States were Dr. Joel Shew, Dr. Russell Trall, and Dr. James C. Jackson. Shew opened his water-cure establishment in New York in 1844, the same year his *Hydropathy, or, the Water-Cure* was published. The book was a primer on the types of baths or treatments offered (taken wholly from Priessnitz's model) and the diseases cured. In addition to sitz baths, the various wraps, and the douche, drop, and plunge baths, Shew described the "oral and nasal bath," in which the patient drew "water up the nose" and expelled it; the head bath, in which a person lay on his or her back on the floor with a pan of water beneath the back of the head ("to disturb the morbid humors"); finger baths, eye baths (with "a small glass made for the purpose"); lip baths, and sweating. All these treatments, Shew asserted, "produce all the effects of both *bleeding* and *blistering*, except the pain."[15]

The list of diseases cured by the various baths and wrappings was long. Syphilis, in all its manifestations—"ulcers, chancres . . . etc."—was treated with "sweating, bathing, douching, fomenting bandages, and drinking water," with a success rate that "naturally destroys our confidence in mercurial treatment." Other diseases allegedly cured by variants of the same formula included sore throat, stiff neck, cough, burns, deafness, earache, toothache, fractures, piles, "hypochondria and hysterics," headache, heartburn, insomnia, epilepsy, paralysis, tetanus, irregular menstruation, fainting, and apoplexy ("sudden loss of consciousness, sensation, and voluntary motion").[16]

Shew defended his methods by distinguishing between nature and artifice. Like Ralph Waldo Emerson and other Transcendentalists, Shew asserted that "the life of every highly cultivated society is highly *artificial*. It is therefore *unnatural*. But can that which is *unnatural* be possibly *proper?*"

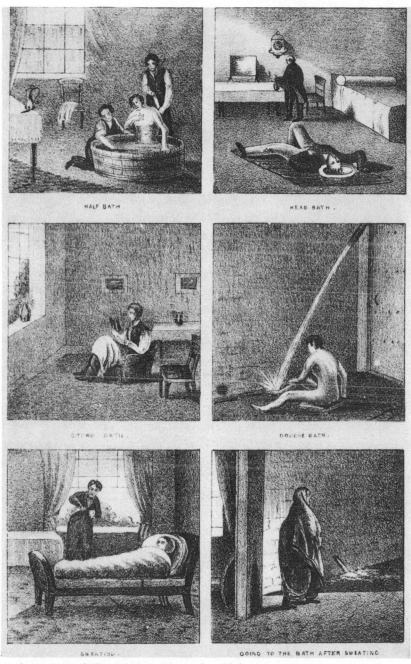

Hydropathists believed that hot and cold baths, sweating, and plunges would provoke a "crisis," after which recovery could occur. Frontispiece, Joel Shew, Hydropathy, or, the Water Cure *(New York: Wiley & Putnam, 1844).*

He equated art and artifice, and asked, "Can art be considered a better judge of that which is fittest for man's welfare than nature? . . . The contrivances of nature are the result of *divine wisdom.*" Shew's distinctions and definitions form part of a continuous distinction between "human ingenuity," as he phrased it, and the world as created by God. Settlers of seventeenth-century New England valued the artifice, or human manipulation and control of an environment that was oftentimes seen as hostile rather than simply rich with food and water, but by the 1840s art and artificiality were results of civilization or cultivation that were problematical to many. For Shew, "the inventions and adaptations of *human ingenuity* . . . entail upon us disease and premature death! . . . What wonder that we should find it impossible to get rid of our diseases while we obstinately persevere in preferring the ordinances and contrivances of art to the manifest ordinances and contrivances of God himself!" For Shew and other devotees of the water cure, art and human ingenuity had their proper places—to discover the workings of the universe, insofar as it was ordained by God that humans should do so, and to apply that knowledge within the divine order. Hydropathic physicians, then, used water as "a Natural influence intensified by art." Thus Shew rejected all "artificial" stimulants, such as tobacco, liquor, and wines, and criticized Americans for their overexcited life, full of the "theatre, the ball-room, music, dancing, gaming, political ambition . . . [and] in the middle classes . . . the cares of business, the anxieties of speculation, solicitude for the welfare of a numerous family, pride hourly contending with poverty, debts, doubts, dangers, and difficulties."[17]

Shew's articulation of the "artificial" nature of his society and his explicit condemnation of "cultivation" is at once a departure from and a reinforcement of the kind of political and social ideology that prevailed at that time in America. By criticizing ingenuity for weakening people, Shew's critique ran headlong into the boosterism of politicians, men-on-the-make, and other aggressive capitalists or would-be entrepreneurs, who looked with great satisfaction upon the "anything is possible" theme emerging in the United States. But his analysis resonated with that strain of American and Western European thought that nostalgically envisioned a simpler and more robust past and people. The optimism of endless material abundance was tempered by the powerful ideology of ministers who favored good, hard work but saw only luxury, decline, and destruction as American society seemed to abandon the values they ascribed to the great heroes and heroines of 1620 and 1776. Shew was a secular revivalist: he was part of the tradition of revival that was current in his time, yet not because he had religious regeneration in mind. The science of medicine and healing, as he knew it, was, in effect, his crusade.

Water-cure establishments proliferated—Shew opened the first in 1844, and within ten years, sixty-two were in operation. Their appeal was particularly strong away from the East Coast: 30 percent were located west of the Appalachians in 1855, and half were there by 1860. In part the increase was a result of the financial collapse of eastern establishments in the Panic of 1857, and in part the result of the rapid westward movement of settlers. Not all were as strictly regimented as Shew's treatment, which also stipulated vegetarianism, but nearly every one of them used the Priessnitz model. Mary Gove Nichols advertised the first hydropathic medical school in 1851.

Like other reformist health groups (especially the vegetarians), hydropathic physicians formed societies and published journals. The American Hydropathic Society (later the American Hygienic and Hydropathic Association of Physicians and Surgeons) was established in 1849, with Shew as president, the phrenologist Samuel R. Wells as treasurer, and Russell Trall as chairman of directors. In 1845, it began to publish the *Water-Cure Journal*, which underwent numerous name changes through the 1860s. The journal had one thousand subscribers by 1848, and ten thousand the year after. Its surprising growth can be attributed to two factors: first, water cures had sprung up throughout New York, New England, Pennsylvania, and Ohio; second, the editorship of the journal was assumed by a more dynamic entrepreneur, Russell Trall.

Born in 1812 in Vernon, Connecticut, Russell Thatcher Trall grew up in an area of upstate New York through which evangelical religious revivals and social reform enthusiasm regularly swept. With an M.D. from Albany Medical College, he was an early convert to the temperance movement and became the editor of the New York prohibitionist paper *The Organ.* In 1844 he opened his "water-cure house" at 15 Laight Street in New York, and soon afterward he organized a college. He had quickly become disenchanted with the common practice of medicine and adopted a program that included hydropathy, gymnastics (a new and untried method in 1845), and strict regulation of diet, sleep, and exercise.

Trall came slightly later to the hydropathic faith than did Shew, but he approached his task more aggressively and with perhaps a better, more interdisciplinary comprehension of his clientele. He quickly opened a medical college for would-be hydropathic physicians in New York, and by 1850 he had taken a full-page advertisement in the New York City business directory. His college was staffed by eminent practitioners, not only of the water cure, but also of other such quasi-medical or pseudoscientific activities —in particular phrenology, one of the other great fascinations of the antebellum era.

By 1854 Trall's school had been renamed the New York Hydropathic and Physiological School and boasted of eight faculty members, including five M.D.'s and one professor of "Medical Gymnastics." Students paid $150 for tuition, room, and board ($100 in summer) and came from as far away as Louisiana, Michigan, and Nova Scotia. Nearly one half of Trall's students were women.[18]

Trall managed or comanaged several hydropathic institutions, mostly in New York and Pennsylvania, and he spent a good deal of his time writing. Among his publications were *The Hydropathic Encyclopedia* (two volumes, 1852), *The Illustrated Family Gymnasium* (1857), *The New Hydropathic Cook-Book* (1856), and *Home Treatment of Sexual Abuses* (1857). Trall considered disease to be primarily the result of "unphysiological voluntary habits," which led to "capillary obstruction, deficient external circulation, and internal congestion." He was part of the tradition of medical pathology that combined a Protestant reliance on human responsibility for disease and for what many analysts termed "premature death." Like others of his medical-reformist bent, Trall argued for a total way of life that could, in his view, prevent disease. Thus he embraced the new fashion of gymnastics, which became popular in the 1850s, as well as dress reform for women, better ventilation in homes and workplaces, and control of the passions, especially sex. He opposed tea, coffee, whiskey, wine, and tobacco but allowed lean meat in the diets of his patients and scholars. He argued that a vegetarian diet was superior to the meats in most Americans' diets, but he held to the principle that those in good health who engaged in active occupations needed meat. Moderation—in passions, exercise, and quantity of food—was his message.[19]

Trall and other hydropathic physicians were not without their critics. The *Boston Medical and Surgical Journal* in 1857 termed Trall's college a "quack institution," and water-curists were outnumbered by botanic, homeopathic, and traditional physicians during the half-century that the technique was popular. In part the preponderance of other forms of treatment can be traced to the difficulty patients had setting aside traditional methods, and in part to economics: To open a water-cure facility involved considerable investment and therefore treatment was expensive.

Trall's school was the guiding organizational genius for the hydropathic movement in the late 1840s and 1850s and was one of the most successful and long-lived of such establishments. Many other less grand water-curists, such as David Cambell at New Lebanon Springs, were driven out of business by the severe recession of 1857. James C. Jackson, the third member of the water-cure triumvirate, survived the economic crisis and ultimately became the most famous water-cure specialist of his day, building the institutional model for the even more successful health-food and sanitarium operators John Harvey Kellogg and C. W. Post.

Jackson combined evangelicalism for health with a sense of corporate organization that was only just forming in antebellum America. He began his career in about 1850 as the supervisor of the business department of a water-cure establishment in Cortland County, New York. He soon assembled enough financial backing to buy the business—called "Glen Haven" —and by 1851 had begun advertising in the *Water-Cure Journal.* He instituted a "women's department" in 1852 and claimed to have treated "six hundred cases [of both sexes] without drugs" in 1853. He offered the unique guarantee of "no cure, no pay," an idea that promptly made him famous. He also advertised a set of fixed rates for treatment: one dollar for advice, three dollars for an office exam, and five dollars for a prescription by letter. He was able to convince his major investor, F. Wilson Hurd, to buy a four-story house in Dansville, New York, in the upland region of the Genesee River valley. Jackson sold Glen Haven in 1858 and, with Hurd's help, began to transform his Dansville structure and the several outbuildings into "Our Home on the Hillside," one of the great spas and health centers of the United States in the nineteenth century.

Patients were segregated by sex in the main house, and each section had four large rooms for treatment, packing, exercise, and resting. They were cared for by two resident physicians and three trained superintendents for packing and bathing, in addition to Jackson and Hurd. The group was powerful enough to attract the "National Health Convention" to Dansville in 1859 and to install themselves and Jackson's relatives in all but one of its offices. At the meeting Jackson's people delivered addresses that showed their drift away from the water-cure-as-panacea ideology of Trall and Shew (the latter had died in 1855) toward a broader concern for health and preventive medicine as embodied in the dress reform and calisthenics and gymnastics movements that had just begun to take hold in America.

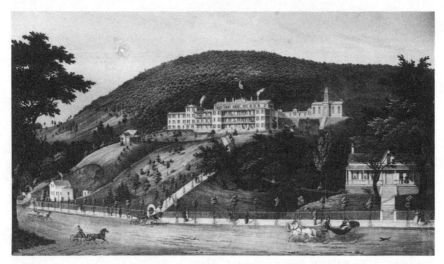

James C. Jackson's sanitarium and health resort, the largest of its kind in the mid-nineteenth century, was a center for the water cure, dietary reform, and ultimately a treatment facility for patients with tuberculosis. "Our Home on the Hillside," Sage Sons and Co., Buffalo, N.Y., lithograph, ca. 1860.

As Graham, Alcott, and Trall had before him, Jackson engaged the printing presses of his area to promote his institution and his way of life and health. He was, as they were, a product of an evangelical and scientific age. His tracts on Christian good health included such titles as *Christ and the Health Reformation, Hints on the Reproductive System,* and *How to Bear Beautiful Children.* Eventually, in 1858, he began his own periodical, *The Letter Box* (later *The Laws of Life*), which he continued for nearly twenty-five years.

Of all the water-cure centers established in the United States, Jackson's was most successful. That of Sylvester S. and Sylvester E. Strong at Saratoga Springs endured as a water cure until it was eclipsed by the gambling and resort life popular there after the Civil War. These two, with the Mount Prospect and Granite State Water-Cures, constituted the "establishment." Each advertised widely and probably survived because they adopted a broad program of treatment, embracing both therapeutics and prevention, as well as a sensitivity to new technology. Unlike some of their more extremist counterparts of an earlier era, none of these practitioners embraced so complete a militaristic regimen as did Graham, Shew, or even Trall. While the four major institutions and their directors favored vegetarianism, they understood that it was neither broadly popular nor necessarily a part of Americans' Christian belief systems.

Both hydropathists and the owners of public baths boasted of the healthful results of immersion in water, but there was a critical theoretical difference between the two groups. Bathhouses, like New Yorker Louis J. Timolat's "Washington Warm Baths" and "Medicated Sulphuric, Fumigating, and Aromatic Baths" (first opened in 1823) were primarily warm or steam baths, which treated the entire body. Public baths were advertised in the 1830 New York City business directory as treatment for "all affections of an internal and chronic or cutaneous nature," whereas hydropathists, recognizing the appeal of the activity but less willing to make therapeutic claims, sold warm bathing as "an indulgence [and] luxury . . . which is considered to be highly conducive to health." They essentially resurrected the ancient and early medieval *thermae,* theoretically based on the warm water immersion idea. Like that of Mason B. Miles and Henry B. May of Boston, their businesses were primarily "Medicated Vapor Bath Establishment[s] and Asylum[s] for the Sick."[20]

Unlike public warm bathing, water cures flourished briefly between 1844 and 1870, to be replaced by other specific and scientifically based (in marketing if not in fact) treatments. Warm bathing slowly grew in popularity until after the Civil War, when, divorced from its moral overtones, it was combined with the attraction of the resort experience, which appealed to a growing middle class. Hydropathists' claims that it was a panacea doomed the treatment's popularity. Like other treatments for which practitioners made extravagant claims, new discoveries of medical scientists made it passé.

Nearly all advocates of warm bathing, water cures, temperance, health foods and dietary reform began from a basically similar theory of the organization of the body. "Stimulation," either in the form of food or drink, or nervous irritability, was harmful, because it "drained away" the body's reserve of energy. The concept of energy was itself defined variously, but it was usually conceived as some sort of "vital force," or "nervous energy." The *Journal of Health* had warned in 1830 that the excitements occasioned by the advent of spring had the effect on people that the sun had on slumbering plants and animals—but not the same positive results. In addition to the "sore throats, coughs, pleurisies, spitting of blood, and rheumatism," more threatening was the allegedly increased incidence of "gout, and apoplexy, excessive mental excitement, and madness itself" that "not infrequently mark the vernal equinox." The "spring fever" many people evidently experienced induced "a great number [of] them to resort to bleeding, or to some active [heroic] medicine," which the *Journal* warned against.[21]

Almost alone in its time, the *Journal* attacked the idea that "weakness or exhaustion is . . . the chief cause, either remote or immediate, of nearly all the physical suffering to which the human system is liable." Hitchcock agreed that "nervous disorders" did "excite a deep interest in the mind of every friend to learning and humanity," but, like the vast majority of commentators on American health, he asserted that the "premature prostration and early decay of students and professional men in our country . . . is no longer doubted."[22]

Sylvester Graham agreed with Hitchcock and concluded that the alleged increase in disease and nervousness was a result of a lessening of control of the passions, especially those of sexuality. He theorized that semen was forty times as potent as blood, which meant that the "loss" of one ounce of semen had the effect of losing forty ounces, or two and a half points, of blood. All forms of sickness, thought hydropathist Joel Shew, were manifestations of different parts of the human organism trying to overcome the "congested condition of the vital capillaries." Curists sought to relieve the congestion by cold water and sweating; Grahamites and other vegetarians, by eliminating meats; and nearly all reformers, by getting rid of stimulating foods and drink.[23]

In spite of the complaint and advice of physicians and lay health reformers, most Americans embraced an alternate solution to the problem of nervous prostration, the reverse of what the "informed" had in mind. If debility or exhaustion was a key to disease, one might profit not from further abstinence from stimulants but by supplementing the body's supply of them —ironically, the same plan as the heroic physicians they claimed to distrust.

Explanations of the nature of this invisible yet obviously powerful "nervous fluid" or "vital force" had been offered for centuries. One briefly popular interpretation was advanced by the Swiss physician Franz Mesmer (1743–1815). Mesmer studied medicine in Vienna, where he learned of experimentation that had been performed with electricity as well as with astrological explanations for human behavior. His conviction that electricity was the key to understanding celestial and earthly phenomena and his financial and social ambition motivated him to write *On the Influence of the Planets upon the Human Body* (1776). In the course of his inquiry Mesmer abandoned the electrical explanation for magnetism, an unseen power like the "vital force." At first he treated people with magnetic rods, assuming that he could restore equilibrium to the system by readjusting or redistributing bodily forces. But soon Mesmer relocated the healing power in his own body.[24]

Mesmer called this internal force he possessed "animal magnetism." He posited that there was some "mysterious agency, allied to the magnetic power . . . a fluid, in fact, through which the heavenly bodies, the earth and animated bodies reciprocally act on one another." Mesmer was careful to point out, however, "that all living bodies are not equally susceptible either of receiving or retaining it. . . . To the operation of this fluid, by its passage from some favoured beings (magnetisers) into the frames of others (the magnetised) was given the title of 'animal magnetism.' By its means, the physician would be able to ascertain the state of health of all persons submitted to his inspection," identify "the origin, nature, and progress of their diseases," halt any deterioration, and ultimately cure the malady. "Mesmerism," as it was called, was also painless.[25]

By 1778 Mesmer was practicing in Paris and had attracted many wealthy patients—including the Marquis de Lafayette—despite opposition from most of the Parisian medical establishment. Even with public denouncements of the theory and practice by Jefferson and Franklin, Mesmerism caught hold of the American imagination, especially when a native son, Elisha Perkins, began to practice a related form of it.

Perkins (1741–1799) was a Yale-educated physician who in 1795 announced to the Connecticut Medical Society that by using metallic rods he could cure internal disease and speed the process of healing wounds. He quickly had manufactured "Perkins' Patent Tractors," two brass and iron rods pointed at one end and round at the other, which he alleged would relieve pain by drawing it to the patient's extremities, at which point it left the body. Perkins's sons made a good deal of money in England selling the devices, but the patriarch died of yellow fever in 1799 after having been expelled from the Connecticut Medical Society three years earlier.

Though disgraced among medical practitioners, animal magnetism lived on in the United States in the form of interest in the power and potential healing effects of magnets and, ultimately, in electromagnetism. In 1844

Theodosia Dunham received a letter from her friend Kate of Wilmington, Delaware, containing her account of being "magnetised."

> It certainly is a very strange and unaccountable thing; we see the effect but know not the cause. I met with a lady and gentleman not long since, who had the power of magnetising and firmly believed in it; the lady magnetised my hand and would have had me in the magnetic state would I have submitted to it, certainly both my hand and arm had a very strange and unpleasant sensation, I thought that was enough. . . . She told me I was a very good subject.[26]

In 1855 Calvin Owen went to two lectures (with demonstrations) on "Magnetic Psychology." Owen thought that "there is a great mystery about it that can't be comprehended by the mass," but he was "satisfied that some persons can be brought under the control of another person in a magnetic state, the whole action and movements are at the will of the operator."[27]

The "magnetic state" Dunham's friend referred to was really one of six separate states of apparent unconsciousness (or "superconsciousness") that practitioners of Mesmerism thought themselves capable of inducing. "Magnetic sleep," sleepwalking (somnambulance), and clairvoyance were conditions produced by magnetizing; the most receptive subjects were thought to be able to see into the future and read the minds of others. Dunham's friend was uneasy about the possibility of being induced into such a condition.

Animal magnetism, Mesmerism, or magnetism—whatever term was used—was proffered as both a therapeutic device and a spiritualist technique. In *A Manual for Magnetizing* (1845) H. H. Sherwood laid out a theory of treatment grounded in the idea that the body was a magnet and that disease occurred when the body's magnetic forces were not in equilibrium. He elaborated various "poles" of the body and argued that the visions of "Clairvoyants in the Mesmeric state" were indicators of this imperceptible bodily system.

> The internal organization of the pole in the centre of the brain, as disclosed in the somniscient state, is, however, the subject of the greatest interest; for the interior inverted cone, described by clairvoyants, is the magnetic miniature *germ* of the form of the brain. The heart, lungs, stomach, and other organs, as well as the limbs,

have magnetic miniature germs of their organizations, which are varied, according to the variations in the forms of the organs and limbs, as seen by clairvoyants. These organizations are also seen to be connected together by magnetic axes and interlacings, irrespective of the organization of the nervous system, and constitute a perfect magnetic, spiritual, or immaterial form, corresponding with that which is material.[28]

Sherwood listed a series of common diseases that he argued were treatable with magnetism and termed most of them "tubercular," which he defined as the result of an inflammation of the mucous membranes. He also discussed the use of magnetic electricity for tubercula of almost every organ from lungs to ovaries. He identified another large subgroup of diseases under the heading of "rheumatism," a condition in which "pressure with the fingers upon the intervertebral spaces of the cervical vertebrae will produce *pain* more or less severe, in proportion to the intensity of the disease." It resulted in dizziness, palsy, or apoplexy.[29]

Sherwood, though a physician himself, was shrewd enough to perceive that Americans' opinion of physicians was ambivalent at best. He therefore marketed his treatment and his vibrating and rotary magnetic machines to the general public as well as to his professional brethren. His advertisements in New York City business directories made no mention of the need of a physician for treatment and stressed that each machine (available in "neat mahogany cases, of several sizes and powers") came with "a complete Manual of the Practice of Medicine, with a very full glossary"[30] as well as diagrams and instructions for home use.

The first machines Sherwood offered consisted of a crank-driven wheel that, when turned, rotated an "armature of soft iron, wound with copper wire," which struck poles of a magnet, generated sparks, and sent electric shocks by copper wires to two brass cylinders held by the patient, one in each hand. In late 1843 Sherwood replaced this machine with his "vibratory magnetic machine," which substituted an electric (wet) cell for the crank-driven power and regulated the current more precisely. By placing the brass tubes or other conducting apparatus (disks or plates) on other parts of the body near the affected organ, magnetizers argued that they could restore the body's health.[31]

Magnetism of this electrical sort and animal magnetism, which was much closer to hypnotism than the mild shock treatment of Sherwood's machines, was extraordinarily popular in the pre–Civil War era. J. Stanley Grimes, an American proponent of the treatments, commented in 1850 that there had been a "lively excitement awakened in all the principal cities of the United States, during the past winter, by lectures upon Mesmerism, and its off-shoots, Pathetism and Electro-Biology."[32]

Animal magnetism offered people a painless way to treat their illnesses, if they could overcome their trepidation at the thought of a trance. It also made people feel special, because not everyone was deemed receptive to the passing of the hands of the magnetizer over the hands and arms of the would-be clairvoyant—and it provided a convenient rationale for failure. Moreover, the magnetizers were termed "favoured beings"; by definition, the patient or subject was less favored. Thus the onus was not on the purveyor of the goods but on the consumer. Theodosia Dunham's friend Kate probably felt gratified upon being told she was a "good subject" in 1844, although she was not interested in a trance. The magnetizers also reinforced a caste or national pride in their sales pitch; "light complexions are considered best" for magnetizing, they wrote.[33]

The magnetism advocated by Sherwood and others did not have the advantage of being painless, as did animal magnetism, but it did not necessitate the trance. It also had the imprint, if not the imprimatur, of "science." The machines used the newly developing technologies associated with electricity, that mysterious agent few Americans understood but nearly all knew had great power. Moreover, the power—sparks and flashes—was visible, if a little terrifying, and it appealed to the American fascination with machines and technology. By contrast, magnetic "lines of force" were invisible.

Not everyone embraced electromagnetic or animal magnetic therapy, however. Sherwood warned readers that "magnetizers should exercise the greatest caution in the use of the Rotary Magnetic Machine, for the drones of the medical profession—the old ladies in breeches, are laying in wait with their *curs* trained to pounce upon you the moment an accident happens of any importance in the use of the instrument."[34]

The literature on both animal magnetism and electricity increased steadily between 1835 and the mid-1850s, when the spiritualist component of animal magnetism began to be discredited in books and periodicals. By mid-century, the theoretical literature of medical treatment for nervous debility was dominated by volumes that were more closely linked to the work of physicians and academic scientists who had been experimenting with static electricity and direct current.[35]

Electricity's credibility as a therapeutic agent profited from the tradition of professional scientific experimentation with it. Galvani's (1737–1798) experiments with electrical stimulation of the muscles of frogs (published in 1791) and the work of Faraday (1791–1867), who in 1831 discovered that "a Galvanic current, at the moment of closing and opening the circuit, generated in neighboring conductors other electrical currents" (which he called "induction-currents"), were the most important breakthroughs in the early history of electrotherapy.[36] Some scientists, building upon this knowledge, theorized that the "nervous fluid," "vital force," or "vital energy" to which so many physicians and lay people referred was identical to, or at least akin to, electricity.

Daniel Davis's *Manual of Magnetism* (1842) was one of the earliest popular scientific publications on the topic. It provided lay and professional readers with clear, complete, and scientific analysis of the different kinds of magnets, electromagnets, and wet cells available, and included 180 illustrations as well as Davis's own catalog of apparatus. In his *Medical Applications of Electricity* (1846), Davis presented a cogent history of the medical use of electricity, "introduced with great effect in the treatment of paralysis." He cited Joseph Henry's successful use of faradic (direct) current for facial paralysis in 1838 and noted that direct current was later "resorted to in cases of nervous prostration, and in all nervous disorders. It is now employed, under continually new circumstances, in diseases of every nature and class, in which the nervous system sympathizes with physical disorder."[37]

Those who took the electrical treatment in these early years of its development experienced the tingling or the pain of electric shocks. As Davis pointed out:

> There may be a slow succession of strong shocks, or a very rapid succession of weaker shocks, producing a cramping or numbing effect, and occasioning strong tonic muscular contractions. These varieties, and the various gradations between them, are of course applicable to different conditions of disease, and will be applied by the practitioner according to the effect which he wishes to produce.[38]

Holding the brass or other metallic tubes or having the pads or plates (of other machines) applied was often painful. Yet electrotherapy—still practiced by only a few physicians out of the great mass of botanic, homeopathic, and more traditional physicians in pre–Civil War America—slowly gained many adherents among the professionals as well as their patients.

Popular medical and pseudomedical entrepreneurs were quick to respond to the new therapeutic and marketing possibilities for a clientele eager to combat "nervous debility" without having to submit to the bleeder's lancet and leeches. Water-curists, for example, began to advertise "electro-chemical baths," and in the April 18, 1857, issue of *Harper's Weekly*, Dr. J. Voorhees, of Brooklyn advertised that "astonishing cures . . . of CHRONIC and NERVOUS DISEASES" were being made "by electricity. Electro-Chemical Baths available at all Hours." Voorhees also offered free consultations. The "Electropathic Institute, 66 West Thirteenth Street, [New York]" offered treatment for "acute, chronic and mercurial diseases, of every description," promising that such illnesses would be "successfully treated without medicines." One bath cost fifty cents.[39]

The typical medicated electrical bath resembled a large electrolysis tank, with one or two bathtublike fixtures and a large galvanic cell. A patient to be treated reclined in a metal tub filled so that only his or her head was exposed. Metal plates were attached to the inside perimeter of the tub walls. One wire of the battery was attached to an electrode held by the patient, and the other wire was connected to the tub. The current was extraordinarily weak.

Promotors of electrochemical baths applied the theory of electrolysis to their therapy and allegedly cured suffering patients by extracting from the body disease-generating metals, as an advertisement for "Dr. Hankinson's Electro-Chemical Baths" proclaimed in about 1860. Hankinson asserted that electricity would "help . . . the victims of industry and the devotees of pleasure, and extract from their bodies, atom by atom, the devastating metal that has fastened on their tissues, and weighed down the springs of life." Hankinson promised to effect the cure on any "unfortunate patient, corroded by lead, mercury, gold, silver, or any other metal. . . . The electrical current precipitates itself through the body of the sufferer, penetrates into the depths of his bones, pursues in all tissues every particle of metal, seizes it, restores its primitive form, and, chasing it out of the organism, deposits it on the sides of the tub."[40]

The diseases "cured" included "Nervous and Spinal Affections, Rheumatism, Gout, Paralysis, Neuralgia" and certain occupational diseases, including those of plumbers and painters (who commonly suffered from lead poisoning), mirror platers and gilders (who were adversely affected by their exposure to silver and gold), and "Paris Green Manufacturers" (who were poisoned by the production of the insecticide). He also assured women that the treatment was unparalleled in its success with "Female Diseases," excluding pregnancy, "in which cases they should be avoided, on account of the certainty of producing Abortion." This last statement was perhaps as much an inducement as a caution: although it was nearly universally condemned in advice literature, abortion was common in nineteenth-century America, and abortifacients (most of which were pure quackery) were readily accessible through the mail.

Nearly all the larger water-cure establishments jumped at the chance to show the scientific and medical astuteness of their methods. Trall's Hydropathic and Hygienic Institute in New York had, by 1860, an electrochemical bath to "extract without pain all the metallic poisons from the system." This bath supplemented the plunge tubs, douches (showers), vapor baths, rubbing rooms, and other accommodations In 1856, T. T. Seelye's Cleveland Water Cure Establishment of Cleveland, Ohio, similarly boasted an electrochemical bath to extract minerals.[41]

Electrotherapy took one other major form in the pre–Civil War era. "Galvanic belts" or rings were introduced in 1801 and remained a minor and often-criticized mode of treatment until their heyday after the Civil War. These belts were basically a series of zinc disks or plates connected together with a copper wire. By soaking the "belt" in some sort of weak acid, such as vinegar, the cells actually generated a tiny current. Great claims were made for these early devices, and great scorn was heaped upon them. In 1845 Dr. A. H. Custee, "a brother of the inventor," promised "a certain Cure and Preventive in all cases of Rheumatism, Gout . . . Indigestion, Paralysis, Stiff Joints, General Debility, Deficiency of Nervous Energy, all nervous disorders" for patients who used his "Patent Galvanic Rings and Magnetic Fluid." The most famous of these devices was probably the Pulvermacher Electric Belt, introduced in the United States as early as 1853.[42]

Detractors such as Daniel Davis dismissed these as quackery, though Davis was critical of the product, not the idea. He allowed that such "belts can be made on scientific principles, by which a constant though slight galvanic current shall pass through the person wearing them, but such are not of the description offered to the public." Less enthusiastic was J. Stanley Grimes, who was himself an advocate of "Etherology," a combination of animal magnetism, phrenology, and Mesmerism. Grimes asserted that "it is evident to anyone at all acquainted with electricity, that the zinc and copper coins now used cannot have the least appreciable effect, except as they may serve to delude the ignorant, by throwing an air of mystery around the process." Such criticism, in Grimes's case, seems a bit strained for an advocate of the powers of clairvoyance.[43]

Like the water cure, with which it was often combined, electrotherapy in the pre–Civil War era promised a cure for nearly every disease, much as vegetarianism had. Electrotherapists tended to be less concerned with overall social and moral reform than were other crusaders, perhaps because their roots were in professional and academic science and not religious and moral regeneration. But as scientific thought increased in its ability to influence average Americans, and as the ferment of millennial reform activity receded after the Civil War, electrotherapy became more popular both as a medical treatment and a quackery designed to prey upon the cultural fears and perceived inadequacies of Americans.

CHAPTER FOUR

"BAD AIR" AND THE "MOVEMENT CURE"

The heyday of dietary reform, animal magnetism, electro-magnetism, and hydropathy saw many other attempts to preserve, heal, or alter the human form and constitution. Like those who tried to change American eating habits, advocates of better sanitation and ventilation in buildings and proponents of gymnastics and calisthenics in schools and homes were more directly concerned with prevention, rather than therapy. They carried forth the first stages of their movements with a fervor often equal to that of their more popular counterparts, and they laid much of the groundwork for the dominant concerns of late-nineteenth-century middle-class culture in America. They differed from vegetarians and critics of various "stimulants" by not trying to force Americans to deny themselves the traditional pleasures of meat or drink, although many combined the reforms. More fresh air and exercise were active therapeutic responses to the threat or reality of debility and in this sense were perhaps more closely allied with hydropathy and electrotherapies. They were painless reforms,

77

executed in changes in architecture or behavior that made visible differences.

"It is probable," wrote the prolific and somewhat hyperbolic Catharine Beecher in 1856, "that there is no law of health so universally violated by all classes of persons as the one which demands that every pair of lungs should have fresh air at the rate of a hogshead an hour."[1] "Bad air" was terrifying because it was imperceptible—invisible, quiet, and usually odorless. In seemingly harmless social activities or living accommodations, it might generate debility or even death. The enemy lurked in three sources: crowded cities and public institutions, overcrowded leisure activities (especially those of the evening), and the American tendency to heat homes with tightly sealed cast-iron stoves, rather than with open fireplaces.

Criticism of city life is at least as old as the European medieval era. In the United States, there had been an undercurrent of discomfiture about urban life since the middle of the eighteenth century, when there were but five cities about which to complain—New York, Boston, Philadelphia, Baltimore, and Charleston. But by the late 1820s, when those five coastal cities had been joined by at least a dozen more urban centers, criticism of the effects of city life on individuals and on the nation's political and religious experiment became more common and more shrill.

Writing in the *American Journal of Education* in 1828, one author argued that cities had "torrents of corruption which flow through the streets . . . [full of] the exhalations of vice which arise from crowded shops and manufactories or the still more infectious atmosphere of . . . wretched habitations."[2] Within this short passage, several of the major political and quasi-medical fears of the era were directly voiced. It restated the medieval notion that vice, corruption, and (by extension) crime were contagious, could be generated by close quarters, and could be passed insidiously to unsuspecting passers-by.

City life's new rewards were attended by new dangers. New entertainments—the theatre, the "opera," and dancing—drew people, not to "crowded manufactories" but to equally dense rooms of "night air." "Persons who are fond of frequenting unwholesome crowds, such as the warm, full theatre, or dancing assembly, ought . . . to be informed that nothing is so indelicate as to breathe *respired* air," the *Journal of Health* warned in 1829. Breathing "respired" air was not merely "indelicate," however; it was dangerous because such air was "rendered impure by the mere act of breathing." Dr. Edward Hitchcock not only supported this warning but also added a frightening aspect to this hazard: the damage was done without the victim's even being aware of it.[3]

The reactions of Beecher, Hitchcock, and the editors of the *Journal of Health* seem to have been less a conservative discomfiture with a new hedonism among the middling sorts and more a part of a consistent pattern of criticism of crowded, unventilated areas. The *Journal of Health* argued that the children of the poor suffered from "the summer complaint" more than any other group because their diets were less healthy, their immediate surroundings dirtier, and their broader environs—"narrow and confined streets, courts, and alleys"—were less able to provide enough room to breathe pure air.[4]

"Used" air was not the only danger for the uninformed and unsuspecting; heated air was also a potential hazard.

> Every half-hour spent out of the carpeted, stuccoed and stoved sitting-room, will contribute its might towards the redemption of the constitution from oppressive languor and sickliness—and to mitigate the propensity to catarrhal affections, or colds or coughs, which are the constant plague of so many individuals during the winter season.[5]

This 1829 *Journal* article, entitled "Hardiness," was actually about "languor and sickliness." It bemoaned life, "below the standard of hardiness" upheld by country folk who, like their forebears, lived in relatively unheated homes.[6] Twenty-seven years later, as wood stoves became even more popular than they had been in 1829, Catharine Beecher was more explicit in her critique of artificially heated air:

> Our ancestors always slept in cold and well-ventilated chambers. And in the family by day, the broad-mouthed chimney and un-corked doors and windows secured a constant flow of cool and pure air. . . . It is the universally-acknowledged fact, that the present generation of men and women are inferior in health and in powers of endurance to their immediate ancestors.[7]

The *Journal of Health* advocated a central cellar furnace with flues or pipes in place of "our common stoves and grates." Beecher wanted no part of furnaces or "close stoves, with tight doors and windows." She favored "open fire-places, that make a constant draught of the air of a room upward and outward," to "insure a constant supply of fresh air from the doors and windows."[8]

Cast-iron stoves had become the most popular mode of heating in the colder climates of the United States by the 1840s. They were more efficient producers of warmth because they used less wood or coal (which meant less

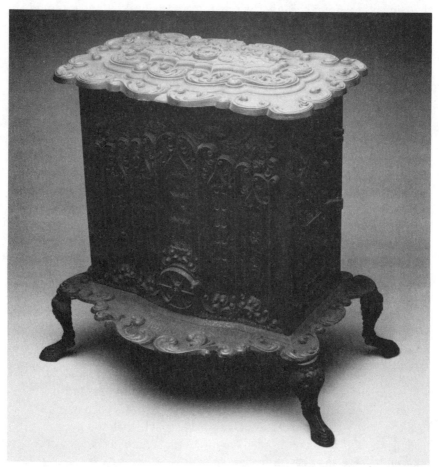

Efficient and inexpensive, cast-iron stoves were popular products, though reformers almost universally objected to the way they restricted the free flow of air in the house. John Kellogg even asserted that air was contaminated as it passed over the hot metal.

hauling and less expense), and were not prohibitively expensive.

Perhaps to combat the obvious consumer preference for these new machines, Beecher couched her resistance to them in the most potentially frightening terms of the era. "The inmates of a room [heated by a stove] will constantly breathe impure air, which will act as a slow poison in undermining the constitution," she warned. "And when the constitution is thus weakened, diseases of all sorts find ready entrance."[9] The damage, she implied, was inevitable, and its course imperceptible.

Scientific discoveries that were only dimly understood and partially known by average Americans made this argument especially powerful. Microscopes and telescopes that revealed worlds beyond the human eye's perception had been available in crude forms for more than two centuries but were not used by the vast majority of scientists until about 1800. But by the 1840s microscopes were more sophisticated and less expensive, and knowledge about what scientists were seeing with their aided eyes began to permeate popular culture. Advertisements began to feature bizarre-looking evil beasts whose existence was only made "known" by the use of a microscope.[10]

The microscope now gave Americans cause to worry about those two elements whose purity had always seemed to be perceptible—air and water. The microscope revealed that even clear water was not clean, and physiologists of amateur and professional status argued that the very conveniences Americans used to heat their homes more efficiently were poisoning them. Slowly and imperceptibly, disease stalked the unwitting American, just as the confidence man or the false lady of fashion duped the innocent and virtuous person. All of society, warned Beecher, was unknowingly, gradually, and inexorably declining.

> But as wealth and luxury have increased, houses have been made tight, windows have been corked, fire-places have been shut up, and close stoves and furnaces introduced. Men work in heated counting-rooms, offices, stores, shops, and manufactories, with brain stimulated and muscles inactive, or with both muscles and brain stimulated, while the fetid effluvia of many skins and lungs are the only fountain of supply to the lungs and the dependent capillaries all over the body. Then they go home and sleep with wives and children in close, unventilated, and sometimes heated rooms. And even when they travel, especially in winter . . . they are packed in

close cars, with a stove burning up the oxygen and thinning the air, while windows are fastened down and every crack made air-tight with frozen breaths.[11]

When she urged abandonment of the cast-iron stove for the open fire-place of her forebears, Beecher anticipated a development that in fact took place after the Civil War for reasons nearly identical to those she advocated. Furnaces, which were just beginning to become popular by the 1850s, offered one partial solution to the "dullness and debility [that] are the certain results of impure air"; a less tightly sealed house also did so. Americans were urged to open a window a crack and have an opening above a door in any room. Like the return to the fireplace, however, transoms over doors did not become common until after the Civil War, when Americans accepted a broader commitment to health and fitness.[12]

Institutional architecture, and in particular that of schoolhouses, was also subjected to rigorous analysis and criticism. Organized activities directed at standardizing the schooling of the young arose, for the most part, after 1830. Armed with the new conviction that children were inherently good and human behavior perfectible, a phalanx of reformers sought to improve American education by developing texts as well as environments conducive to education.[13]

The most important alteration in institutional architecture involved ventilation. William Alcott, remembered now for his many self-help and advice books, rose to prominence with his *Essay on the Construction of School-Houses* (1832). A stinging rebuke of the schoolhouse architecture of his day, the book called school buildings "dark, crowded, and . . . disorderly huts," ill-lit and unpainted. Alcott also charged that "playgrounds [were] . . . scarcely known." He advocated large windows, building sites far from roads, and fenced-in spacious playgrounds. To instill good habits and to control disease, he urged schoolmasters to have their buildings washed frequently, to allow "free" ventilation, to provide desks with backs, to offer different-size desks for different-size children (which would develop good posture), and to allow time both for exercises and for a short recess "once an hour."[14]

Arguments about proper architecture and the proper mode of schooling continued unabated for the next half-century, although good intentions often lost to the efforts state and local legislators made to keep taxes down and thereby stay in office. Beecher was particularly aware of the irony of teaching "physiology" (an improvement in curriculum, at least) in an environment "where two or three hundred live, month after month, breathing chiefly impure air." This situation was particularly destructive in the schoolroom, where "the young inmates have their brain and nervous system on a constant drain by intellectual activity and moral responsibility." The result of these crowded conditions was that "year after year . . . fevers and various diseases sweep off the young inmates by death." But schoolchildren were not the only sufferers from "air famine," as it would later be called. "So in our manufactories and shops of labor, thousands of the young congregate to labor in poisonous air, till their constitutions are undermined, and then return home to remain invalids for life."[15]

Even if youngsters and adults managed to avoid crowded shops and unhealthy, unventilated schools and managed to demonstrate their concern by opening windows an inch or two, they might yet unwittingly defile their lungs by some traditional American habits and comforts, especially "the downy couch" and other accoutrements of sleep.

> In youth especially, feather beds, like every other species of luxury, by causing a premature development of the system, without strength proportionate to the rapidity of its growth, often lay the foundation for many of those diseases by which multitudes are consigned to an early grave.[16]

"Luxury" provoked "premature" growth; it was not only "the bane of republics," as Andrew Bigelow would point out in 1836, but also the bane of individuals.

Feather "comfortables" or quilts, which caused profuse perspiration during the "milder seasons of the year," would thus "enervate the constitution, and lay it open to serious impressions from trifling degrees of cold." Mattresses were to be made of "hair or moss," which were "soft and elastic material[s]." For similar reasons, feather pillows and nightcaps, "excepting in the instance of females who are accustomed to wear a cap during the day," were condemned. So too the common practice "of placing the children's bed beneath another bedstead during the day, cannot be too severely reprobated," since the smaller bed restricted "free ventilation."[17]

"Sleeping apartments" were equally baleful influences on health. The ideal bedchamber in 1830 had one bedstead. "There cannot be a more pernicious custom, than that pursued by many families, of causing the children, more especially, to sleep in small apartments, with two or three beds crowded into the same room," the *Journal of Health* declared in 1829. Bedchambers were most healthful, the authors argued, if kept at fifty degrees or colder; and they asserted the shock of climbing into a bed with frigid sheets would not be "the least inconvenience, even in the severest weather" for "a person accustomed to undress in a room without a fire." By guarding against a dependency on "external warmth," individuals would be able to steel themselves against "colds, coughs, and consumptions."[18]

Material evidence suggests that Americans probably took some chances with "colds, coughs, and consumptions." Architectural plans and surviving buildings indicate that fireplaces were usually included in nineteenth-century homes, and the sheer number of extant quilts, coverlets, and other forms of bedcovers indicates a predisposition for warmth and comfort, but only to a point. The long-handled brass bed-warming pan so fondly displayed in nearly every historic house or restored village in the late-twentieth-century United States had disappeared from regular use by the 1830s or 1840s, and most accounts of life in the northern states in the pre–Civil War era acknowledged that unheated bedchambers were common. Whether this practice was a result of economy, fear of house fires, or concern about disease is unknown.

Reformers occasionally offered solutions more enterprising than open windows and activity in the outdoors. Entrepreneurs tried to market filters that would economically solve the problem of foul air, just as they had done with water. The chief impetus for such improvements came from England, where the "sanitation movement" first gained strength and government support in the 1830s. In 1855 John Stenhouse made a case for charcoal powder as a filter appropriate for deodorizing air as well as for removing "miasmata" and "decay." He promoted charcoal air filters, which consisted of "a thin layer of charcoal powder interposed between two sheets of wire-gauze," which he maintained could "be readily applied to buildings, to ships, to the gully-holes of sewers, to respirators." He even recommended pillows and coverlets stuffed with powdered charcoal.[19]

English physicians such as Stenhouse managed to convince city, county, and national officials that disease could be traced to the vapors produced by the decaying refuse that was all over the streets and yards of the cities of industrial England. Although they were unable to link the transmission of disease to contaminated water supplies or insect carriers, they were instrumental in the formation of sanitary commissions whose goal was to clean up the cities, as well as, not surprisingly, the morals of the inhabitants of the more wretched dwelling areas. There were only a few sanitary commissions established in the United States before the Civil War. (Massachusetts had a state commission by 1850.) The few reports published, such as John Griscom's *The Sanitary Condition of the Laboring Population of New York* (1845), were reviewed with due concern in the newspapers and periodicals of the day, but there was little tangible change in sanitary conditions until more formal reform activities began during the Civil War.[20]

Although British reform of unsanitary living conditions did not rapidly cross the ocean before the Civil War, one European reform did make a successful passage to the United States. As large numbers of German immigrants fled the economic and political dislocation in their country following the revolution and counterrevolution of 1848, they brought with them calisthenics, sports, and gymnastics. Before this, only a few physicians and educational reformers were interested in exercise and physical education, and nearly all of them had studied in Europe or were aware of trends in German or other European systems. Long life—or at least the avoidance of "premature death"—was tied to sports, but the suggestion was that these activities were reserved for the young. Edward Hitchcock concentrated on a different group in 1830, maintaining that "there is scarcely any individual among the sedentary and the literary, who does not acknowledge, in general terms, the necessity of exercise." The expansion of sport and fitness to all ages was to be a discovery of the post–Civil War era.[21]

Hitchcock and the *Journal of Health* advocated regular exercise—walking, running, leaping, dancing, gardening, and various mechanical occupations—"with the mind . . . at the same time pleasurably, but not too intensely occupied." Sailing, "swinging, and riding in carriages or on horseback" were acceptable forms of exercise, though they were considered "passive" and therefore less useful to the individual who wished to become or remain hardy. Hitchcock considered walking "the very best" exercise for retaining health.[22]

"Gymnastic exercises," however, were recommended with even more enthusiasm. As defined in 1830, these activities resembled what late-twen-

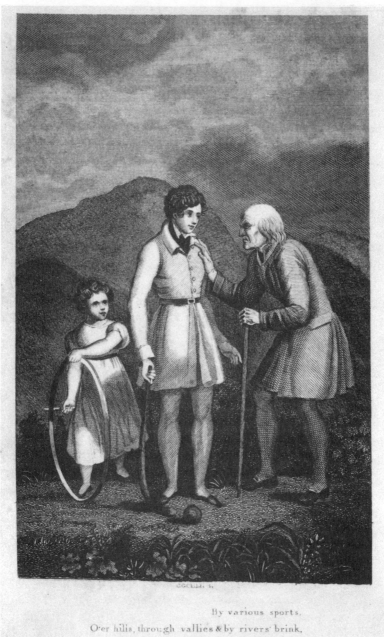

By various sports.
O'er hills, through vallies & by rivers' brink,
Is life both sweeten'd & prolong'd.

This frontispiece from the first volume of the Journal of Health *asserts the importance of sports and fitness to general good health and longevity, symbolized by this meeting of the generations. Engraving, G. C. Childs, American, ca. 1829.*

tieth-century Americans think of as sports and games. Dancing was acceptable, if done in moderation, but the *Journal of Health* carefully admonished its readers to avoid the late hours, liquor, and crowded rooms associated with most dancing parties. "We need not be surprised that spitting of blood and consumption of the lungs should be frequent among the votaries of the ball-room or the midnight assembly," the *Journal* noted. "Running and leaping" were only for those already in a strong condition, not for those suffering from "palpitation . . . shortness of breathing, or cough . . . [or] spitting of blood."[23]

Games and sports were thought particularly beneficial because "they allure the sedentary forth into the fields—while in their prosecution, the mind and muscles are both excited to an extent sufficient for the purposes of health." The most favored games among both the populace and the doctors were tennis, bowls, quoits, and golf, a game popular in the British Isles but virtually unknown in the United States until the late 1880s.[24]

Activities that by the 1850s were known as gymnastics and calisthenics —primarily indoor exercises, rather than sports and games—had been criticized by the *Journal of Health* in the 1830s as "a miserable substitute for activities in the open air." They were thought to be "seldom productive of any good effects," and to "bear pretty much the same relation to health, as the castigations of the penitent do to piety or virtue." The favored exercises were those which "engage the mind, at the same time they call the limbs into action."[25]

Edward Hitchcock, who favored most of the positions taken in the *Journal,* thought indoor gymnastic exercises "extremely valuable." He defined calisthenics as "the classical name for female gymnastics" and thought them "the most effectual means ladies could employ for giving freshness and fairness, and a rosy glow to their countenances, and permanent vigor to their constitutions." But Charles Caldwell, who, like Hitchcock, lectured on physical education, was concerned that "some of the violent gymnastic exercises . . . are better calculated to do harm than good," and thought that "the manual-labor system connected with some schools, is not only more useful in its objects, but better fitted to subserve health, than the common gymnastic one." Caldwell approved of football and handball and acknowledged that "the moderate and graceful gymnastic exercises are so useful . . . elegant, invigorating, and manly."[26]

The case for gymnastics and sports in 1830 was roughly the same as the case for dietary reform, ventilation of houses and public buildings, and abstinence from alcohol and tobacco, regardless of the gravity with which they were imbued by any given critic. Americans and Western Europeans were dying young, or so it seemed. After the customary acclamation of the healthy ancient Greeks and Romans (before they discovered luxury, lust, and debauchery), the common theme of those who touted gymnastics was "the undisputed fact . . . that mankind, generally speaking, are, at the present day, inferior in bodily strength to their ancestors of a few centuries back." The wages of this decline were a shortened life, especially among children. Drawing upon the fragmentary evidence of European urban government records, the *Journal of Health* asked, "Whence is it but from this cause [neglect of health] that of all the children born in large cities, particularly those of Europe, nearly one-half die in early infancy?" In "the earliest of ages," they claimed, with no evidence to substantiate their assertion, ". . . human life was protracted to a very large extent." The villains in this degeneracy were Americans' "artificial modes of life," behavior that contrasted feebly with "those indicated by nature." Anticipating hydropathist Joel Shew's argument by nearly fifteen years, the *Journal of Health* argued that this unnatural life-style presented "one of the strongest reasons why instances of longevity are so very rare, amid the refinement and luxury of a large city."[27]

In their support of gymnastics and calisthenics these critics combined the most powerful and popular metaphors available. Their critique of urban areas and of the life of a civilization that had discovered "luxury" rang in unison with extraordinarily powerful cries of ministers for a republic of virtuous, pious men, women, and children who would not only carry forward the promise of the generation of 1776 but would also rescue their civilization from the debility and degeneration that seemed to be everywhere. This critique—a secular one with decidedly religious overtones—was the intellectual framework from which the movements for the physical and moral reform of Americans would arise for the next century.

The need for exercise and good ventilation was further advanced by the seemingly sudden increase in the number of cases of consumption, or "phthisis" (tuberculosis) that occurred in the 1830s. This phenomenon was, for critics of American health, a sure sign that the populace was degenerating. Sylvester Graham and William Alcott were both victims of the terrifying disease, which was characterized by the coughing of blood, weakness, and slow death. Unlike the epidemics of cholera, diphtheria, scarlet fever, typhoid, and other virulent diseases that swept through American cities periodically between 1830 and 1900, consumption was always there, always threatening the unsuspecting with an "early grave." Fresh air and exercise —horseback riding or riding in "carriages over rough roads"—were the cures most recommended.[28]

Physical education—teaching physiology, gymnastics, sports, games, and, by 1850, calisthenics—did not immediately attract many devotees among the general populace. Edward Hitchcock established a program of regular classes in physiology and physical education at Amherst in 1830. William Alcott called physical education "the lever by which we are to raise the world,"[29] and worked hard for its inclusion in the Massachusetts common school system curriculum. But Alcott was only partly successful, even with the support of the nation's most prominent educator, Horace Mann. Mann's 1842 statewide survey for the Massachusetts Board of Education showed ten thousand taking American history, two thousand enrolled in algebra classes, fifteen hundred in bookkeeping, and only four hundred and sixteen in health courses.[30]

Organized exercises became a common part of the American common school system and urban adult life after 1850. The movement began in Germany under the leadership of the intensely nationalist Friedrich Ludwig Jahn (1778–1852), the literate son of a Protestant minister who was deeply affected by Napoleon's defeat of the Prussians in 1806. Jahn was an ardent supporter of the reunification of Prussia, and in 1809 he organized a militaristic school in which he taught a combination of courses that attempted to unify exercise and sport with German history, tradition, and customs. Jahn's calisthenic and romantic German nationalism were carried to America in 1824 by one of his most charismatic students, Charles Follen (1796–1840), the author of the seminal book on German gymnastic societies, *Die deutsche Turnkeise* (1816). Forced to leave Prussia after one of his followers assassinated journalist August von Kotzebue, Follen was welcomed in America as part of the new generation of young Europeans throwing off the decadent order of the Old World.

Follen was appointed Harvard's first teacher of the German language, a course of considerable interest at the college since the first decade of the nineteenth century. Many of Harvard's scholars, such as Edward Everett and George Ticknor, had studied in Germany and had returned to America full of the romantic idealism current there. Professors George Bancroft and J. G. Cogswell were enthusiastic about German educational forms and theory—and so disenchanted with the comparative lack of discipline at

Harvard—that in 1823 they established the Round Hill School, dedicated to "a systematic and thorough course of early instruction and mental and moral discipline, combined with means for promoting health and vigor of constitution." As more and more academies were founded to promote the total education of boys and girls (there were more than eight hundred established in the 1830s), physical exercise became a more common part of the curriculum.[31]

To teach calisthenics at Round Hill, Bancroft and Cogswell hired Charles Beck (1798–1866), who had come to the United States with Follen in 1824. Beck set up a a gymnastics area, complete with parallel bars, ladders, and climbing ropes, and an exercise program that required students to participate three times each week. Meanwhile, Follen was working toward establishing the first college gymnasium in the United States. Opened at Harvard in 1826, the gymnasium was a success, and Follen was asked by Dr. John C. Warren, the head of Harvard Medical School, to run a public gymnasium in Boston. Follen took over the new institution in the autumn of 1826, but its appeal was short-lived and it closed by the early 1830s.

Gymnasiums in America declined rapidly in part because the enthusiasm for German idealism had waned. Other European revolutions—especially that of the Greeks in 1830—attracted the attention of Americans of a romantic bent. In addition, with no public governmental support, physical training for health had a narrow base of support in a city and culture only just beginning to industrialize. Gymnastics, for such German idealists as Follen and Beck, was a way for all classes of society to mingle and find a common, democratic ground, as well as a convenient way to train a militia. But American workers were not particularly interested in additional physical exertion in the 1820s and early 1830s, and the educated middle class was not certain that it was desirable to join the working class in activities of any sort. Moreover, the unifying quality of interest in the *Volk*, or folk culture, which characterized the intensity of German gymnastic activities, was absent in the United States. Rather than a composite cultural commitment, as it was for German émigrés, gymnastics for early-nineteenth-century Americans was a means of regeneration. As such, it competed with other forms of care and consideration for the welfare of body, mind, and country —religion, dietary reform, and temperance. The integration of these social, medical, and hygienic activities with the broader cultural enthusiasm for ethnic identity and history would not occur in the United States for more than half a century, when many middle-class Americans sensed that their culture was again threatened, from without as well as from within. In addition, the militaristic and regimented quality of German calisthenics or gymnastics troubled Americans. Sarah Josepha Hale, writing in *Godey's Lady's Book* in 1841, was "decidedly in favor of Calisthenics, but exercises of this sort should never be insisted on when they grow irksome." Like nearly all supporters of exercise, she advocated play "in the open fields" for girls and boys until fourteen or fifteen years old. In contrast to those who fretted about girls injuring themselves while exercising, she thought that they "should be allowed to run, leap, throw the ball, and play at battle dore [badminton], as they please."[32]

The small amount of organized physical activity that occurred in the United States between 1830 and 1850 was concentrated in colleges and academies, and especially in those for young women. Round Hill had closed because of financial difficulties in the late 1830s, and Hitchcock continued his program of gymnastic and calisthenic exercises at Amherst, which, like nearly every other college, was for men only. Exercises and calisthenics for women had been a part of the educational program at Emma Willard's school in Troy, New York, since 1821; at Catharine Beecher's school in Hartford, Connecticut, since 1824, and at Mount Holyoke since its founding in 1837. Teachers in girls' schools considered the gymnastic exercises of the German teachers to be too strenuous—even dangerous—for young American girls, but they rapidly accepted and modified the English and French systems of calisthenics to their own use in about 1830. The publication in 1831 of *A Course of Calisthenics for Young Ladies, in Schools and Families,* which is attributed to Catharine Beecher, and the 1831 review of *Calisthenie ou gymnastique des jeunes filles* in the *Annals of American Education* marked the beginning of popular interest in calisthenics, at first for girls and ultimately for both sexes. *A Course of Calisthenics* was also significant because it asserted that calisthenics were not necessarily reserved for the gymnasium or school but were appropriate for the privacy of the home as well, an idea that has remained popular to the present.

In *Physical Education and the Preservation of Health* (1846), John C. Warren carefully distinguished between mental and physical education. He linked mental enrichment to the "culture of the mind," which required "the early, constant, and well-directed efforts of an artificial system." "Physical faculties," he argued, were "fully effected by the powers of nature," which to be healthy needed to be left "free and unconstrained." Nature and culture were here set in opposition to each other, as they had been by hydropathists, and the implicit conclusion was that culture, "artifice," or "artificiality" in some way hampered physical development and well-being.[33]

Warren advised his readers—whom he thought would primarily be women—to relax their ambitions for academic competition and achievement and concentrate on physical acitivity instead. He recommended walking in the open air and dancing at home, either alone or with friends or family, even for the women "in our manufactories" whose work had become monotonous and relatively sedentary. Like other reformers of his day, he found fault with American diet and American clothing, especially men's cravats and women's corsets, which he thought hindered their ability to breathe and most certainly their ability to exercise.[34]

The custom of tight-lacing, or corseting, can be traced to the courtly houses of Europe in the fifteenth century. Women of high social rank commonly laced themselves into corsets that shrunk their revealed waist size to approximately nineteen inches. Criticism of this practice had been voiced sporadically since the inception of the practice, but it became intense in the middle decades of the nineteenth century. "Corsets! Corsets!," a 1829 article in the *Journal of Health,* cited the case of an unidentified eighteen-year-old French woman treated at a Paris hospital for a variable-size tumor on her throat that her physicians insisted was caused by her use of the corset. In 1833 Dr. Charles M. Caldwell similarly condemned corsets, calling them "an alarming evil" and asserted that indigestion and pulmonary consumption were caused by the severe constriction corsets provided.[35]

Many women took to the lecture circuit to fight the century-long battle against the hated device. Antoinette Brown Blackwell, the first woman to graduate from a traditional medical school (1849), Mary Neal, Paulina Wright Davis, Mary Gove Nichols, and others tramped throughout the Northeast and Midwest, speaking against a variety of evils; all agreed on the absolute hideousness of the corset. Nichols's Boston lectures for women on anatomy and physiology usually drew approximately four hundred listeners, and she once attracted almost two thousand women.

The most vociferous critic of tight-lacing, however, was Catharine Beecher. In each of the multitude of advice and how-to books she wrote between 1837 and the Civil War, she indicated her extreme displeasure with corseting, tight shoes, and all other "unnatural" forms of dress. The constraints and abdominal breathing and muscles produced "the most terrible suffering, especially on the female sex." Corseting also caused "curvature of the spine," "dull and wandering pains," dyspepsia, constipation, "dreadful ulcers and cancers."[36]

Beecher also argued that the corset had been disfiguring women for generations, so that "from parent to child . . . a large portion of the female children now born have a deformed thorax, that has room only for imperfectly formed lungs." Her argument that acquired characteristics such as a waist deformed by a corset could be transmitted to future generations was ultimately destroyed by Charles Darwin, but it held great power for much of the nineteenth century. Beecher's warning of the danger to future generations was calculated to provoke fear into a populace already shaken by the seemingly rapid upsurge in the gravity and number of cases of pulmonary consumption and caught up in the belief that their generation had declined precipitously from the sturdy stock of the nation's first settlers.[37]

Beecher also faulted American women for the way they exposed some parts of their bodies to the cold while overheating others. "They dress the upper portion of the body so thin, that the spine and chest are exposed to

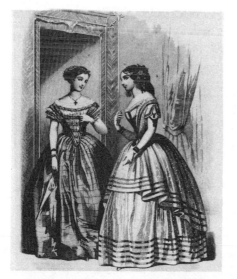
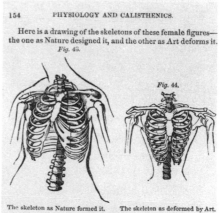

Fashion called for heavy skirts and corseted waists, but critics of corseting, or tight-lacing, presented startling images of the deformities they thought the practice caused. Left: fashion plate from Godey's Lady's Book, *June 1854, p. 574. Right: illustration from Catharine Beecher,* Physiology and Calisthenics *(New York: Harper and Brothers, 1856).*

sudden and severe changes of temperature," which Beecher argued "tends to weaken that portion." To compound the error, women overdressed their lower halves, weakening the spine and pelvic organs "by excess of heat." Citing the American horror at the "efforts of the Chinese mother in binding up her child's foot," she termed it "wisdom compared to the murderous folly thus perpetrated . . . by thousands of mothers and daughters."[38] Ironically, while many of the popular ladies' magazines often carried articles condemning corsets and heavy petticoats, their constant visual message was that the slender-waisted woman with heavy skirts and broad hips was the fashionable ideal.

For Beecher, the changing character of American life was the ultimate cause for the decline she saw occurring all around her. Specialization in work, not simply between intellectual and manual tasks but between heavy and light labor, had created a tendency to debility. "One portion of the women have all the exercise of the *nerves of motion*, and another have all the *brain-work*, while they thus grow up deficient and deformed. . . . And so American women every year become more and more nervous, sickly, and miserable, while they are bringing into existence a feeble, delicate, or deformed offspring."[39]

What could be done about this "general *decay of constitution*"? A radical change had to occur in America, but one which was not really new at all: the introduction of calisthenics. Beecher's detailed list of movements and exercises, a synthesis of the German-influenced gymnastics of the 1820s and the French and English calisthenics of the 1830s, was also strongly influenced by a phenomenon known as the "movement cure," described as "a methodical application of well-defined and appropriate rhythmical movements to the human body." First developed in Sweden, it was used to treat a variety of diseases and afflictions, among them gout, "nervous affections," congestion, constipation, "delicate chest," and "affections of the heart." The movement cure provided relief because it would "increase the vital and nervous power . . . by driving the blood towards those parts of the body where it is wanted, and thus to restore equilibrium and harmony in the whole organism." The technique involved various bending, stretching, twisting, and rotating movements, as well those "movements independent of the will . . . friction, vibration, pressure, percussion, ligatures, etc.."[40]

The movement cure gained some adherents among the more dynamic health-care entrepreneurs of the era. Russell T. Trall, quick to seize upon new answers to persistent problems, enlarged his hydropathic institution with areas for "motopathy," "kinesipathy," "calisthenics," "vocal gymnastics," and "movement cure" by 1855. At least one enterprising inventor came up with a gimmick advertised in 1845 with a full page of testimonials. With levers in the front and on either side of the arms, and a tufted-hair cushion seat (evidently on some sort of spring attachment), "O. Halsted's Patented Exercising Chair" was "eminently calculated as a substitute for carriage, horse, and many other forms of gymnastic exercise . . . [and] adapted to a great variety of diseases in all seasons."[41]

The nature of the evolution in American attitudes toward both physical exercise and the ideal of the human form was articulated in the introduction to Beecher's *Physiology and Calisthenics*. Beecher's goal was to "promote health, and thus to secure beauty and strength." Health, as she defined it, was not only the avoidance of disease, but also the more positive uplifted spirit and attitude toward life. Beecher's assertion of a causal relationship between "health" and "beauty and strength" seems almost axiomatic to twentieth-century minds, but it was a breakthrough for the nineteenth century. Physicians concerned for the moral, mental, and physical well-being of their patients and the human race in general had suggested such a connection before, but Beecher was one of the first popular commentators to suggest that a subjective and culturally determined attribute—beauty— was a function of health. Her equation indicated a fundamental shift in emphasis consistent with other critics' conception of "nature" as an opponent of "culture," or of "art" or "artifice." As it had for many of the era's painters, nature came to be regarded as a realm in which the hand of God was most clearly evident. Just as the human body ceased to be characterized as a sinful prison for the soul, the Easterner's vision of nature had evolved from the howling wilderness of the seventeenth century to the sublime gentle place of the nineteenth century.[42]

To Beecher, the ancient Greeks, "the wisest and most powerful of all nations," exemplified health and beauty. Yet, she pointed out, "they were a small people, in a small country." By the mid 1850s Americans had already begun to regard great physical stature as an important component of beauty and power. Beecher departed from the once pervasive equation of portliness as a sign of beauty and identified the Greeks "as the most perfect forms of human beauty."[43] The muscular ideal—most famously manifested in Horatio Greenough's toga-clad statue of George Washington (1847)—was perhaps as much a paean to a rediscovery of that particular type of human form as it was to Greek democratic politics.

To achieve this muscular ideal in men, Beecher touted the benefits of gymnastics, or those exercises that used parallel bars, climbing ropes, and other such equipment. They imparted "courage and . . . independence and presence of mind, . . . and diminish the craving of the taste for sensual pleasures." Calisthenics, however, offered nearly all of these advantages to both men and women. Mid-nineteenth-century mores did not permit young women to enjoy the sensation of daring that young men were allowed. Gymnastics could be dangerous, as anyone who has ever missed a vault or dismount can attest. The calisthenic system Beecher and others outlined "contained all that either sex needs for the *perfect development* of the body" and was "adapted to mixed schools, so that both sexes can perform them together." In addition, everyone could "practice it without aid from a teacher, and in any place. The members of a family in the parlor, the children in a nursery, the invalid in the chamber, the seamstress or milliner in their shops, the student or professional man in his office, study, or counting-room, can open a window twice or thrice a day, and have all the 'fresh air and exercise' needed for *perfect health,* by simply following the directions in this work."[44] Advocacy of quick exercise for the sedentary office worker—from Beecher's calisthenics through Bernarr Macfadden's risqué exercises to isometrics for those chained to their computer terminals —has been a constant in American culture, changing only in the form and nature of the movement.

Beecher's calisthenic system was directly descended from the Swedish movement cure. The typical class began with participants dressed *"loosely,* [with] all their clothing suspended from the shoulders" in the "military position." With head erect, shoulders back, knees straight, and chest thrust forward, participants began the first of fifty separate exercises. Beginning with a thorough but not violent beating of the chest (to "enlarge the chest and lungs"), exercisers young and old did six very specific arm activities— basically stretches and extensions—followed by extension exercises for fingers and forearms and a variety of bending and stretching exercises done from the waist. Deep knee bends, toe raises, semideep knee bends, leg raises and extensions from a standing position, and high stepping completed the regimen. For the more energetic and well-developed pupils, the same exer-

EXERCISES FOR THE CHEST AND LUNGS.

EXERCISE 1.

LET all the pupils take a given station, and at such distances that they can throw out their arms without touching each other. Then let the teacher give words of command as here indicated.

Word of Command—"Military Position!"

The directions here given are the same as those used by drill-sergeants in training military men, and therefore it is called the *Military Position.*

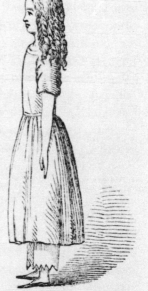

Fig. 1.

Let the heels be half an inch apart, and the feet turned out so as to form *an angle of sixty degrees.*

Let the knees be straight.

Let the shoulders be thrown back, the arms hang close to the body, the hands open to the front, the elbows turned in and close to the sides.

Let the chest be advanced, and the lower part of the body drawn back.

Let the head be erect, and the weight of the body be thrown onto the front part of the feet, as in *Fig.* 1.

This position brings the ear, shoulder, hip, knee, and ankle into a line, as is illustrated in this figure.

The "Military Position" advocated by Catharine Beecher who, like other advocates of calisthenics, adopted a military model for students' exercises and published detailed instructions for every bodily movement.
Illustration from Physiology and Calisthenics *(New York: Harper and Brothers, 1856) p. 10.*

cises could be done with small weights, or dumbbells, usually made of cast iron and weighing between three and five pounds.[45]

Beecher proposed that such activities might profitably take place in a "Calisthenic Hall" or "Temple of Health," which she hoped cities and towns might construct. Surrounded by "pleasant walks, and shades, and flowers," the building was to contain all the necessary space and apparatus for both gymnastics and calisthenics, especially those exercises that "could be performed *in measures and to the sound of music.*" "Scientific and medical men" were to head such institutions, and they would examine each prospective participant "in regard to their daily avocations, their diet, the ventilation of their sleeping and business rooms, the defects of their physical system, and any diseases they might suffer." Individual exercise plans would then be developed.[46]

Many American educators just before the Civil War evidently agreed with Beecher's contention that "children in school-houses, or on Sunday in the churches . . . [once] had rosy cheeks and looked full of health and spirits. But now . . . a great portion of them, either have pallor or pale complexions, or look delicate or partially misformed."[47] Yet the enthusiasm for re-forming bodies could have deleterious effects if carried to an extreme. Overexertion, Beecher argued, might also reduce the size of muscles because "the decay made by exercise exceeds the supply of nourishment furnished by the blood." She traced the tendency toward such excess to a too-literal application of German practices, which she thought "needed modifications to adapt it to the excitable, sensitive, and worn-out constitutions of the American people."[48]

The great mass of Germans who began emigrating after the revolutions of 1848 settled throughout the United States, and in particular in the Midwest. The first of their gymnastic institutions, called *Turnverein,* was the Cincinnati *Turngemeinde,* established in November 1848. Some of the twenty-two groups formed by 1851 took political stances advocating socialism, whereas others argued for apolitical institutions. Their outings—which consisted of picnics, games, gymnastics, and much beer drinking—provoked suspicion among Anglo-Americans. The gatherings were celebrations of German culture—participants were intent on keeping their own language, and they often dressed in foreign military uniforms and almost always carried arms. To what or to whom was their loyalty? Confrontations with swaggering young native Anglo-American men occurred; they often resulted in bloodshed and the destruction of equipment, and they politicized the

Turnverein. In 1855 the central committee of the groups, the *Turnerbund*, announced its opposition to slavery, to the prohibition of alcohol, and to the racist and hostile Know-Nothing Party. The Civil War and changing American educational ideas helped change the *Turnverein* into a less aggressive organization for the preservation of German culture. Moreover, many German soldiers fought in the war, nearly all on the Union side; thus assimilation increased, and the fear of alien insurrection declined. Finally, American schools began to adopt the German system of gymnastics. Some wealthy families, such as the Higinbothams of Oneida, New York, adopted the system for home use in the indoor gymnasium of their house.

For adults and children who did not get enough physical education in the schools, there were plenty of opportunities for gymnastic exercises of all sorts by the mid-1850s. Two gymnasiums, those of Charles Ottingnon and George Weyprecht, were advertised in *Wilson's Business Directory for New York City* for 1855; there were seven in New York City by 1860. People in Albany, New York, could exercise at the Albany Gymnasium, organized in 1853, for five dollars annually, three dollars for six months, or one dollar per month. The gym also offered bowling on "five of the finest alleys in the city."[49]

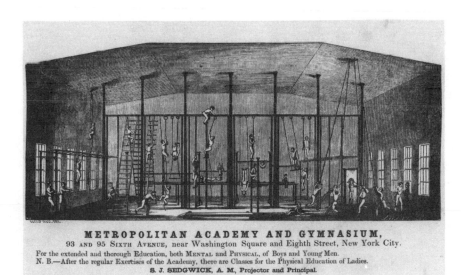

METROPOLITAN ACADEMY AND GYMNASIUM,
93 and 95 Sixth Avenue, near Washington Square and Eighth Street, New York City.
For the extended and thorough Education, both Mental and Physical, of Boys and Young Men.
N. B.—After the regular Exercises of the Academy, there are Classes for the Physical Education of Ladies.
S. J. SEDGWICK, A. M., Projector and Principal.

Metropolitan Academy and Gymnasium, advertisement from a New York City business directory, ca. 1855.

Gymnastics and calisthenics were significant alterations in the American approach to health in the mid-nineteenth century because they implied that Americans could and should shape the form of their bodies in an active way. Unlike vegetarians or such critics as Russell Trall, who condemned the roundness and great girth of many people, the advocates of exercise asserted that a different body shape—modeled after muscular Greek and Roman statuary—was the ideal. Their arguments dovetailed tightly with the more pervasive idea that human action was essential for improvement of the race and the nation, and calisthenics of gymnastics joined with other new cures —vegetarianism, water cures, animal magnetism, electromagnetism, and electricity—to lay the ground work for a new era of health reform that began after the Civil War ended.

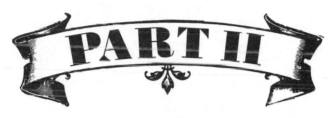

PART II

THE PRICE
OF CIVILIZATION,
1860–1890

CHAPTER FIVE

THE SANITATION MOVEMENT AND THE WILDERNESS CURE

B y 1860 the radicals of the 1830s were either converts to another faith, too aged and infirm to carry on as public figures, or dead. The millennial dynamism of perfectionist reforms declined precipitously in the aftermath of the War between the States, but it did not completely dissipate. Americans were still concerned about the future of their nation and still believed in the potential of human action to realize a better society. But by the 1860s the connection between religious and physical regeneration was less clearly articulated. More than any other factor, the increasing force of scientific thinking and the communication to the public of scientific knowledge about the cosmos—both the extraterrestrial and the microscopic—enabled Americans to take a more secular approach to individual and social health. The synthesis of the prewar years had broken apart.

American hostility to physicians had not extended to practitioners in the natural and physical sciences. Though nearly all laymen and women resisted the implications of Charles Darwin's theory of evolution as put forth in *On the Origin of Species* in 1859, they were receptive to the ever-increasing discoveries of researchers and to the growing number of museums, or "cabinets of curiosities," that were established in large and small towns and cities throughout the nation. Popular periodicals such as *Harper's Weekly* carried regular columns that reported the scientific news of the day, and *Scientific American,* which began publication in 1845, was from the start a popular journal.

Scientists—geologists, physiologists, biologists, chemists, and physicists —also altered the way Americans defined the diseases that plagued them, and they identified new ones. In 1830 Edward Hitchcock had lumped together nearly all internal diseases under the general heading of "dyspepsy." The affliction included mental disturbances from severe depression to indecisiveness, as well as heartburn and other forms of indigestion. His was the majority opinion about the nature of disease, and the solutions of the pre–Civil War era logically devolved from that set of theories. But by the 1860s physiologists had begun to distinguish between different sorts of internal afflictions. Dyspepsia—still a plague—was identified as solely a digestive problem; "nervousness," which could affect digestion, was analyzed more closely by, among others, Dr. George Beard and was identified as a separate, new disease. Beard and others linked nervous exhaustion —what they termed *neurasthenia*—to the social and economic conditions of the United States and often nostalgically compared the later nineteenth century with the dimly remembered colonial past. Research and mortality statistics—which were kept in a more sophisticated manner than before— also identified consumption, or tuberculosis, as the third great affliction of the age. It had been a problem before the war but became even more serious afterward, perhaps because cholera and other epidemics seemed to visit less frequently.

The 1860s were also characterized by a shift in emphasis in the solutions Americans chose in order to gain or regain health. The movement to improve the ventilation and sanitary conditions of American homes and cities became much more powerful in the 1860s, a result of the increasing sophistication of microbiological analysis of the causes of disease and of the creation of the sanitary commissions that were active during the Civil War. The water cures of the Priessnitz, Shew, and Trall model began to disappear, to be replaced by an increasing American enthusiasm for bathing in warm springs and for both bathing in and drinking mineral waters. Resorts and spas flourished in this period, meeting the demand of an ever-enlarging middle class that took advantage of one of bureaucracy's characteristic benefits—the vacation. Dietary reform, and in particular vegetarianism, continued to be a cause for some reformers, but with little success, while temperance gained in strength.

Most Americans of the postwar era did not opt for a single form of cure or prevention. Almira MacDonald of Rochester, New York, typified this medical heterogeneity. In September 1871 she took a "blue moss" for "biliousness" after a visit from her doctor. She figured that "balsam, copperas [iron sulfate, used as an invigorator], and the use of hot wet flannels and Elixir Opium" did her the "most good," however. Apparently having trouble with constipation, she took "sedlitz powder" (an antacid) and an "injection" (enema) which produced an "opperation [*sic*] from the bowels." Thus in one night, she combined "heroic" medicines (opium), water cures (hot wet wrap), mineral powders, and flushing of the system. When she still felt unwell three days later, she again used a variety of treatments —an "injection," castor oil, "new milk" (fresh raw milk), morphine powders, and "a local application to fevered parts of Bella Donna" (a poisonous plant).[1]

Over the next few years, Almira's choice of treatments included a "blue pill" and "congress water" for a cough and sore throat, quinine for "weakness"; calomel, "Dover's" (a mixture of gum arabic and rock candy dissolved in water), and peppermint; and applied "the blister" (for headache) and poultices of bread and water and ground slippery elm. She was still taking laudanum in 1879, even as she was getting regular treatments at a "medical electrician."[2]

MacDonald was clearly receptive to new ideas and treatments, but her attitude was at its base pragmatic. Fear of smallpox in 1871 pushed her to have her family vaccinated, a treatment that was still controversial at that time. She probably learned about the procedure through the local papers or through such periodicals as *Harper's Weekly,* which in 1870 reported on "Vaccination at Paris." "There is much smallpox in the cities," she wrote in December 1871, "and it is advisable to be protected."[3]

Anxious to learn about new health remedies and advice, she eagerly attended (or tried to attend) lectures given by the many itinerant advisors who passed through the city. In January 1880, she was advised by a speaker to "breathe only eighteen times a minute." She went again three years later to hear the same lecturer on her return to Rochester.[4]

MacDonald's eclecticism in her selection of medical treatments demonstrates the power of scientific discovery in the postwar era as well as the lasting imprint of prewar medical thought. Born in 1836, she came of age when calomel, bleeding, and blistering were the norm. She appears to have rejected the lancet, as most other patients and physicians had, and found some hope in new methods of treatment, in part as a result of the well-publicized work of medical scientists during the war.

The Civil War was reported to Americans as no other event in world history had been, primarily because of two revolutionary developments in communications technology. Many newspapers regularly advertised "the latest news by telegraph," and some papers were even titled "Telegraphs." Photography, which had been used to record certain aspects of the Crimean War in the mid-1850s, became a widely used tool for seemingly "real life" (or death) reportage. Few were aware that the daguerreotypes were often "posed" shots; Mathew Brady sometimes even moved corpses to obtain the dramatic effect he desired. Engravings in newspapers and books were made from daguerreotypes and, to heighten their authenticity, were promoted as having been so made.

The image of war and its horrors presented to Americans was therefore of tremendous evocative power. They saw the slaughter to which the photographer bore witness, and illustrated newspaper and magazine stories provoked their disgust and anger about the horrible conditions under which prisoners of war lived at Andersonville and other prisons. They also learned of the overwhelming number of soldiers who died not from their wounds but from disease.

At the same time, they read of the triumphs of the field doctors, many of whom used some of the latest scientific treatments and compounds to save soldiers' lives. Collodion, a combination of gun cotton and ether, was announced as a "new invention for surgeons" as early as 1849. Quick drying and transparent, it enabled a surgeon to cover and protect a wound or incision with "no irritating quality."[5] Though it was used increasingly for the preparation of photographic plates, news of this and other novel field techniques helped bring physicians more to the center of the debate on health and hygiene.

Reports of the heroic and vital work of field surgeons and of their need for help led to the creation of civilian-staffed sanitary commissions. Based in part on the English model of two decades prior to the war, federal and state commissions were formed to help clean up the filth that many observers were convinced was carrying disease. The United States Sanitary Commission was established in 1861. It was staffed primarily by women (and a few physicians, merchants, bankers, and other male community leaders who volunteered to look after wounded and ailing Union soldiers). Well financed, by the middle of 1861 it had enough political power to secure permission from the War Department to investigate the sanitary conditions of field and camp hospitals, as well as the condition of healthy troops in the field.

The commission's investigation led to a congressional order that reorganized the army medical department. After the war the sanitary movement in the United States slowly gathered force, first as an effort to relieve the problem of cities congested with refuse and human waste, and later in the century as a broad-based plan of attack on American architecture and personal habits.

One of the earliest thorough critiques of the structure of American cities and of the individual living quarters within them appeared in 1858, with the publication of David Boswell Reid's *Ventilation in American Dwellings*. Reid was a trained physician with strong intellectual ties to the English sanitary reform movement, which had for at least two decades sought to rid English cities of the filth physicians were convinced led to disease. Reid and Elisha Harris, who contributed an "Introductory Outline" to the book, joined the core of English reform theory to the American context. Harris maintained that "the homes of the people, or the conditions of domiciliary life, furnish most reliable indices of the state of intellectual and moral advancement in any community." This was not a particularly new concept, but in the context of developing biological and pathological theory, it took on new meanings for those concerned with the preservation of health in America.[6]

Harris asserted that there was a direct correlation between physical surroundings and "moral elevation." He was careful to point out that though environment was not the sole determinant in morality, "neither intellectual progress nor moral social refinement can long be maintained where the requisite conditions for physical health and comfort are not suitably provided." Harris echoed the earlier millennial-minded evangelicals in linking physical form in dwellings and moral condition, but now was concerned with more modest, and more explicitly secular, goals.[7]

Anticipating the Progressive reformers of some fifty years hence, Harris and Reid argued that urban crowding led to the development and spread of disease. They found fault with "the close, uncleansed, unventilated residences of the poor" because they became "the homes of disease and pauperism." The equation is significant. Writing before the development and popularization of the germ theory of disease, the authors identified the fact of crowding with the generation of disease, in a sense a midcentury recapitulation of an ancient and medieval idea—spontaneous generation. Moreover, there was a social dynamic to Harris's and Reid's equation: they were convinced that "the crowded narrow tenements to which avarice drives poverty, in filthy streets and noisome courts, become perennial sources of deadly miasmata that may be wafted to the neighboring mansions of wealth and refinement, to cause sickness and mourning there; and when once the breadth of pestilence becomes epidemic in any city, commerce and trade are driven to more salubrious marts."[8] In the mid-nineteenth century, "urban flight" was induced by the fear of disease, arising from the crowded conditions in which the poor were forced to live. They would continue to be blamed for disease for the ensuing seventy-five years.

There were some encouraging signs, however, especially in American architecture and in the "ample supply of pure water" in most American cities and towns. But Harris also found economic concerns had engendered a disregard for sunlight, fresh air, and drainage.[9] Like pre–Civil War American Protestants, Harris still identified "luxury" (and its corollary, greed) with sin (and filth). His thinking also illustrates the ambiguous and ambivalent nature of reform. At the same time that Harris castigated the greed of certain wealthy individuals, he condemned the poor for generating the diseases that caused business to flee and the more "refined" to die. The equation appears nonetheless to have been a popular one: the August 1860 issue of *Godey's Lady's Book* carried two short entries, one entitled "Ventilation" and, immediately below it, another called "Dangers of Wealth."[10]

By 1860, a sophisticated plumbing network reached nearly all urban middle-class homes and even some working-class housing, if only on the first floor of many-storied tenements. In an article in the November 30, 1878, issue of the *American Architect and Building News*, George E. Waring bragged that "plumbing, as we know it, is essentially and almost exclusively an American institution." In providing a labor-saving device even for those classes unaccustomed to luxury, "we have carried the possibilities of the industry to its utmost limit."[11]

But if the water was "ample," it was hardly pure. In a more popular magazine of the same era, *The Household,* Dr. J. H. Hanaford advised his readers (most of whom were women at home) that their luxurious tap water carried "many, many ills," among them typhoid, "diarrheas," and various forms of indigestion. Hanaford complained that many houses were so positioned that runoff and seepage from cesspools and sinks could easily find their way into drinking water.[12] John Harvey Kellogg, by 1876 an established physician and hygienist in Battle Creek, Michigan, advocated filtering even rainwater, and he advertised a device for this purpose that could be "obtained at reasonable rates." No slave to the principle of amassing wealth, Kellogg also provided instructions for making one's own filter out of a clay flowerpot, charcoal, sand, and a white flannel cloth.[13]

Nearly every writer who tackled the impure-water issue advocated filters. In 1879 the editors of *The Household* criticized lead and galvanized pipes because they corroded easily and recommended ceramic tiles and filtration in their place, although they allowed that iron, gutta-percha (a hard rubber-like compound), glass, and even wood pipes were acceptable. Similarly, in a series entitled "The Art of Preserving Health," *The Household* linked impure water to "diarrhea, dysentery, cholera, [and] malarious fever" and strongly advised filtration.[14]

Filters had been available since the mid 1850s but did not become common items in the home until the 1870s. Hardware dealer W. L. Ingraham, of Rochester, New York, advertised his 1867 improvement of Kedgie's original 1856 patent water filter as capable of "rendering all soft Water Perfectly Pure and Clear as Crystal." The device was simply an oak cask (open at the top) with a spigot at the bottom that the owner packed with "pure prepared charcoal," thus avoiding "insidious diseases."[15]

By the 1880s Americans could choose from a variety of brands of filters for home and institutional use. John C. Jewett and Sons of Buffalo, New York boasted of their "more than a quarter of a century" of experience "in the manufacture of Filters," and their stock ranged from four-and-a-half-quart portable tin devices to fourteen-gallon stationary iron and porcelain mechanisms, as well as "ornamental" and "landscape" styles.[16]

Larger and faster-acting filters for larger buildings became available in the 1880s and were usually plumbed directly into the water supply route of a building. "The Celebrated Cummings Water-Filter" of about 1890 summoned up fears of the recent past for Americans when their advertising pamphlet asked "If the Cholera Comes, Are You Ready for it?" Cummings, a Philadelphia-based firm, warned that its home city was "to-day the same as Hamburg last winter," when the German city was afflicted with the

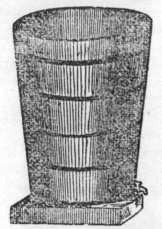

IMPROVED WATER FILTER.

THE accompanying cut is a representation of one of the greatest and most useful inventions of the age—*Kedzie's Improved Water Filter.*

Its mechanism is so perfect that it accomplishes all that could be expected or desired of a filter to accomplish, and without the bestowal of more than the slightest amount of attention. It removes from water all those products of decay and disease which are the most prolific causes of sickness and death.

THOUSANDS USE THEM

And admire them, and all are ready to testify to their efficiency and utility. No family should be without one; for it is impossible to obtain from springs or wells water which is, in all respects, so free from injurious properties as is soft filtered water.

Five sizes are manufactured to suit the wants of all. The following table gives their dimensions :—

No. 1,.................... 25 inches high, reservoir holds 2 gallons.
" 2,.................... 27 " " " " 2½ "
" 3,.................... 29 " " " " 3 "
" 4,.................... 31 " " " " 3½ "
" 5,.................... 32 " " " " 4 "

Prices. No. 1, $9.00 ; No. 2, $10.50 ; No. 3, $12.00 ; No. 4, $13.50 ; No. 5, $15.00. Orders promptly filled.

Address, *Health Reformer, Battle Creek, Mich.*

As Americans began to learn that their health could be endangered by organisms they could not see, clean water became critically important, and water filters for the home became popular. The decoration on water coolers sometimes reflected American ideas about exotic places and their allegedly healthier peoples. Left: illustration from John Harvey Kellogg, The Household Manual *(Battle Creek, Mich.: Good Health Publishing Co., 1882), inside back cover. Right: illustration from advertising pamphlet, Buffalo, N.Y., ca. 1875.*

dreaded disease. The firm predicted "a Cholera harvest" without proper filtration. These water filters were expensive: the Loomis in-System filter cost between seventy-five dollars for a five-gallon-per-minute unit and two thousand dollars for a system that filtered two-hundred-and-fifty gallons per minute. Most people, therefore, continued to rely on the pour-the-water-through variety, which the Simmons Hardware Company of St. Louis,

Jewett's Water Filters.
JEWETT'S PORTABLE FILTER AND COOLER

Patented November 16, 1869; Patented October 15, 1878; Patented September 23, 1879.

COMBINES:

1st.—A Separate (Galvanized Iron) Vessel, containing the Filtering Medium.
2d.—An Outer Case, fitted to receive said vessel, with Cover.
3d.—A PORCELAIN-LINED COOLER.

The whole exterior is finished in harmony, and will last a life-time. Whenever the Filter fails to satisfactorily perform, a new filtering vessel can be obtained at small cost (no more than the expense of re-packing, as formerly), which will make the whole complete as when first purchased.

It is intended that the filtering vessel and outer case should fit tightly together. To separate them, remove same to the floor, then take hold of the side handles, press down hard enough to slide the case down.

Acknowledged to be the only Complete FILTER and COOLER in the World.

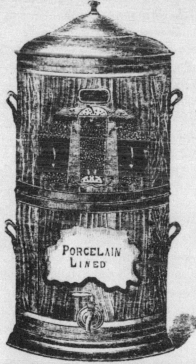 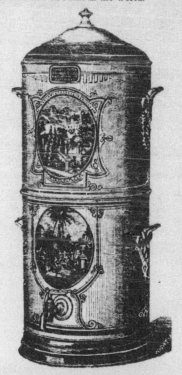

Portion of front removed showing interior of Filter, also of
Porcelain-Lined Cooler.

GRAINED OAK.	ORNAMENTAL STYLE.
No. 161—Reservoir, 4½ quarts, $ 6.75	No. 171—Reservoir, 4½ quarts, $ 7.25
No. 162—Reservoir, 7½ quarts, 8.75	No. 172—Reservoir, 7½ quarts, 9.25
No. 163—Reservoir, 11 quarts, 10.50	No. 173—Reservoir, 11 quarts, 11.00
No. 164—Reservoir, 16 quarts, 12.50	No. 174—Reservoir, 16 quarts, 13.00
No. 165—Reservoir, 26 quarts, 15.00	No. 175—Reservoir, 26 quarts, 15.50

FILTERING VESSELS ONLY.

For No. 161 or 171, ... Each, $2.00	For No. 164 or 174, ... Each, $3.75
" " 162 or 172, ... " 2.50	" " 165 or 175, ... " 4.50
" " 163 or 173, ... " 3.25	

Missouri, for example, advertised in the late 1880s. Decorated with paintings, line drawings, and designs consistent with the prevailing Anglo-Japonesque or "Aesthetic" Styles, these filters sold for between ten dollars (for the one- to two-barrel size) to fifty dollars (for the ten- to thirteen-barrel size).[17]

Plumbing, as historian May Stone has observed, was a paradox for Americans. It was not only an index of wealth and technological superiority, but it was also a source of dreaded microbes, poisonous gases, and disease. Improperly vented water supplies and waste removal systems could easily send sewer gases back into the house, as articles in popular household magazines continuously explained. The result of improper plumbing, wrote E. G. Cook in the October 1887 issue of *Demorest's Monthly*, was that "the deadly poison is manufactured in silence and darkness, to worm its hydra-head into our sleeping-rooms, giving the fatal potion to the dearest and most helpless, who have the least power to resist it."[18]

One way to avoid the poisonous possibilities of the kitchen sink drain was to disinfect chemically the waste water in the pipes. Kellogg suggested one compound composed primarily of carbolic acid. The editors of *Godey's* not only explained the connection between typhoid and the "foul gas" of sinks and sewers but also advised women about the ways they might disinfect their drains, warning them to instruct servants carefully so they would not be "extravagant" with chemicals.[19]

For the problem of the privy, thought to be a threatening source of contamination for the up-to-date house of the 1870s, Kellogg offered another solution, the "dry-earth system." Widely manufactured after the Civil War, earth closets, or commodes, consisted of a hinged wooden seat cover that lifted up and back (against a backboard and "tank" for dry earth) to reveal a boxed-in chamber in which a pan filled with earth rested. In 1873, earth closets could be had in chestnut or pine from the Earth Closet Company of Hartford, Connecticut, for twenty-five dollars, or in black walnut for "$5.00 to $15.00 extra, according to finish." In addition to its ability to reduce the chance that sewer gas would develop, the company asserted, "there is no waste of fertilizing material, and NO POSSIBILITY OF INFECTION, even in CHOLERA."[20] For those who wished to make their own, Kellogg once again offered instructions.

> Have made at the tin-shop a sufficient number of pans of thick sheet iron. The pans should be about two feet square, and two

inches and a half deep. Each should be furnished with a long bail, and a strong handle at one side about a foot in length. In using these pans, fill each half-full of fine dry dirt—not sand—or ashes, and shove it into position, allowing the bail to fall back upon the handle behind. By the addition of a little dry dirt several times a day, all foul odors will be prevented.[21]

Earth closets were popular only till the turn of the century, by which time contractors and sanitation experts became more proficient not only at designing and building plumbing systems but also at policing building projects.

Plumbing and drainage introduced new problems and new conveniences in American architecture, but older problems relating to air breathed and overall ventilation remained. Beecher's complaints about houses that were too tightly sealed to permit the free flow of air were echoed throughout the latter nineteenth century. Kellogg argued in 1882 for openings at the bottom and tops of rooms. Anticipating criticism for recommending opening windows in frigid northern climates, the doctor sternly noted that "cold air is not poison. Plenty of air and a rousing fire are cheaper in the long run than foul air and less fire." In 1887 Mrs. E. G. Cook argued similarly in a continuing series of articles in *Demorest's Monthly* entitled "Sanitarian." She wrote that "the best authorities" believed "that about forty per cent of all deaths are due to the influence of impure air."[22]

Reformers in both England and America argued that "pulmonary consumption, or consumption of the lungs, has been largely promoted by the presence of unchanged or impure air in the dwelling house." As consumers considered the architectural style of the home they might purchase or have built, they were urged to choose those designs that included the most windows. English architectural reformer Shirley Murphy recommended Italian architecture in particular. "Not only is it compatible with English notions of comfort and convenience, but it admits of the most ample amount and the freest distribution of light and air." Murphy was quick to point out that "whatever style is adopted, a first and foremost necessity is to adapt that style to the best-known rules of health and convenience of the present, and not to reproduce the imperfect and unsanitary arrangements of the past ages as necessary accompaniments of the style."[23]

English architect Robert W. Edis, in his essay "Internal Decoration,"

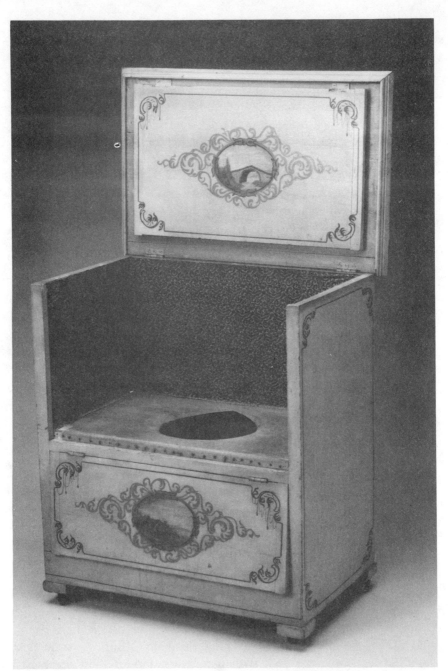

Earth closets solved the problem of containing and disposing of human wastes without the inconvenience of the outhouse or, advocates said, the smells and difficulties of chamber pots. Commode, American, painted pine and poplar, 1870–90.

specifically made the connection between "reform" and health in the home. He argued that "simplicity of form without the unnecessary and unmeaning overlaying of bad ornament . . . is not only useless but costly, liable in the glass, china, or pottery to be easily chipped and broken, difficult to clean, and as a rule, utterly useless." As for furnishings, Edis thought, "it must be evident to common-sense people, that all furniture which collects and holds dust and dirt which cannot easily be detected and cleaned; that all window valances and heavy stuff curtains with heavy fringes which cannot be constantly shaken; and that all floor coverings which are fastened down . . . are objectionable and unhealthy."[24]

In "Floors and Floor Coverings," Edis traced what he considered to be the process of "reform" in a house burdened with the aesthetic and hygienic mistakes of the past. First, he urged people to "send away cart-loads of . . . rubbish," including "carpets . . . window-curtains . . . [of] muslin which people hang across the lower halves of bed-room windows, all books and pamphlets which were not really required, all anti-macassars." Then, home-owners could begin "the work of reform." First, they were to check the condition of water supplies and drainage, making certain all soil pipes were properly vented. The next step was "to cover the old floors—which . . . by their cracks and unevenness are among the worst possible forms of dust-traps—with thin oak parqueterie both in living-rooms and bed-rooms." Edis recommended "a few small Oriental rugs" on the oak floors, small enough to be "taken up and shaken in one hand."[25]

In 1874 Anna Holyoke, a regular contributor to *The Household*, agreed with the English reformers. "Carpets are an evil," she maintained, "inasmuch as they absorb impure air, gases and contagious effluvia, and in the attempt to cleanse them so much foul dust is thrown into the air." She recommended "wood carpets." Kellogg agreed, noting that "great care should always be taken to avoid dust as much as possible. In sweeping carpets and dirty floors, a person is exposed to injury unless some precaution, such as sprinkling the floor or moistening the broom, is taken to prevent filling the air with dust."[26]

Edis and other reformers reserved their most vitriolic commentary for the European-influenced furniture and wall coverings favored by so many Britons and Americans after the Civil War. He criticized the furniture's bad design as well as its impracticality. "The gold or metal work in the ornaments [on furniture] soon got black and shabby," and fashionable "fluffy" upholstery collected and held dust and other impurities, which no amount

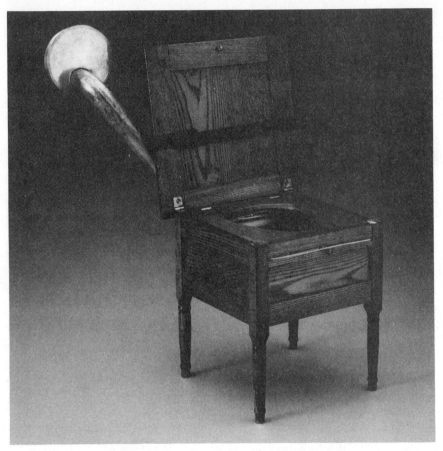

Here was one inventive alternative to the chamber pot and water closet. L. R. Damon decided he could solve the venting problem by ducting the fumes of the earth commode into the stove exhaust. Unfortunately, Damon neglected to consider the results of a backdraft. Merchandising model for a "parlor commode," L. R. Damon, Dexter, Maine. Oak, metal, pine. Patented September 16, 1902.

of brushing or cleaning could entirely get rid of. "Everything about us," Edis complained, was "trashy, vulgar, and commonplace."[27] "Reform"-style furniture (commonly referred to as "Eastlake" in the United States) had restrained, flat ornamentation; Eastlake houses were usually built with oak strip or parquet floors, moldings with slightly sloping top edges (so that dust

PARLOR COMMODE

❧ Ventilated, Portable. ❧

ABSOLUTELY ODORLESS.

No Deodorizing of Sick-room Required.

PATENTED SEPT 16, 1902.

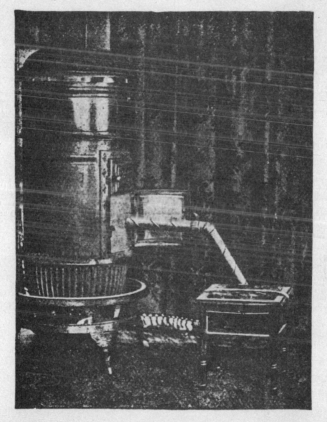

PERFECT VENTILATION.

No dust. ❧ No chemicals required.

NO SICK-ROOM EQUIPMENT

COMPLETE WITHOUT IT.

Upholstered top. Highly finished. Neat, Attractive.

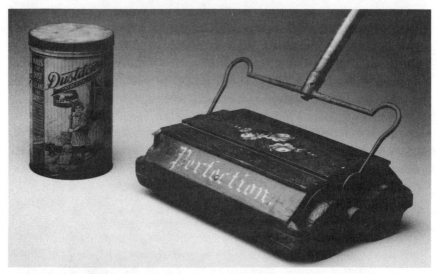

"Dust" described any invisible or tiny particles thought to carry disease. Rug-cleaning powder, the Fitch Dustdown Co., Cincinnati, Ohio, painted tin, ca. 1910. Carpet sweeper, Bissell Carpet Sweeper Co., Grand Rapids, Mich., ca. 1890.

would not collect), and different-colored woods rather than ornate carving for decoration. Eastlake kitchens commonly had maple floors and painted wainscoting. Popular by the 1880s, such homes had high ceilings, furnaces to heat them, lots of windows (often a bay window among them), and at least one fireplace.

Reformers also took aim at the wallpapers that were the fashionable order of the day. First, they argued that the heavy, flocked papers absorbed dirt, dust, and "unhealthy vapours," or condensation from the air. Moreover, some of the dyes used were poisonous. "Many cases of poisoning," wrote Kellogg, "some of which were fatal, have been traced to the arsenic contained in several of the colors of wall-paper." Because it usually contained arsenic, green was particularly dangerous in both papers and curtains, Kellogg warned; reds might also contain arsenic, he said, because manufacturers of aniline dyes commonly used the poison.[28]

Poisoning was only half the problem with richly colored wall papers. Perhaps recalling an old problem for pre–Civil War dietary reformers, Edis and other critics discovered that the gaudy and vulgar designs employed by

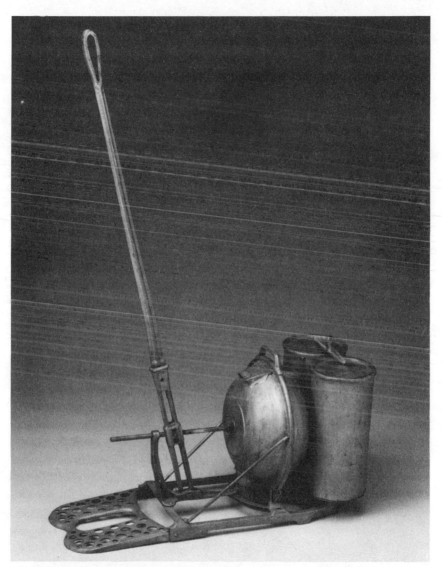

Moving the handle of this machine in a reciprocating motion produced a decreased pressure inside the drum, which in turn caused some of the dust and dirt on floors and carpets to be lifted up and conveyed into the canisters. This machine saved only a small amount of labor, but was a status symbol of sorts. Vacuum cleaner, Automatic Vacuum Cleaner Co., Bloomington, Ill. Cast iron, tin, cardboard, 1905–15.

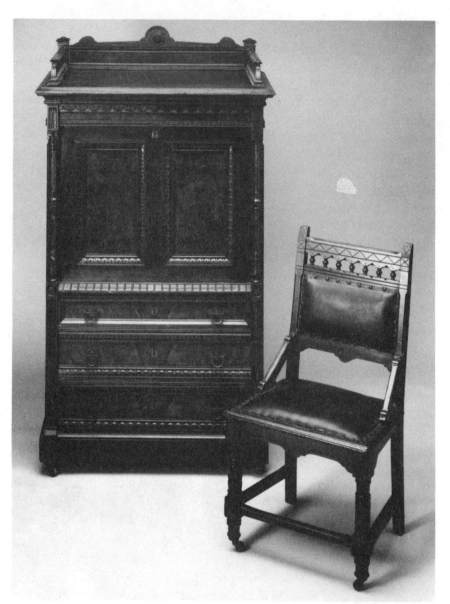

The flat surfaces and leather seats of "Eastlake" or "reform" style furniture were popular because they were easily cleaned. Secretary, American, walnut and burled walnut veneer, 1871–85; side chair, American, mahogany with leather seat, ca. 1885.

interior designers and manufacturers were too stimulating, in this case to the mind rather than to the digestive tract. "Inartistic and subversive of that mental enjoyment or pleasure which good and harmonious colouring tends to produce," Edis observed, papers and carpets were often designed with "little regard to the mental effect of jarring colours and patterns, or the nervous irritability which almost unknowingly is excited." The "endless multiplication and monotony" of "strongly-marked patterns . . . [is] a source of infinite torture and annoyance in times of sickness and sleeplessness, [which] could materially add to our discomfort and nervous irritability, and after a time have a ghastly and nightmare effect upon the brain."[29]

Proper decoration and coloring consisted of "warm, quiet tones." Halls and stairways, especially, were to be painted in such tones, since "the eye on entering a house is generally fatigued by the strong glare of daylight." For the "drawing room, a good all-over decorative pattern, such as Morris blue pomegranate" was recommended, and "dull reds or warm russet-browns" were thought best for dining rooms and libraries.[30]

Ways of heating the home continued to be scrutinized. Most homeowners who could afford it heated their homes with cast-iron stoves as airtight as possible, hoping to eliminate the drafty fireplaces that wasted as much heat as they supplied. But as early as the 1850s, medical writers such as Reid and lay authors such as Beecher began to question the advisability of abandoning the open fireplace. While simple conservatism or nostalgia for the colonial hearth may have stimulated some critics, others viewed the stove as unhealthy, depriving residents of a supply of ever-changing fresh air. Reid argued that so much attention was paid to ventilation because, among other things, the use of powerful stoves and other heating apparatus—to the exclusion of open fireplaces—had caused a ventilation problem.[31]

The problem of the cast-iron stove was judged more acute in the post–Civil War era, as public consciousness about ventilation and health in general increased dramatically. In the April 1873 issue of *Godey's*, the editors stated that "it will be a happy day for our households when the 'stove demon' . . . is exorcised from them." In 1882 J. H. Kellogg was more optimistic. "The old-fashioned fire-place was a most efficient ventilator," he maintained. "It is a good omen that fire-places are again coming into use. The most fashionable parlors in the large cities are now heated by them." He warned readers that they could be poisoned by "carbonous oxide" from their stoves. According to Kellogg, the gas was "often found in air-tight stoves" and was especially dangerous because it could "pass directly through cast-iron, especially when it is heated." Here was another undetectable poison lurking in the background of modernity, and another home improvement that could kill as well protect.[32]

Five years later, in 1887, Mrs. E. G. Cook took a slightly different approach from Kellogg's, arguing that the heat from fireplaces was more healthful because "it more nearly resembles the sun by radiation." Moreover, Cook maintained, cast-iron stoves were an evil because "the organic condition of the air is changed by passing over hot iron," which allegedly increased the concentration of iron in the air and thus injured health. More strident in his criticism of stoves was Marc Cook, whose book *The Wilderness Cure* (1881) was a popular guide to curing lung diseases. Cook celebrated mountain air, "with no noxious odors, no defective drains or gas-pipes, no miserable furnaces, no double windows to shut out the oxygen . . . but in place thereof cherry-wood fires, open chimney-places, and a surrounding atmosphere of absolute purity." Stove manufacturers responded to these charges by producing a new sort of apparatus, or at least a newly christened stove, usually called a "ventilator." In 1889 Albert Well of Rochester, New York, advertised the "Sterling Ventilator" stove as capable of "perfect hot air circulation," with "the best foul air combustion." Such stoves remained popular past the turn of the century and were often the main source of heat for families that could not afford cellar furnaces.[33]

The gases and substances that threatened Americans ironically were products of the very technological and scientific successes by which they marked their progress from the unenlightened people of earlier centuries. Usually beyond the boundaries of human perception, these new threats to health seemed especially menacing because they were generated inside the house, where one sought security, rather than in the outside world of strangers. Even more insidious than the sewer gases, carbon monoxide, and ozone, which the plumbing or the hearth could produce, were those impure and potentially poisoning gases that were generated in the most secure room of all—the bedroom. Here people were most vulnerable, unaware of the diseases that were silently, slowly, and imperceptibly attacking them.

Health reformers of every persuasion and professional level broadened the attacks they had begun in the 1830s on American sleeping practices. Much to their chagrin, they found that softer feather beds had replaced lumpier and harder corncob or animal-hair mattresses as the standard for most middle-class Americans. In 1876 Kellogg considered feather beds "very unhealthful" because they underwent "slow decomposition . . . thus evolving foul and poisonous gases" while absorbing "fetid exhalations from the body which are thrown off during sleep." Eventually, he concluded, "the featherbed becomes a hot bed of disease." He recommended the "hair, cotton, straw, or husk mattresses of the rural past" and urged his readers not to "cling to the old feather-bed because it is an heir-loom. The older it is, the worse it is." Kellogg was supported in his condemnation of feather beds by the editors of *The Household*, who in 1874 referred to them as an "atrocity," defiled with the "atrocious effete animal matter which has escaped from the sleepers that have sought repose here for generations past." The arguments against feather beds were countered, if a bit feebly, by those who simply asserted that they could be aired. In 1871, *Godey's* urged that rooms be ventilated all day, and that the feather bed be shaken each day, and, if possible, hung outside for at least two hours. But by 1880, perhaps convinced by the reformers' arguments, the editors reversed their position.[34]

The "modern" replacement for the feather bed was the tied-spring mattress. Spring steel had been perfected in the 1830s and was used by many furniture makers and upholsterers by the early 1840s. Within a few years of its inception, there were attempts to integrate spring-steel technology with the production of mattresses for home use. In 1857, for example, Thomas Tolman, of West Townsend, Massachusetts, obtained a patent for a "ventilating spring mattress."

Particularly dangerous poisons lurked in the air that sleepers or their chamber partners had exhaled. Contemporary physiology explained the respiration process as one in which pure air was inspired, taken into the bloodstream through the lungs, and impure air expired, full of poisons of which the body was ridding itself. Kellogg called it "organic *poison*" and "another enemy of life more potent" than the other "gases, germs, and dust . . . which attack man from the air."[35]

Shirley Murphy thought unventilated sleeping rooms were "like so many experimental boxes for the synthetic development of pulmonary disease." *The Household* linked small bed chambers with "frightful dreams . . . the spectral nightmare, the fearful groan, the terrible shriek." These horrible conditions or phenomena were a result of reinhaling air already exhaled. "Each inhalation of pure air is returned loaded with poison; one hundred and fifty grains of it is added to the atmosphere of a bedroom every hour,

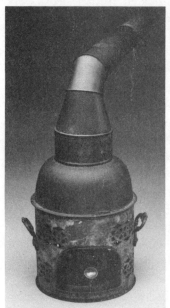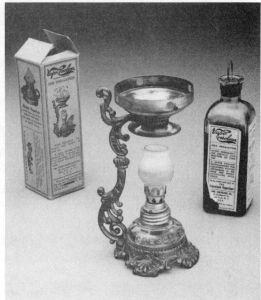

Vaporizers fired with kerosene burners were commonly used to promote healthy breathing and ease lung congestion. Electric models were available by 1915. Left: herbal vaporizer, American, tin, ca. 1890–1910. Right: vaporizing lamp and vaporizing fluid, Vapo-Cresolene Co., New York, N.Y., brass, cast iron, pressed glass, 1888–1920.

or 1200 grains during a night." Even P. T. Barnum, who was about as far from health reform as one might have gotten in the nineteenth century, had nothing good to say about the cramped and unhealthy sleeping conditions of America's forefathers and mothers, and, by implication, most of his contemporaries. In *The Art of Money-Getting* (1859) he asserted, "Our ancestors knew very little about the principles of ventilation . . . [or] oxygen," and criticized "their houses with little seven-by-nine feet bedrooms [in which] these good old pious Puritans locked themselves up" each night. They gave thanks each morning for living through the night, "and nobody had better reason to be thankful," he noted sarcastically, since their lives had been inadvertently saved by "some big crack in the window, or in the door [which] let in a little fresh air."[36]

Overloading the bed with covers was also condemned because, like the feather bed, they could cause the unsuspecting sleeper to perspire and thus exacerbate the already polluted condition of the bed. "Neither the unhealthful covering called a comfortable nor the unsightly covering known as a patched quilt should be seen on a bed in this day," wrote *The Household* in 1874. Washing these articles was difficult, and it was unlikely that people did so very often. Thus, as the article pointed out, the "comfortable," or quilt, would carry forever the filth of generations of exhalations.[37]

The perfect bedroom of the latter one-third of the nineteenth century was well ventilated and painted or papered with warm and relaxing colors. It was large, with many windows and no heavy curtains. Floors were of oak strips, covered only with small hearth rugs. The room had a fireplace, and the modern decorator had dispensed with heavy bureaus in favor of walk-in closets with hooks and poles for hanging clothes. The ultimate closet had built-in drawers and was painted for easy cleaning. Homeowners with no indoor plumbing used a dresser set and a chamber pot—kept scrupulously clean and discarded if chipped or cracked—in the bedroom. The ideal bed had a mattress of the "ventilating" spring type, and only scant covers. Healthful pillows were filled with straw or sea grass and, if of feathers, were aired out and shaken daily. Such was the regiment and environment necessary for sleepers to get all the "lung food" they needed.

The prevalence of lung diseases—"colds," bronchitis, and the great killer of the age, consumption—was a frightening fact of life. Explorations of the nature and range of consumptive affections were scattered in the early nineteenth century, and the first scientifically researched comprehensive tract on the disease was probably Henry Ingersoll Bowditch's *Consumption in New England* (1862). Bowditch (1808–1892) systematically analyzed the pathology of pulmonary consumption, employing the precise methods of French physician Pierre C. A. Louis (1787–1872), who pioneered the use of mathematical and statistical accuracy in pathological and epidemiological research.[38]

The potential causes of consumption were many. Gymnastics advocate Dioclesian Lewis ascribed "those numberless diseases of the lungs and heart, including that depopulating disease, consumption (which carried away its millions) to a contracted chest, which lessens the space for the play of those organs contained within it." Lewis argued that exercise would help Americans fend off the dreaded disease. "As the size of the chest is increased by

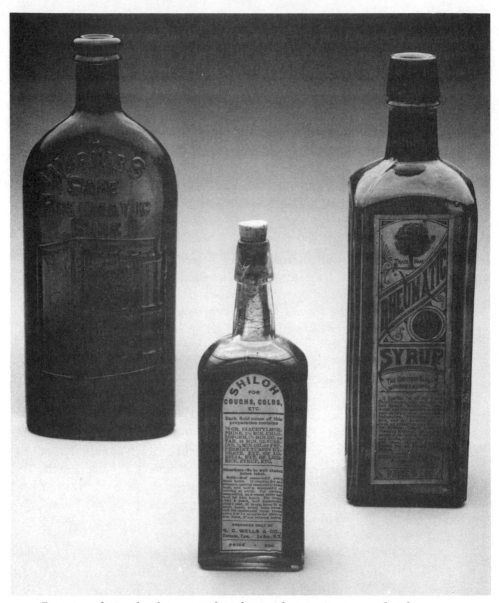

Patent-medicine hucksters produced countless tonics to combat lung ailments. Alcohol was the active ingredient in them, and they offered little relief. Rheumatic Syrup Co., Rochester, N.Y. Mold-blown glass, 1882.

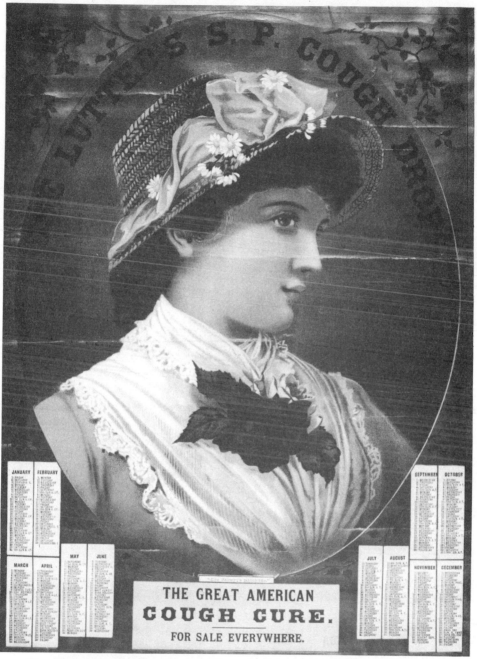

Cough drops were a convenient. if ineffective, treatment for the persistent American problem of bronchial irritation (popularly linked with tuberculosis). Advertising calendar, American, chromolithograph, ca. 1885.

these [gymnastic and calisthenic] exercises, so is the size of the lungs augmented, respiration perfected, and a susceptibility to those insidious diseases lessened."[39]

By nearly all accounts, the best treatment for consumption for those who could afford it was to get out of the city or village, or even sometimes away from the farm, and head for the mountains. Exercise and mountain air (especially if tinged with balsam and other evergreen scents) were thought to be the best way to heal a damaged set of lungs. "If a consumptive were to 'live in the saddle,' and sleep out of doors, taking care to keep the feet dry and warm, and to live upon good, nourishing food, in short, to 'rough it,'" wrote the editors of *The Household* in 1882, "he would recover his health in a few months, even if the disease had made considerable progress."[40]

The *Household* article appeared a few months after the publication of an important and popular little guide. Marc Cook's *The Wilderness Cure* offered a readable and comprehensive analysis of what to expect, of how to go about the curative trek, and of life in the mountains. The book begins with a parable about a young New Yorker whose health suffered under the "strain of a reporter's life and boarding house fare"—a sedentary, nerve-wracking job and the absence of good home cooking. He eventually developed a persistent slight fever, "night sweats," a declining appetite, and a high (over 90) pulse rate. "All this time," Cook wrote, "cod-liver oil, whiskey, and a diet of special nutritive qualities were continued perseveringly. And so was the cough."[41] A brief stay in upstate New York and then in the White Mountains gave temporary relief, yet, after he returned to New York, he suffered a severe relapse. Reasoning that his health was in danger from the perils of urban life, Cook journeyed to the Adirondacks. From a state of near death he rallied to the point where, by December, about six months after his arrival in the north country, he was able to go "for a seven-mile ride over the glistening snow." The near-zero-degree air was by that time no threat to the ever-strengthening Cook. It "might freeze your dainty city ears," he scoffed, "but it is nothing to the hardy backwoodsman."[42]

Cook slept in a tent in the summer months of his first year in the woods. "Patience, atropine (a drug), and the pure air of the tent" rid him of the sweats in two months. Physicians, he thought, had too often prescribed "going to the mountains" without having the slightest idea of what that meant. Reverend W.H.H. Murray's immensely popular book of 1869, *Adventures in the Wilderness*, an almost nostalgic evocation of the sublime qualities of the woods and waters, with little or no mention of the rugged character of the mountains, was geared for the already healthy middle class or wealthy urbanite who by the 1870s was looking for a vacation away from the city. It offered little useful information for invalids or other health-seekers, unlike some of the popular "railroad guides" of the 1870s. In contrast, Cook offered for the fainthearted and fearful (as well as for the ignorant) the comforting thought that camping could include "all the comforts and nearly all the luxuries" of city life, especially if one's camp was near one of the many major hotels that were built after 1870.[43]

Cook was no modern backpacker or woods-wise mountain man like the legendary Kit Carson or fictional Natty Bumppo. His "camp" was a comfortable little home in the wilds. He had a tent, a bed with sheets, three "bark" buildings (a kitchen and storehouse, dining room and sitting room, and guide's cabin) and an arbor. His structures (including the tent) had wooden floors, and his furnishings included a stove, tables, chairs, books,

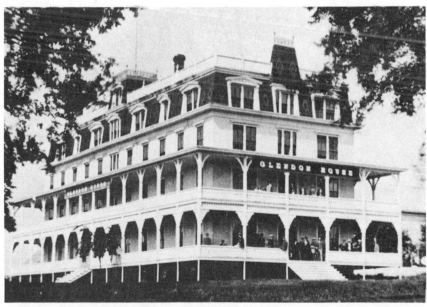

Glendon House typified the massive, airy hotels of an era that sought the healthful effects of mountain air. Their large verandas served the needs of the breeze seekers and the social desires of vacationers. Stereograph, American, ca. 1885.

writing utensils, and a clock. He purchased and had delivered a supply of "good and diverse food," wine, beer, and—of all things—cigars, and he purchased or had made a small boat. In short, Cook had made and supplied *a camp*, but he was not "camping out" in the modern sense.[44]

Cook dismissed the annoyance of insects. He insisted that a good mosquito net was all the protection a camper needed. Troublemakers of a larger variety—bears—were indeed present in the woods, Cook admitted, but they were few and were unlikely to bother humans. Fish and game were abun-

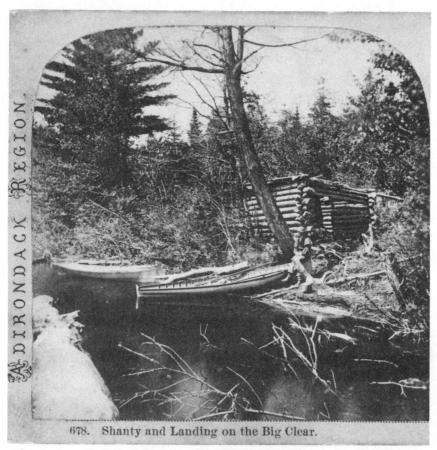

678. Shanty and Landing on the Big Clear.

The perfect abode in which to take "the wilderness cure." "Shanty and landing on the Big Clear," stereograph, northeastern United States, ca. 1870–80.

dant, "but they are not to be had for the asking"; one had either to hunt and fish for oneself or to pay a native for the service. He assured wary city slickers that physicians, mail, telegraphic service, and newspapers were available at any of the hotels.[45]

For those wishing to plunge ahead with the "Wilderness Cure," the interior reaches of the mountains could be reached with relative ease by train and stage. To get to the Saint Regis Hotel or to "Paul Smith's" in the northern Adirondacks, invalids took a twenty-mile train ride from Plattsburg, New York, to a stage depot, where a forty-mile ride over reasonable roads brought them to their destination. Once there, Cook advised people to hire a guide and then to find a suitable spot to establish camp. The best locations, he suggested, were on high ground near water, trees ("balsamics . . . purify the atmosphere"), and a hotel. "If the guide possesses the usual ingenuity of his class, he will be able to build tables, chairs, a lounge, and many other useful articles of furniture" of unfinished limbs or roughly sawn wood. This "camp furniture" graced not only camps but many of the big and small hotels as well.[46]

Cook evidently ate well and was careful to point out that a sound diet was of great importance to the man or woman who would be cured. He urged health-seekers to stock "flour, oatmeal, hominy, canned vegetables, potatoes, butter, eggs, sugar, tea and coffee." From the hotel conveniently located nearby, he secured beef, mutton, ham, and pork, "the later two meats for the guide." Local farmers supplied him with eggs, as well as fresh vegetables in season. He proposed elaborate menus for all three meals, including a summer dinner of roast venison or lamb, corn, canned tomatoes, potatoes, squash, beets, frog's legs or game, salad, blueberry pudding, and a cigar to top it all off. The only problem was the quality of the beef in the Adirondacks. "Even at the best of the hotels, the best of their beef would surely be criticized in a fifteen-cent city restaurant. . . . I speak particularly of this matter because of the large dependence which the physicians place upon nourishing beef in the diet of the consumptive patient."[47]

Cook figured that four months' regeneration in the woods could be had for a minimum of $152 for two people—$25 for a canvas tent, $10 for a bark building, $15 for camp equipment (pots, pans, a used stove, crockery, tin pails, forks, knives, baskets, candlesticks and candles, and a canteen, an axe, a saw, a hammer, and a hatchet), and $102 for "food and all necessary expenses." The well-to-do could spend $2,317 with elaborate tents ($100), buildings ($250), equipment ($250), wages for one female and five male

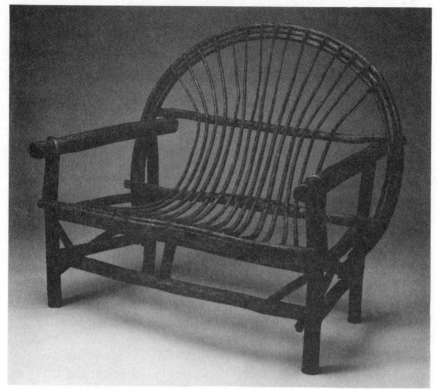

*"Rustic" or "camp" furniture could be found in resorts and camps in
mountain and other vacation areas. Settee, American, spruce, 1900–1940.*

guides, ($1,200) and miscellaneous "running expenses." The cost of travel-
ing from Plattsburg inland ($4.50 per person) and the cost of getting to
Plattsburg from New York, for example (slightly more than $9 in 1877),
were additional. Guides usually cost $2.50 per day, and the services of a
hired man about the camp could cost another $1 per day.[48]

For those who wanted to experience the salubrious effects of cool and
clean mountain or country air but who needed the regular attention of a
physician, camping was an untenable option. They turned instead to
sanitariums such as John Harvey Kellogg's or James C. Jackson's, great
edifices designed for the medicinal treatment of disease. Unlike the resorts

of the era, they were often rigidly run according to the founder's or principal manager's ideology. In most cases, alcohol and tobacco were forbidden, and Kellogg maintained a strict vegetarian diet. They were often closely tied with religious ideologies, and the Battle Creek Sanitarium in particular held to certain aspects of the Seventh-Day Adventist tenets for at least a few years after Kellogg took over from Ellen White in 1876.

James C. Jackson was closely allied with the dominant northern Protestant belief system, which rejected alcohol, dancing (except vigorous daytime

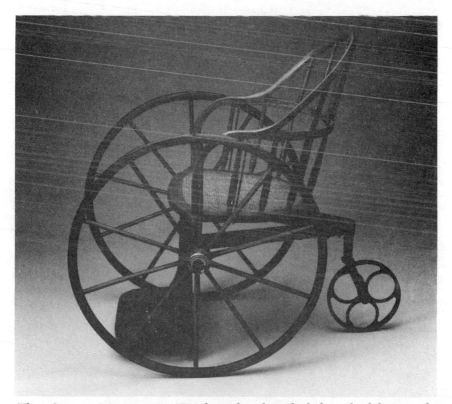

The 1894–95 Montgomery Ward catalog described this wheelchair as the "most popular model." This particular chair belonged to Dr. John Curtis of Richfield Springs, N.Y. An English physician who chose a spa village to practice medicine, Curtis needed the chair because of a stroke he suffered early in life. Wheelchair, New Haven Folding Chair Co., New Haven, Conn. Oak wicker, iron, ca. 1885.

activities for health), and any sort of sexual conduct not oriented to procreation only. Like the resorts, the sanitariums contained the latest in medical-
physiological gear for treating illness, including various baths (since many
developed out of hydrotherapeutic institutions), exercise machines, electrical and magnetic machines, and calisthenic apparatus. Unlike the resorts,
however, medicine and curative work were priorities, and they were usually
staffed with physicians. Entertainment and "vacation" were not usually part
of the package.

   In 1870 Jackson advertised "Our Home on the Hillside" in Dansville,
New York, as "the Largest Hygienic Institution in America," and there is
little evidence to counter his claim. "Our Home" had departed from its
early hydropathy-centered concerns to a more diversified treatment center
that was particularly marketed for consumptives. Jackson also promoted a
series of small health tracts, as well as his *magnum opus,* the four-hundred-

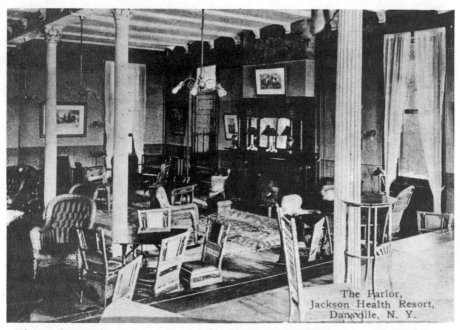

The Parlor,
Jackson Health Resort,
Dansville, N. Y.

*The parlor at the Jackson Health Resort in Dansville, N.Y., was carefully
decorated with warm tones and furniture that was harmonious with
prevailing notions of a healthful environment. Postcard, American, ca.
1910.*

page tome *Consumption: How to Treat It and How to Prevent It* (1862). Priced at $2.50, the book offered the usual litany of social evils and human errors that caused the malady as well as ways to cure it, many of which Cook was to outline nineteen years later in *The Wilderness Cure.* [49]

Jackson's chief competition among the myriad of sanitariums founded after the Civil War was the Battle Creek Sanitarium, built by Ellen White, a "prophetess of health" who saw between five and ten "visions" annually —initially religious experiences that, after 1848, became increasingly health-oriented. She became convinced that a variety of common human habits and consumption patterns must be changed before the Second Coming could occur: Americans had to forgo tobacco, tea, coffee, meat, gluttony, greasy foods, drugs, physicians, corsets, "unnatural" sexual practices, and artificial hair.[50]

A Seventh-Day Adventist, White rejected much of hydrotherapy and sought to establish an institution consistent with her beliefs that would implement her cures. She operated the institute without much success in her first ten years and then appointed a twenty-four-year-old physician—John Harvey Kellogg—to run her medical department. Kellogg had contracted tuberculosis when younger, and in 1866 he converted to vegetarianism after reading Sylvester Graham's works. He studied with Trall at the Hygeia-Therapeutic College in 1872 and took his M.D. at Bellevue in New York City. Kellogg advocated "biologic living," defended vegetarianism, and attacked those who consumed alcohol or who engaged in "sexual misconduct."

Kellogg's impact was immediate. In 1876 only twelve patients visited "the San," as it came to be known, but his aggressive marketing and broad-based regenerative techniques dramatically increased visitation. In 1882 his advertisements boasted that it was "the largest of the kind in the West." By 1890 thousands were coming annually, and Kellogg (whose own vigor and longevity were great promotions for his way of life) ultimately was host to such luminaries as William Howard Taft, John D. Rockefeller, Jr., Alfred duPont, J. C. Penney, Montgomery Ward, and Edgar Welch (of grape juice fame).

The sanitariums of the post–Civil War era were emblematic of the growing rapprochement between "regular" physicians and many of their critics. Many of the vestiges of the rebellion of earlier decades lingered in some of the institutions, such as Kellogg's, but the increasing sophistication of biological and, in particular, microbiological research had led to a renewal of at least a modicum of public faith in physicians. This was especially true for the treatment of the very ill; many of those afflicted with tuberculosis were spared the inevitable early death with which the disease had traditionally been associated because of the treatments that "regular" physicians introduced.

The extended activity of the sanitation movement and its corollary drive for better ventilation also helped return physicians to a central place in the American effort to restore and maintain health. These reformers also benefited from the laboratory work of microbiologists and represented a secular counterpart to the pre–Civil War millennialist efforts to reform individuals and society to ready them for the Second Coming. But this coterie of reformers was of a different cast from their compatriots of decades before. Perhaps the carnage of the war made it clear that the millennium was so far in the future that needs more immediate had to be tended to without concentrating on their cosmic potential. Or perhaps the revelations of the microscope and of medical research turned the gaze of Americans away from the Godhead to a celebration of human potential for solving problems. Religion was not dismissed, but it was defined slightly differently; more was left for the human race to discover.

Still, physicians were not without their detractors in the new age of science. Those who condemned all of the profession—as Sylvester Graham and Charles Grandison Finney had in the 1830s—were fewer in number, but more and more middle-class and wealthy Americans were becoming concerned with what they might do themselves to improve and to maintain their health. These individuals did not need sanitariums, and many gradually accepted the canons of "reform"-style furnishings and architecture as good for human well-being. As primarily urban workers in an expanding bureaucratic economic structure, they began to feel the need to escape from the vicissitudes of the sedentary and tension-producing jobs they held. If they eluded or survived tuberculosis and the other diseases visited upon the population, many still suffered from dyspepsia and "nervous exhaustion," maladies that better ventilation and sanitation might alleviate to some degree but could not prevent. For some of them a new concept in an increasingly sedentary bureaucratic society—the vacation—might be an answer. And they, not the tubercular types, would find the regeneration in the woods and mountains that Reverend Murray extolled in *Adventures in the Wilderness*. At resorts and spas—new institutions created for the health-seeking vacationer—many turned to a newer version of water treatment to relieve their dyspeptic discomforts and their nettled nerves.

CHAPTER SIX

THE NEW "AMERICAN NERVOUSNESS"

Exhaustion of the brain and nervous system," as an advertisement for the Strong Remedial Institute of Saratoga Springs, New York, called it, was a newly identified but pervasive disease of the expanding class of bureaucrats and professionals in post–Civil War America. Physicians and some lay analysts of the three decades prior to the war had pointed to it as a malady with which to reckon. Edward Hitchcock had identified the problem, albeit in a general way, in 1830, and Dr. Charles Caldwell worried about the "commotion" of American politics and religion in 1834. In 1844 hydropathist Joel Shew maintained that "all diseases have exhausted nervous influence as their cause," and physiologist Augustus Georgii cited several cases of "nervous debility" in his book of 1853. But nervousness—or, as it came to be known, "neurasthenia"—became a problem better defined and more attended to as the nation became more urbanized and more men and women became subject to the pressures of office work and the increasing domestic and social pressures of middle-class life.

Neurasthenia was first identified as a result of "over brain-work in business, literary or professional pursuits." Its symptoms were "sleeplessness, despondency, anxiety, weariness, nervousness, debility, neuralgia, and pain in the head, back, or groins."[1] As early as 1830 "nervousness" was characterized by Hitchcock as a particular problem for men of a literary persuasion. In 1860 a brief article in *Godey's* commented on "the hurry of the country" and the "excitement of life" as being "too stimulating to the brain and nervous powers; [and that] the constant speculation, projecting, and inventing wear out man much faster than the severest physical toil." Dio Lewis, in the introduction to his path-breaking *New Gymnastics* (1862), similarly commented that the "American people" were singularly afflicted with "imperfect growth, pale faces, distorted forms and painful nervousness." Lewis's litany of decline was seconded by a variety of patent medicine hucksters, including one advertiser in the *Harper's Weekly* who attributed "the broken down and shattered constitution" of American males to the *"wear and tear* of business life, which makes such tremendous drafts on the body and mind."[2]

The great popular and professional theorist of "American nervousness" was New York City neurologist George M. Beard. In *American Nervousness* (1881), he maintained that neurasthenia was a by-product of socioeconomic progress beyond hand and field labor to more advanced societies with high numbers of intellectual or "brain workers." He was careful to distinguish this condition as a malady affecting men in the work force. He thought that women used their brains "little and on trivial matters" and went so far as to assert in 1871 that women's cranial capacity was 90 percent of men's.[3]

Beard undoubtedly drew some of his information and inspiration from several other studies, including George M. Schweig's "Cerebral Exhaustion," published in *The Medical Record* in 1876. Schweig figured that men were more likely to be neurasthenic because they did more "brain work," and that "physicians, lawyers, inventors, etc. furnish proportionately the largest contingent to this class of patients." He identified the major symptoms as a "disinclination for mental labor," and "disturbances of the heart's action, the functions of the stomach, liver, intestinal canal, etc." His opinions were seconded in the popular press. *The Household* asserted in 1880 that "head-workers need more rest than hand-workers" and advised readers that they should get adequate sleep for "recharging with vital force the nerve batteries," terminology Schweig also adopted.[4]

For Beard, neurasthenia was not a negative phenomenon but an indication of the superiority of American and northern European cultures. Roman

Catholic cultures were relatively free from it, as were such "primitive" groups as Afro-American, African, American Indian, Asian, and South American peoples. He alleged that the former were lacking in individualism, intellectual challenge, and social intercourse of the type characteristic of Protestant cultures; he thought other civilizations to be essentially childlike, composed of peoples "who have never matured in the higher ranges of intellect . . . living not from science or ideas, but for the senses and emotions." Beard's condemnation of the "lesser" peoples of the world was accepted by some and rejected by other American intellectuals and by a broader-based group of consumers who came to see the primitive peoples and their mores as somehow richer and more rewarding than the bustle of American business culture. But if the "primitives" were seen as somehow better off for their lack of civilization, their condition was not sufficiently better to impel the middle class to defect from the national ethos of accumulation. Instead, Americans surrounded themselves with goods either made by or copied from the preindustrials even as they participated in the economy of the "brain-worker." The home, resort, vacation cabin, and even sometimes the office (in the case of "American colonial" goods, especially) were so organized and outfitted to suggest a therapeutic antidote to bureaucratic, machine-age culture that was no threat to that environment.[5]

Beard was certain that neurasthenia would be "oftener met with in cities than in the country, [and] is more marked and more frequent at the desk, the pulpit and the counting-room than in the shop or on the farm." Its symptoms included tenderness of the scalp, spine, teeth, and gums, itching, abnormal secretions, flushing, "fidgetiness," palpitating pulse, sensitivity to weather changes, insomnia, dyspepsia, depression, timidity, dry skin, writer's cramp, chills, heat flashes, sweaty hands, deficient thirst, spermatorrhea, dilated pupils, yawning, hopelessness, and headaches. In short, just about any symptom might be an indication of neurasthenia.[6] How convenient a disease it was! Since "brain workers" allegedly had to endure more anxiety and stress than the laborers who were fortunate enough to work in the coal or other mines or in the cozy heat of the steel or textile mill, brain workers ought not only to be paid more, but the state and manufacturers could guiltlessly forbid combinations of workers who sought shorter hours, shorter weeks, and safer working conditions. It was as much an ideology as an illness—an indication of urban middle-class and wealthy arrogance and status aspiration while at the same time an expression of hostility toward the working class and farm.

But what of the middle-class women who increasingly complained (or who kept silent) about their "nerves"? Most of them, like Almira Mac-Donald, stayed at home and raised a family, while her husband, Angus, worked as a lawyer—one of those "brain-work" professions. In January 1875 she called herself "nervous—not irritably nervous, but the weak condition of the lower part of the spine and other lower parts produces suffering enough to make [me] more nervous, exhausting the system." She was certain she had "*no* organic disease," but was "sensitive." Her lungs were strong, but her blood was too thin. She figured that her "chest needs expansion" and that she "must eat much."[7]

Beard would have seen MacDonald's condition not as neurasthenia, nor as nervous exhaustion wrought from an occupation that made demands upon the brain, but as a manifestation of her debilitated urban condition. "Nervousness" in women in the home was far from a positive cultural attribute. It indicated, as Doctor Moses T. Runnels asserted in 1886, that women had fallen behind in the evolutionary development of the human race, and that they were being outstripped biologically by the growing numbers of nonneurasthenic immigrant and working-class women, who were more vigorous.[8]

"Nervousness" and "neurasthenia" ultimately gained at least as much attention as any other malady of this period. Elixirs, nostrums, and "tonics" continued to be popular home remedies, and it is possible that many men and women felt better with their forty- or fifty-proof "medicines." But for those with the money and the will, one of the most popular "cures" was that offered by the hydropathists. "For general nervous irritability or nervousness," wrote Kellogg in *The Uses of Water in Health and Disease* (1876), "the *warm* full bath may be applied with uniform success."[9]

Two forms of water-related therapy lingered on after the Civil War. Hydropathy, in much the same form as it was in the 1850s, continued through the war but began to decline by the 1870s. "Taking the waters," or bathing in and drinking various mineral waters, replaced hydropathy as a means of increasing or maintaining health. Baths and spas were marketed as cures for many of the diseases with which hydropathists had contended, but as business ventures they were most successful as therapeutic centers for the wearied neurasthenic businessmen and women who used them as respites from the stress of their lives. The new disease brought forth a new type of cure. Drinking mineral waters by the middle class and the wealthy —the poor could not afford such luxuries—was one of the chief ways Americans treated dyspepsia and "auto-intoxication," a problem that was, by 1890, a part of most discussions of American health. In 1862 more than seventy water-cure establishments were in operation in the United States; over half had disappeared by 1874. The ill patient seeking the water cure could find it almost anywhere—in, for example, New York City, Saratoga Springs, Peoria, Iowa City, Sacramento and San Francisco, and Saint Anthony Falls, Minnesota.

The Remedial Institute of Doctors Sylvester S. Strong and Sylvester E. Strong, located in Saratoga Springs, New York, was a vital hydropathic institute that lasted well into the latter decades of the nineteenth century. Situated in an area with mineral springs of great renown and adjacent to the Adirondack Mountains, the institute enjoyed an active business from its first days in 1855. Like nearly every other legitimate institution and quack patent-medicine huckster, the Strongs maintained that their primary focus was "the diseases of WOMEN," yet they were careful to include overworked professional men among the populations they could help. The proprietors were careful not to offend their brothers and sisters in the field who had continued to prescribe medicinal cures, but for those exceptional cases "discouraged with long and fruitless use of medicines only," the Strongs offered their institutional cure.[10]

The institute's treatments were varied, in keeping with the most avant-garde treatments available. They advertised "in addition to the ordinary medical and surgical agencies, Turkish, Russian, Electro-Thermal, and Sulphur-Air Baths, Hydropathy, Equalizer or Vacuum-Treatment, Movement Cure, Oxygen, Inhalations, Calisthenics, etc." The four-story facility was described as "elegant in all its appliances and appointments," with "running water and water closets on all the floors." These amenities were supplemented by "an organ, pianos, and various means of entertainment"— comforts that perhaps more than any other reason, enabled the Remedial Institute to survive. Because they diversified beyond the rigid regimen of ideologically pure, quasi-religious, and narrow commitments to stern virtue, the Strongs were able to attract the increasing numbers of the middle and wealthy classes who sought health unencumbered by total spiritual regeneration or the millennial fervor of other hydropathy institutions. The Strongs served meat at their "tempting" tables, arguing that "the sick, much more than the well, need nutritious animal and vegetable food." Treatment there meant being well treated, in a manner that people with leisure had come to expect. In fact, the Strongs made a point of stressing that "not only invalids but persons of wealth and leisure" lived in the Saratoga area, summer and winter.[11]

In the extensive list of diseases successfully treated at the institute, the most space was devoted to "diseases of the chest." Stating that "the quiver of death has no arrow so deadly as Consumption," they described both the symptoms and the progress of the disease, assigning its infection to "an enfeebled state of the system, or a vitiated condition of the blood." They warned that most patients visited the sanitariums or health institutes when it was too late and the disease had entered its incurable stage. Since they thought consumption began in the same way and manifested the same symptoms as lesser, more easily cured diseases, such as colds and bronchitis, early treatment seemed the only "guarantee" of recovery. But the "early treatment" of tuberculosis may have alleviated those other, lesser diseases, thus resulting in a much higher percentage of "cures" for tuberculosis than actually occurred. Given their assumption that colds and other pulmonary maladies were directly linked to consumption, however, the physicians and institutional healers were probably sincere in their proclamations of cure ratios.[12]

The Strongs promised to cure what were by 1870 the usual list of "diseases of women," including "irritation of the nervous system." Without treatment, the Strongs warned, "its victims are made unhappy, domestic life embittered, [and] years of suffering endured," relieved only by "premature death."[13]

"Chronic diseases" afflicting primarily or exclusively men were also detailed, with special emphasis reserved for spermatorrhea ("seminal weakness which exhausts the nervous system") and brain exhaustion. Like other litanies of common maladies, the Strongs' combined painful physical symptoms ("limb injuries") with character traits ("melancholy," "inclination to solitude"), demonstrating the tendency of medical and popular scientific thought to blend together physical, social, and mental processes as well as the theoretical construct that linked overall male energy and behavior patterns to the genital region.[14]

Going to a water cure was a dramatic and expensive step, and often middle-class people went only when their condition had become too serious or too complicated for local physicians to treat. Elida Works, the twenty-six-year-old wife of a professor of mathematics and natural science at the Fort

Edward, New York, Institute, suffered from a "bad cough" for a few years and had been feeling generally weakened. Finally in 1868, at her husband's urging, she boarded a train and by herself traveled through Rochester to the Castile Water Cure.

The institution, like the Strongs', combined the latest technologies with a consistent—if not radical—philosophy of health reform. Medical electricity in the form of the "Battery"—probably a large galvanic cell from which patients received mild doses of electric current—was combined with a primarily fruit, vegetable, and cereal diet (with some meat), gymnastics, fasting, Bible study, and lectures on dress reform. Entertainment and music do not appear to have been offered, as they were at the Strongs' Remedial Institute, but the Castile treatment program was so popular that Works had to rent a room in the nearby village. Her physical examination revealed that "it is not owing to one thing but several things that causes my trouble." She suffered from "female weakness," but "not much displacement of the womb." Her examining physician, a Miss Green, also diagnosed an "enlarged liver," which she discovered in the course of administering a thorough "pinching-thumping." To make matters worse, Works was told she "was dyspeptic too."[15]

Treatment at the Castile Water Cure cost $8.25 for one week—$4 for the treatments, $0.75 for a room, and $3.50 for board. Her six-week stay cost $49.50, plus rail fare. Since even skilled workers usually made less than $1.50 for one day's work, this was a treatment reserved for the middle and wealthy classes. For her seventy-five cents, Works got a little eight-by-ten bedroom, in which she was "thoroughly homesick" and full of guilt and remorse about her condition.[16]

Works began her treatment on July 24—"my initiation day," she wrote. "Breakfast at seven. We had Graham bread (*very nice, you* would love it, I know). Butter, Baked Potatoes and Raspberries (red and black). Tea and coffee," she remarked, "are not to be seen here, much less drunk, and they [the patients] are not allowed to drink water during eating and not within an hour after." Midday dinner included meat, potatoes, vegetable, and dessert, with a lighter evening supper. The dietary regimen avoided the "stimulation" of too much meat and the dyspepsia-producing fried foods of which Americans were so fond. Vegetables and fruits were clearly important at Castile, and butter was allowed, but such stimulants as tea, coffee, and condiments were not. The meal pattern was constant, with slight variation in specific vegetables or meats.

After breakfast Works took her first cold bath. "I undressed," she wrote, "then Nettie my Bath girl poured some cold water over my head. Then she took a tub of water at 70°, a coarse towel and went over me from head to foot, then a dry towel and rubbed me until I was dry, then she rubbed me with her hands until I was all *aglow.*" At three P.M. Works took "what they call a "Sit [sitz] Bath." After completely disrobing, she described sitting "in a large bath tub half full of water at 82° for 12 min. . . . As I sat down, they covered me with a flannel blanket. I was to rub my limbs and chest what I could while sitting." Nettie gave her "another rubbing," and the whole experience left her feeling "weak and tired," though, she admitted, that "I rather enjoy it."

Miss Green referred to Work's condition as a "scrofulous affection of the stomach and liver," an affliction roughly equivalent to an enlarged and ulcerated condition of one or both organs that Green attributed to her dress. "Do you know what Miss Green says about *corsets?,*" she asked Adam. "She says I must get some Water Cure Waists made as soon as possible. You would laugh to see the style. Every garment of underclothing, even to drawers must be buttoned to this waist, so as nothing shall hang on the *hips* but from the *shoulders.*"

On July 29, Works began to have a fifteen-minute morning "sweating bath." That evening she wrote her husband that she "was stripped naked . . . then a thick quilt was spread over a chair, over that a flannel blanket. Then I sat down and they were wrapped closely around me. Then a tub of water 114° in which I placed my feet. I thought certainly the skin would peel off when they came to be rubbed." She was made to drink cold water, and the perspiration "ran in streams down my body." After removal and another rubbing, "I did not cease perspiring for 1 1/2 hours."[17] The hot sweating bath "makes me feel rather slimey," she wrote her husband, but "Miss Green says that is to draw the poison from my system."[18]

By July 31, with five weeks to go. Works began to plan her return home. Green told her she needed to stay for as long as two years and, since she was unwilling to do so, advised her to stay "long enough to get well acquainted with the manner of treatment . . . and then go home and treat myself. Then . . . she wants me to get the *Vermont Spring* water and make very thorough use of it."

By August 4, Works was on the second day of a three-day fast, during which she was allowed to drink only "Sulphur Water." The baths continued —sweating in the morning, sitz bath and "hot forment" in the afternoon, "what she [Green] calls 'heavy treatment.' " Works felt "thoroughly wilted" but was comforted by Green's assertion that it was "the natural result of getting my system stirred up." After her fast Green put Works on a "bread and fruit diet—just Graham bread and fruit—*no butter . . .* she says Graham bread, fruit, and vegetables should be my principle [*sic*] food for the next year." By August 24, one month after she had entered the Castile Water Cure, she wrote, "I am a thorough convert to the Water Cure style of diet. Have not tasted any *pepper* for four weeks and three days."[19]

Works left Castile after six weeks and apparently maintained much of the regimen. In October 1868 Adam Works noted in his diary that "Elida's second box of Vermont Spring Water" arrived, and in January of the following year her mother-in-law worried about her "bread and fruit" diet. Elida Works died in 1869.[20]

Many of the large hydropathic institutes had complex machines and appliances to treat patients. Based on the assumption that apparently localized maladies were the result of constricted capillaries, "the Equalizer" was a set of airtight devices that encased various limbs or the entire body of a patient and reduced the atmospheric pressure around the afflicted part of the body by means of a crank-driven piston. By reducing the pressure in one area, the capillaries were thought to enlarge and thus to deliver sufficient blood to that area.

The "Electro-Thermal Bath" (also called the galvanic or faradic bath) was still in common usage in the 1870s, essentially unchanged from its form of the 1850s: the patient was treated with small amounts of electric current while reclining in warm water. Like the equalizer or vacuum treatment, it was intended for "nervous debility or exhaustion" and was billed as "a marked restorative to professional or business men, who are broken down by over-work."[21] The sulphur bath was employed for its allegedly therapeutic effects on the skin, since "the value of sulphur, as a remedial agent in many diseases, is so generally appreciated that . . . but a few words" were thought necessary to explain it.[22]

More familiar were the Russian (steam) and Turkish (hot air) baths offered by hydropathy institutions and by the growing number of pay-as-you-go urban bathhouses all over the country. Miller's Turkish Baths of West Twenty-sixth Street in New York were advertised as "refreshing, rejuvinating [*sic*], recuperative, a necessity and a luxury." Turkish and Russian baths were common all over Boston by 1870, as the business directory for that city demonstrates. In Rochester in the 1880s, Almira MacDonald frequently

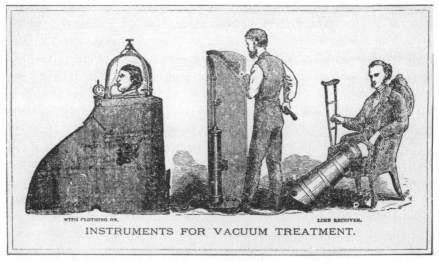

WITH CLOTHING ON.   LIMB RECEIVER.

INSTRUMENTS FOR VACUUM TREATMENT.

These vacuum treatments allegedly aided in the removal of infection to the skin, where water could alleviate the problem. Illustration from "Dr. Strong's Remedial Institute," advertising pamphlet, Saratoga Springs, N.Y., ca. 1875.

visited "Mrs. Dr. Clinton's for a steam bath" and "Mrs. Greenleaf's room [where I] . . . took a vapor bath." She continued visiting Greenleaf for twenty years.[23]

According to the Strongs, the Russian bath required three rooms. The first was the steam room, where bathers sweated profusely; then they proceeded to a general shampooing and rinsing room, and finally to a cooling room, where bathers might rest, sleep, and finally reclothe themselves. In more elaborate Turkish baths, bathers changed from street clothes to bathing clothes in a dressing room, proceeded to the "Tepidarium or warm-room, where the temperature is from 115° to 130°," and remained there "until gentle perspiration starts." They then went into the "hot-room," or Caledarium, which was kept at 140° to 175°. Bathers then left the heat of the Caledarium for the shampooing room, where a masseur or masseuse shampooed and massaged them. The final step was a shower or plunge bath, after which bathers undoubtedly felt clean and refreshed.[24]

Health-seekers might also partake of related health activities—the "Swedish Movement Cure," "vibrators, and other instruments," "Medicated Inhalations" using inhalators made of glass or ceramic ware, "Compressed Air Baths"; "the Health Lift," a stationary weight-lifting device; and "Therapeutical Electricity," or small shocks of electric current. Rates at the Strongs' establishment in 1875 were twelve to twenty dollars per week between July 1 and September 15, with "reduced prices [for] . . . clergymen, physicians, and their families." Examinations, which the doctors urged all

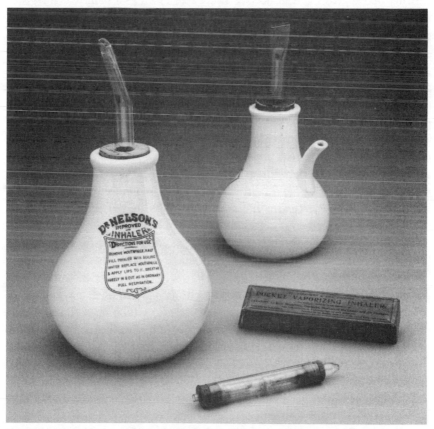

Used both at home and in hospitals and sanitariums, inhalers used hot or boiling water (in the case of the ceramic pieces) or chemical distillates to relieve congestion. Clockwise from left: Inhalers, England, transfer-printed earthenware and glass, ca. 1880; pocket inhaler, Donaldson and Co., Philadelphia, Pa., glass, paper, cork, rubber, ca. 1880.

to have, cost another ten dollars. Prices went up after September 15, since the autumn was evidently the most popular time to take the cures.[25]

John Harvey Kellogg's *The Uses of Water in Health and Disease* (1876) outlined the late-nineteenth-century conception of the water cure's place in contemporary medical cures. Unlike his predecessors of a quarter of a century before, Kellogg did not see the water cures as a panacea; the great benefits of external water application included the cleansing action of the baths. Where Trall and Shew had assumed that internal disorders could be and were "drawn out" or otherwise manifested on the skin, Kellogg based his philosophy on his knowledge of the utility of perspiration as a flushing agent for the pores, which he called "minute sewers." By drinking great quantities of pure (not mineral) waters, Kellogg maintained, the body was rid of poisons.[26]

Kellogg tried to convince the public that water alone was superior to drugs, calling it a better "sedative, tonic, anti-spasmodic, laxative, and astringent," among other things.[27] "Heroic" water treatments—such as diving into frozen lakes and cold baths on cold days in cold rooms—were also criticized. These treatments shocked the system so much that they might ultimately lead to the very debility people were trying to avoid. He was especially vitriolic about the water-curists' notion that patients had to endure "a crisis" before they could be freed of their malady, a theory that he believed indicated ignorance of the body's vital functions and of contemporary medical science, which had moved away from such notions. "No account was then taken of the immense waste of vital energy during these painful morbid processes," Kellogg asserted, and he attempted to shame his readers by comparing the effects of "the crisis" to a "condition similar to that produced by the old process of depletion by bleeding, antimony, mercury, and purgatives."[28]

Kellogg's assumptions about bodily energy and the human constitution were significantly different from those of physicians of the pre–Civil War era. They had feared overstimulation of the body—from bad diet, alcohol, nervousness, or other causes—and had sought to relieve the "pressure" by draining the body through bleeding, blisters, and minerals. But by the 1870s that physiological theory was being challenged, and it was ultimately replaced by the notion that the body had a limited amount of energy, which could be dissipated by "bad habits," sexual release, sedentary work, and "brain-work" and that Americans of especially English and northern European origins were most susceptible to this loss of vitality. Though horrified that patent-medicine hucksters had seized the idea of a limited amount of energy that was dissipating, postwar physicians and health reformers nonetheless also sought to preserve and rejuvenate patients, not to drain energy away from them. For the general public, the cries of the tonic and elixir maker made even more sense in this framework; if energy was depleted, then why not build it up with a tonic?

While Kellogg was a purist about water as a therapeutic device, many middle-class Americans were not. The post–Civil War era was witness to the growth of another form of health-related use of water—the spa or resort, marketed as both a haven for the health-seeker and as a vacation. Less regimented and dogmatic than sanitariums and water cures, they were often staffed in part by physicians, and they stressed the enjoyment and recreation offered by both drinking and bathing in their waters. They were often located near natural hot or mineral springs, and eventually formed the core around which the late-nineteenth-century American's fascination with water revolved.[29]

Europeans first rediscovered the relaxing effects of hot bathing in the eighteenth century and developed a minor subculture of devotees to mineral baths, which were thought simultaneously to cleanse the skin and to provide vital minerals that could be absorbed through the skin into the body. Americans with enough money and faith in the waters' healing powers, or with little faith in treatments they had been receiving, visited Europe—especially Germany, where they encountered the springs, or *Bads*. In 1880 Julia Felton (1842–1884) traveled to Germany, noting in her diary that "one can find a new path every day, either leading to some mountain lake, or 'Bad,' where people crowd to bathe in the waters."[30] In the United States, the sulphur and other mineral and hot springs that were scattered all over the country were quickly developed by enterprising health reformers and other businessmen into new and exclusive resorts, aimed not only at the increasing number of middle-class Americans who had aspirations to be fashionable (and the leisure time and money to go on a vacation) but also at the growing concern for health and vitality in an urban, "nervous" country.

By 1877, there were so many spas that D. Appleton and Company,

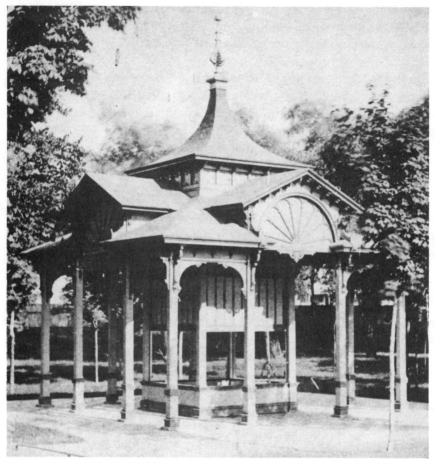

Decorative structures like this spring house were often built over places where the spring was tapped and served as advertisements for the waters sold commercially. "Pavilion Spring," stereograph, American, ca. 1885.

publisher of "railroad guides" detailing the American railway system, issued in 1877 *Appleton's Illustrated Hand-Book of American Winter Resorts for Tourists and Invalids.* In addition to a "Table of Railway Fares" from New York to points of departure for nearly every resort in the nation, the book contained a brief description of major and minor resorts in each state. Belying the American concern for consumption as a major health threat, the editor aimed "to furnish invalids and physicians with *all* the facts as to climatic and local conditions necessary to enable them to choose a resort intelligently and confidently." The book described resorts from Bermuda and Florida to California and the Sandwich Islands (Hawaii), as well as in more well known areas, such as the Adirondacks and the White Mountains.[31] The entries were elaborately detailed; Green Cove Springs, Florida, was described as "one of the most frequented resorts. . . . The spring discharges about 3,000 gallons a minute and fills a pool some 30 feet in diameter with greenish-hued crystal clear water. The water has a temperature of 70° Fahr.; contains sulphates of magnesia and lime, chlorides of sodium and iron, and sulphuretted hydrogen; is used both for bathing and drinking; and is considered beneficial for rheumatism, gouty affections, and Bright's disease of the kidneys."[32]

Glen Springs and Limestone Springs were South Carolina's big attractions, and in Arkansas, Hot Springs—where "the entire town, indeed, is simply an appendage to the sanitarium"—was the most important area to obtain the waters' benefits. At Hot Springs waters were taken both internally and externally, and "a great number of bathing houses have been constructed. . . . The *vapor baths* start at 112°; the *douche,* a spirit-bath, at 120°; the *saving bath* at 116°." The nearby creek was warm enough to bathe in during midwinter, owing to discharge from the springs, and the spring waters, "when taken internally . . . have an aperient [laxative] and tonic [invigorating] effect, [and] are rapidly absorbed into the circulatory system." The waters were credited with "wonderful cures of rheumatism, rheumatic gout, stiffness of the joints . . . malarial fevers," but consumptives and others "suffering from pulmonary or throat diseases" were urged to stay away from Hot Springs because "the air is warm and very moist." Other popular hot springs were in Manitou, Colorado; White Sulphur Springs, West Virginia; Las Vegas, Nevada; and Paso Robles, California.[33]

Neurasthenia and other forms of nervous debility were high-status maladies, and the resorts, with their swank accommodations and dining rooms for "the waters," catered to these victims of their own success. Kellogg and Jackson, who died in 1881, would have objected strenuously to the fashionable displays at these institutions, where one might even find alcohol tolerated along with smoking and meat. The resorts were more expensive than workers could afford; in the opinion of Beard and his followers, laborers were not burdened with such problems anyway. The middle and upper-middle classes may have been troubled—or even somewhat smug—about a problem that was exclusively theirs. But in solving it, they were still concerned enough with comfort and status to seek a cure that was pleasing as well as healthy. Recreation—croquet, tennis, bowls, and the like—was important, and that some of these institutions later became exclusive country and golf clubs is not surprising.

A social transformation had occurred. The sanitariums of reformers such as Kellogg—whose ideology was faithfully and elaborately realized in his Battle Creek institution—would endure, but only because they were well run, well reputed, and diversified. The hot and mineral springs, which

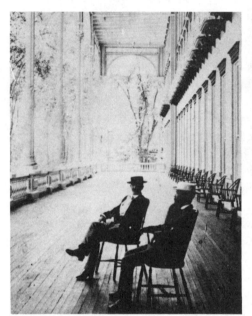 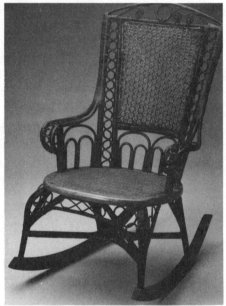

Left: The Grand Union Hotel, one of the most famous of the grand Saratoga Springs hotels. On verandas such as this, vacationers and health seekers enjoyed the country air, in this case in appropriately virtuous Windsor chairs like that of the nation's allegedly healthy founding fathers and mothers. Stereograph, Charles Bierstadt, Niagara Falls, N.Y., ca. 1885.

Right: Inexpensive and lightweight, wicker furniture was also the favorite of reformers because, since it was not upholstered, it could be washed easily. Rocking chair, American wicker and maple, ca. 1880.

functioned as vacation spots and play areas, were, by contrast, popular with middle-class and wealthy Americans with no particular committment to reform. Saratoga, with its gambling, horse racing, hotels, and springs, was perhaps the best example of the genre. For the purists, the spas were centers of sin and scandal, the antithesis of "rational" hydropathy and health. But for many middle-class Americans, they were a comfortable compromise, with just enough health-related content to assuage any possible guilt about the costs of rising social status. The completely prostrate needed the help of physicians, and everyone knew it. But the vaguely uncomfortable, occasionally dyspeptic, and somewhat tired or "fagged" businessman or his

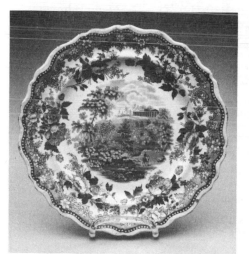 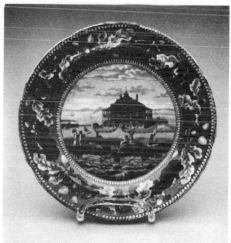

Left: The benefits of mountain air and scenery were the chief attractions of the Catskill Mountain House, which, like the Nahant Hotel, had a national and even international reputation. "View of the Catskill Mountain House, N.Y.," Job and John Jackson, Burslem, Eng., transfer-printed earthenware, 1830–43.

Right: Built in the 1820s, the Nahant Hotel was a famous and popular seaside resort for those who wanted the allegedly salubrious effects of sea air. The wide surrounding verandas functioned as intermediate spaces between seaside and inside. Plate, "Nahant Hotel, Boston," Ralph and William Stevenson, Cobridge, Eng., transfer-printed earthenware, ca. 1830.

spouse needed only a taste of the regimen prescribed for the very ill, and "taking the waters" satisfied that requirement.

For those who could not or would not make the trip to the spa during the "season," and for the fortunate during the rest of the year, the bath and the drink could be brought home. But bathing was troublesome and tiresome in the early nineteenth century; not only was there no indoor plumbing, but wood had to be hauled so that water could be heated. Total-immersion commercial baths were not available for homes, and prevailing middle-class attitudes toward modesty, especially among women but also among men, kept some people away from commercial establishments.

After the Civil War, in part as a response to changing attitudes about personal cleanliness and in part due to the greater accessibility of piped water in the cities, a new industry—bathing appliances—was born and began to flourish. Mass-produced soaps, hot water, and bathtubs became facts of life, as did regular bathing. Catharine Beecher's prewar urgings to keep clean were now seconded by nearly every postwar advice writer in both books and periodicals. Kellogg, for example, argued that clogged pores were a cause of kidney problems, dyspepsia, "rheumatism, gout, hysteria and other nervous problems." Anticipating the more pervasive fears of the turn of the century, he maintained that physical activity produced poisons as nutrients were used and that the most abundant and dangerous toxin was urea, which "must be hurried out of the system with great rapidity."[34]

The solution was a daily bath, "the most agreeable and efficient of all cosmetics." The cosmetic argument responded to widely held notions of feminine beauty in the middle and late nineteenth century. A clear, white, almost translucent skin was prized, and cosmetic and soap manufacturers claimed that their wares could produce such effects, reinforcing the cultural association of beauty with cleanliness. By the middle of the century mass-produced soaps were within easy economic reach of nearly everyone living off the farm, and many farmers or their wives readily forsook the bother of soapmaking as soon as they could.[35]

Still, many Americans were resistant, especially in winter. They were certain bathing produced chills that made one "take cold," a rational fear given the belief that a cold could become bronchitis or consumption. Kellogg argued conversely that baths protected people from colds by invigorating and cleaning out the skin, and he urged families to buy one of the newer

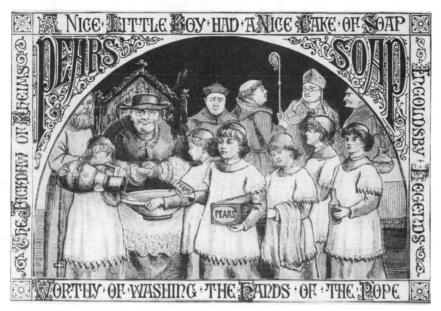

Here, Pears Soap is marketed using the era's enthusiasm for medieval tales. Trade card, American, lithograph, ca. 1900.

scientific gadgets of the day, a microscope, so that they could see for themselves the parasites and dirt clogging the body's flushing systems. In 1871 *Godey's Lady's Book* claimed that in due time "every good housekeeper will think . . . [a microscope] necessary."[36]

Finally, after decades of resistance to their work physicians saw their credibility rise. Pathologists began to link specific diseases with causes, often using evidence gained by the use of microscopy, and antisepsis became an accepted preventive for postoperative infection, thus laying the foundations of modern medical science. Bacteriological investigation was aided immeasurably by improvements in microscopes, and the popularization of knowledge about microorganisms (often called "animalculae") in the press and in books helped convince Americans that they should buy the bathtubs and fixtures to cleanse themselves.

One of the least expensive and most popular early forms of bathing apparatus was the "Universal Bath," which consisted of "a firm, continuous rim of wood, from which is suspended a sack of heavy drilling [heavy, coarse cotton], which is coated with a thoroughly refined and vulcanized rubber compound." The flexible "tub" could be converted into two baths, for children, or a combination sitz (hip) bath and foot bath. Bathers could even have different water temperatures for hips and feet, or mineral waters in one bath and pure water in the other. Since it folded up and weighed only fifteen pounds, it eliminated the need of heavy stationary appliances that cost hundreds of dollars to install and that could not be moved to a sick room when needed. Bathers could use it for the "medicated baths . . . now deemed almost invaluable in scores of ailments," because mineral salts would not corrode the rubber Universal Bath as they would metal tubs. For twenty dollars it seemed a bargain.[37]

For between fifteen and thirty-five dollars, depending on the type of wood and counter surface, Americans could purchase a "portable wash stand," which from the outside looked like a sink set into a cabinet base. In the cabinet below were a small hand-pumped reservoir of water and a large bucket for waste. Patented in the 1870s, portable washstands were marketed as an improvement over the pitcher-and-basin method of washing because they were neater ("no slopping of water over the carpet") and

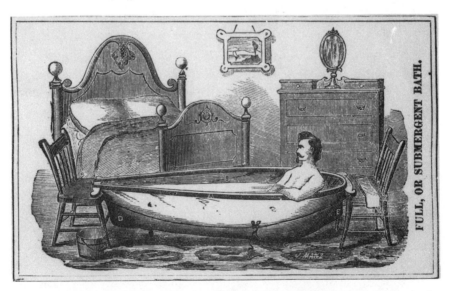

The cheapest possible indoor bathtub was the "Universal," which used rubber and a couple of chairs to provide a portable tub for bedroom or other use. Advertising pamphlet, American, ca. 1870.

more sanitary than plumbed sinks ("no sewer gases in bedrooms"). They also eliminated plumber's bills and could be easily moved to other rooms whenever necessary.[38]

For a little more money (forty-five to sixty dollars), consumers could buy "portable folding bath tubs with instantaneous heaters." When closed, this gadget looked like a tall cabinet; it measured two-and-a-half feet square by six feet high. To open it, the top was pulled down, extending the tub and revealing the heater and reservoir that remained in the vertical section. Convertible furnishings—such as folding tubs, beds, and chairs—were popular in the late nineteenth century and were ideally suited to a culture in which living space was becoming expensive. As more and more people began to live in apartments, portability and collapsibility became important qualities in furnishings.[39]

Among the middle and wealthier classes, permanent, stationary bath tubs and fixtures were more popular than washstands. More expensive to install, they were both a proclamation of status, and a rejection of the outdoor privy. Isolating the bath and the toilet in a room of their own banished these functions from the bedroom (where they were inconvenient, potentially harmful to the furnishings, and productive of noxious scents) and inextricably linked the cleansing of the body's exterior with that of its interior. In the "modern" combination bathroom and toilet room, all waste eventually met in hidden pipes. Clever plumbing manufacturers ignored the potential problems of sewer gas and promoted the stationary tub and separate bathroom as more conducive to health. They shrewdly marketed attachments that could transform humble iron tubs on feet or more elaborate wood-encased metal tubs into the baths found at expensive spas.[40]

Home consumption of mineral waters—the other half of the spa's offering—became popular after the Civil War, when advances in bottling technology coincided with Americans' belief that mineral waters contained chemicals that helped flush the system, and that were missing from public water supplies. The enthusiasm for mineral spring waters was part of a more general American concern for ridding the body of "incipient forms of disease" by easing the burdens of constipation and dyspepsia. As the century drew to a close, other ingredients of mineral waters—alum, strontium, bromides, and lithium—were hailed as curatives for depression, headache, and the tendency to retain potentially harmful uric acid in the system.

"Excelsior" spring water, bottled and sold after the war by A. R. Lawrence and Company of Saratoga, was one of the most famous and popular bottled spring waters. Like so many others, Lawrence and Company advertised widely—in periodicals, trade cards, and pamphlets—with such ploys as testimonials from eminent physicians (including Oliver Wendell Holmes), a chemical analysis, and a diagram of the spring. Excelsior water was sold to stores by the barrel and came with a trade-marked tap. Apothecary shops and general stores viewed the opportunity to offer the various spring waters on draught as a promotional advantage. In 1870 Boston apothecary Charles H. Hovey advertised three varieties of Saratoga Spring Water—"Congress, Empire, and Star"—on draught. Hovey advertised his "cold soda water, with pure fruit extracts" for those who either did not care for the taste of the plain waters or who wished to turn the drink into a confection. Women could now buy some of the more aggressively alcoholic tonics and elixirs by the "dose" and obtain a "mixer" in a socially acceptable way. In the nineteenth century no woman of estimable reputation would go to a saloon, and they were not allowed in men's clubs.[41]

The combination of mild alcohol and mineral waters was also a common retail and marketing strategy. Nearly every urban producer and distributor of mineral waters also dealt in porter, ale, cider, and other malt or hop drinks, all of which were thought to be almost nonalcoholic, and, in the case of malt, healthful. In 1888, Greenaway's India Pale Ale, for example, was advertised as "recommended by our best physicians, for family or club use."[42]

The dominant chemical salt found in nearly all the spring waters was sodium chloride, or common table salt. Usually the concentration of this compound was twice or three times as high as that of calcium or magnesium bicarbonate, the next most prevalent minerals, and ten to one hundred times as much as that of potassium chloride or lithium bicarbonate. Lithium or "lithia" waters were popular in the postwar era because of the compound's allegedly invigorating effect not only on digestion, but also on the nervous condition of the patient. Buffalo Lithia Springs of Mecklenburg County, Virginia, was probably the most famous lithia water of the period, but springs boasting of lithium's effects were located all over the country. Lithium compounds are still used in the treatment of some mental disorders such as manic-depressive reaction, and thus it is possible that claims of treatment for mild depression may have had some basis in fact.[43]

"White Rock Lithia Water," bottled in Waukesha, Wisconsin was a "still," or noneffervescent, water that traded upon long-held fears of unsafe "city" water. It was "pure" and "healthful," the bottler claimed, and especially useful "during the seasons of the year when LOCAL WATER IS UNSAFE TO DRINK, and in localities where the water is unsafe to drink the year 'round." The White Rock Company claimed also that "men of sedentary habits and those who have passed middle age can retain or regain their health more surely through proper elimination than by any other means, and the efficiency of White Rock Water as a solvent for Uric Acid and gravelly accumulations, which are the forerunners of stomach and kidney troubles renders it . . . an INVALUABLE PREVENTIVE OF THESE FATAL MALADIES."[44]

Since quantitative and qualitative analyses of mineral waters were not only possible but were also commonly published, enterprising chemists and entrepreneurs quickly realized that they could produce and sell the waters in a form more convenient than in bottles. Mineral salt mixtures—which consumers could buy and dissolve themselves—were immediate successes in the marketplace. Warner and Company of Chicago, New York, and Philadelphia sold a variety of "granular, effervescent salts of mineral waters" in the 1880s and advertised that "a bottle of these salts represents many bottles of the natural water," since only one teaspoonful of the compound was recommended for each glass of water. Obviously lighter, smaller, and easy to use, the mineral salts were popular and cost between twenty cents and a dollar per bottle.[45]

In addition to the various salts allegedly evaporated from the more famous mineral waters, such as Congress, Vichy, and Kissengen (Bavaria) springs, Warner and other firms offered their own mixtures, such as "Bromo Soda," "Bromo Lithia," and "Seidlitz Mixtures." Sodium bromide was advertised as a way to get "speedy relief of nervous headache and brain fatigue," as well as being "useful in nervous headache, sleeplessness, excessive study, over brainwork, nervous debility, mania, etc." "Bromo Lithia," which contained lithium salicylate and sodium bromide, was advertised as effective "in the treatment of gouty diathesis," a disease linked to uric acid retention. It was the most expensive of the compounds, costing a dollar per bottle.[46]

Much of the strength of the mineral water manufacturers' claims for their products as medicinal agents was borne of their alleged diuretic and cathartic qualities, which promised to "invigorate" the system. This was thought essential because dyspepsia, or chronic indigestion, was so prevalent in the United States. In *The Hygienic Cook Book* (1876), J. H. Kellogg summed up many of his contemporaries' feelings about American dietary patterns in

the postwar period when he termed "modern cookery . . . the greatest bane
of civilization at the present time. . . . men and women are subject to few
diseases whose origin may not be traced to the kitchen." The editors of
Godey's Lady's Book similarly criticized American cookery in 1876, asserting that "the prevalence of dyspepsia among Americans is simply the result
of a century of bad cookery."[47]

Widespread agreement about the breadth of the dyspepsia problem in
the United States was matched by an equally broad disagreement about
solutions to it. The pre–Civil War criticism of spices was carried on by many
analysts, chief among them Kellogg. "Every day a hundred thousand dyspeptics sigh and groan in consequence of condiments." His critique hinged
upon the assumption that these "stimulants" irritated the digestive system
and "clogged the liver." Condiments and spices "poisoned" even the ordinarily healthful foods Americans ate, a category that in Kellogg's opinion

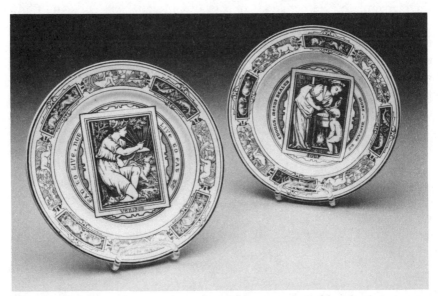

*The moral lesson of overeating was seldom put more bluntly than in
these plates. The mottoes "Eat to Live, not live to eat" and "Enough
means health, more—disease" reflect the increasing concern for excessive
weight that began in the late nineteenth century. Dinner and soup plates,
"The Courses of a Meal," J. Wedgwood, Etruria, Eng., transfer-printed
earthenware, 1878.*

consisted primarily of fruits, vegetables, and grains.[48] He went on to condemn tea, coffee, and any hot liquid at a meal, including soups, stews, and gruels because they introduced too much hot water into the system, stalling the digestion of more solid foods.

This idea had been partly absorbed by household advisors on manners. In the *Bazar-Book of Decorum* (1870), Robert Tomes suggested that readers not "ask twice for soup," arguing that such forbearance was "a very sensible ordinance, justified by the laws of health." This was a critical area of disagreement among dietary advisors during the postwar decades. Tomes maintained that mineral waters and "aperients" would "aid digestion," "cure constipation," and "regulate the liver," as an advertisement for Tarrant's Effervescent Seltzer Aperient claimed in the mid 1880s. Americans who bought Excelsior spring water were advised to drink between one and four glasses and a cup of hot coffee before breakfast "to accelerate [the waters'] cathartic action." Others advocated limiting water intake—especially soups and another popular drink, ice water—based on the assumption that it was absorbed into the bloodstream first and therefore provided no nourishment.[49]

Kellogg's views on condiments and spices were also resisted by the American populace. Recipes commonly called for black or cayenne pepper and sometimes both. Kellogg thought vinegar "more injurious than alcohol" but in "The Art of Preserving Health" in *The Household*, a columnist not only thought vinegar was acceptable but also recommended "black and cayenne pepper . . . [as] a powerful stimulant to the digestive organs, [which] may be taken in smaller quantities to advantage." Kellogg's philosophies did not gain broad acceptance until the turn of the century.[50]

All these "stimulants" had, for their critics, a darker, more dangerous effect than even the discomfiture of dyspepsia: They were thought to create the thirst for alcohol. Nearly all reformers among the middle and well-to-do classes opposed drink, some of them completely, others in immoderate amounts. "No well man," wrote Kellogg, "can habitually use wine, beer, brandy or any other alcoholic drink, without becoming diseased." In the strongly prohibitionist *Demorest's Monthly*, Mrs. E. G. Cook asserted that "it is one of women's rights to help cure intemperance in drinking by removing excitants from the food. By constantly stimulating, in early life, an unnatural appetite for condiments and dainties, the foundation of intemperance is often laid." The struggle against drink was a mighty one throughout the late nineteenth and early twentieth centuries. In 1885 Kellogg was

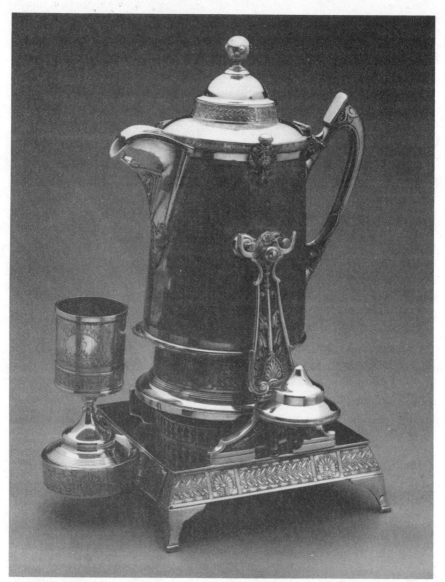

Elaborate ice water pitchers became accessible to the middle class after the Civil War, when silver-plating technology was adopted by silver manufacturers, but many advocates of health reform feared it produced "too much stimulation." Ice water pitcher, Reed and Barton, Taunton, Mass. Silverplate, ironstone, 1881.

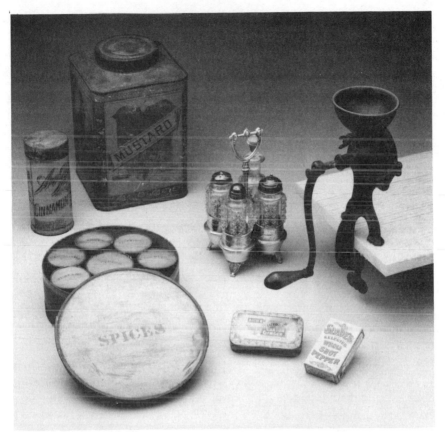

Most Americans used spices in spite of reformers' warnings. Not only did they improve flavors, they also masked the taste of meats that were spoiled. Clockwise, from lower right: spice packages, American paper, sheet metal, wood, ca. 1860–1920; caster set, Aurora Silver Plate Manufacturing Co., Aurora, Ill., pressed glass, silverplate, ca. 1880; spice grinder, Enterprise Manufacturing Co., Philadelphia, Pa., ca. 1910.

named to head the new department of social purity of the most powerful group to oppose drink, the Women's Christian Temperance Union. The "cold water army" of the early nineteenth century had become the "mineral water navy," fighting dyspepsia, drunkenness, and other diseases of the age with its new discovery. Like diet and physical exercise, the temperance movement was ideologically broader than a set of reforms organized to heal or preserve the body; it was a total cultural reformation. It endeavored to end American decline, preserve the family, and hold onto a culture being irrevocably altered by the growth of the city and the changing nature of both immigration and the economy.[51]

Reformers who thought meat eating was the cause of dyspepsia had a difficult time convincing Americans to adopt vegetarianism, yet the undercurrent of support for a meatless diet was still present in the thirty years following the outbreak of the Civil War. Proponents of vegetarianism were up against strong foes. In his experiments of the 1850s and 1860s, biochemist Justus von Leibig (1803–1873) seemed to have proved that eating meat was necessary for strength. He found that carbohydrates and fatty acids were energy producers, and he reaffirmed the belief that high-protein diets were necessary for athletes. Defenders of meat eating like Edwin Temple asserted that "animal food contains no more urinary and fecal matters than vegetable food" since vegetable crops were fertilized. Doctor E. C. Page argued by contrast that flesh eaters got more "colds" and lived shorter lives. The debate continued through the century, and athletes seemed to be the test cases for the competing theories. The famous Yale crew coach, Wilbur Bacon, fed his teams the sort of foods Cook listed and did not allow them to drink any liquids while rowing or at the table. E. G. Cook also recommended "plenty of liquids and fat meat" to those "who have little muscular exercise and much brain-work."[52]

Even the objections raised about slaughterhouses and the purity of their products were not enough to cause Americans to alter their meaty diets. Kellogg ranted about the dangers of pork especially, but it was not until Upton Sinclair's *The Jungle* (1906) that public outcry grew loud enough to galvanize action.[53] The more broadly conceived movement against adulteration of foods that was to culminate in the Pure Food and Drug Act of 1906 had more success in altering middle-class eating habits than did vegetarianism's complaints about unclean meats.

Adulteration of processed foods, rather than the inherent qualities of a particular type of food, was perhaps a greater stimulant to change after the Civil War. Revelations that candy makers were using poisonous paints to color their products and that candies often contained worm larvae caused scandal from 1865 through the turn of the century. Dyspepsia and even death could ensue from eating "worm candy" or "the unseen enemy," as

The Household termed adulterants in 1887. Bakers were similarly suspect. "The introduction of alum in flour . . . has been a trick of the baker for the past one hundred years," the magazine stated, and indifference to this practice "resulted in Americans earning the title of 'a race of dyspeptics.' "[54]

Whole grain, vegetarian, and "health foods" made their greatest inroads among those who selected food for children and among those for whom dyspepsia was so extreme that a meatless diet became imperative. For thirty-six cents, the Our Home Granula Company of Dansville, New York, sent boxes of its goods, "unsurpassed for [relief of] constipation and dyspepsia," anywhere the mail went in 1887. Even *The Household*, a middle-of-the-road magazine for women, published articles praising "health foods." "Even if roast beef be the regulation dinner," the magazine maintained in 1879, "a breakfast of oat flour . . . a cup of cereal coffee and buttered gluten gems . . . would be easily prepared and easily digested, leaving behind no weariness and no nausea."[55]

Vegetarians ran counter to four formidable arguments in their effort to eradicate meat from the American diet. First, most of the nation's increasingly respected professional physicians were opposed to it. Like Dr. Hanaford in *The Household*, most doctors recommended "lean meats, fish, and eggs" and a mixed diet, reduced in butter and sugar.[56]

Second, many biologists countered the evolutionist argument that humans, like other primates, should be herbivores by asserting that the broadened diet of the human race signified its elevation above the apes. As George Beard put it in *Eating and Drinking: A Popular Manual of Food and Diet in Health and Disease* (1871), "The gulf that separates Shakespeare and Newton from the Papuan is wider than that which separates the Papuan from the gorilla and the chimpanzee; and therefore it is easier for the lowest order of human beings to live after the manner of the apes than for the highest order of humanity to live after the manner of the savages." Like neurasthenia, meat eating could be identified with human progress and racial nationalism.[57]

The third obstacle in the vegetarians' path was that more and more Americans believed that the decline in national health was best halted by increasing physical activity and sport, and that athletes needed meat for their rigorous training regimen. Athletics, amateur and professional, became a popular pastime of the middle and wealthy classes after 1860, and "training" and "training tables" were sources of great interest and debate, prompting exchanges in popular as well as professional literature. Wilbur Bacon's low water-lean meat table drew fire in *Harper's Weekly,* for example, where a columnist compared the body to an engine and attacked the "dry meat diet" of "many trainers, on the supposition that it makes the flesh firm, and keeps the blood from being watery." Not until vegetarian athletes began to triumph in large-scale competitions at the turn of the century would even the smallest crack appear in the fortress held by proponents of meat eating for athletes.[58]

Finally, the powerful physiological arguments that dyspepsia was "a disease entirely of the brain and nervous system, in which the stomach only sympathizes . . . [and that] overwork of the brain . . . is a leading cause of the disease" weakened the vegetarians' case for their cure. In "Hints to Dyspeptics," published in *The Household* in 1881, the link between neurasthenia and dyspepsia was presented with a convincing and even comforting lucidity. Building upon Beard's earlier association of advanced Western civilization with meat eating, the argument seemed to void any claims of vegetarianism as the cure for dyspepsia. In fact, as their promoters were quick to maintain, mineral waters cured both dyspepsia and neurasthenia.[59]

Mineral waters, vegetarianism, water cures, patent medicines, and the baths all failed as panaceas for the ailments—nervousness, weakness, biliousness, dyspepsia, and colds—of such families as the MacDonalds. Perhaps they and other Americans were eclectic in their choice of treatment methods because they were frustrated. Physician's prescriptions worked at some times and not at others, and many Americans were still skeptical of the physicians' craft. So on May 14, 1877, Almira MacDonald "rode down town . . . and called at Dr. Whittaker. He gave me a prescription to strengthen, but feel anxious to try magnetic treatment for [my] head, as I have suffered so long and tried medicine prescribed." Faced with no sure cure, she turned to another of the era's great new discoveries for healing and health—electricity.[60]

CHAPTER SEVEN

ELECTRICITY, ENERGY, AND VITALITY

Almira MacDonald evidently suffered intermittently from severe headaches from the mid 1870s until the end of the century. On April 16, 1877, she "arose with a severe headache and was obliged to lay down." Powders and poultices must not have relieved her because she "went to Mrs. Greenleaf and she gave me electricity twice today." The next afternoon her physician came to see her and left "powders for every three hours." Nothing seemed to help. On the eighteenth she was "yet with fearful head trouble," so she "went over today for electricity." Still in pain a week later, she took some traditional medicines: on April 27 "Doctor ordered blistering for the back of [my] head, as there is irritation of the spine."[1]

MacDonald had learned, perhaps for the first time, about the use of electricity in the treatment of disease in 1875, when she had attended "a lecture by Mrs. French" on the subject. An itinerant speaker on health and hygiene, French was extremely popular, and discussed, among other topics, how to arise in the morning, how to bathe, how to rid oneself of "whites" (leukorrhea), and how to stimulate breast milk when pregnant. Greenleaf was a neighbor of Mac-Donald and was listed as a "medical electrician" in the 1880 *City Directory* for Rochester, New York. With Mrs. M. S. Sanford, Greenleaf ran a medicated bath and electrical practice there for at least twenty-five years, and, as was the case with many other women medical electricians, her patients were primarily, and perhaps exclusively, women. MacDonald was a faithful customer, taking a "vapor bath" and "electricity" in July, 1880; during a five-week period in July and August, she "took electricity" every day except on Sundays. Twenty years later, in 1900, she was still going to Greenleaf.[2]

Popular enthusiasm for medical electricity blossomed after the Civil War for three reasons. First, more traditional "heroic" physicians were unable to counter the public tide of disbelief and anger with their methods, in part because of the continuing rancor within their own profession. Homeopathic and, to a lesser extent, botanic physicians continued to thrive in the late nineteenth century, and a public intoxicated by new scientific discoveries interpreted the profession's internal disagreement as weakness. Second, the new diseases of the era—in particular neurasthenia—seemed particularly unresponsive to traditional treatments. Third, the small coterie of informed and semi-informed scientists of the pre–Civil War era who thought the human body electrical or magnetic in nature became much larger as chemists, physicists, and biologists unraveled the mystery of electricity.

Many thought electricity and electromagnetism were, like magnetism, somewhat magical forces. Even if they could not be seen, they were present, able to penetrate some of the densest materials (such as iron) through which light could not pass. Moreover, these were natural forces of great power, as anyone in a thunderstorm could attest. As they learned of Galvani's experimentation with the muscles and nerves of frogs, more and more physicians and patients accepted the identity of electricity and nervous energy or force. "All disease," W. R. Wells asserted in *A New Theory of Disease* (1869), had "but one grand cause . . . a loss of balance of the two forces of electricity in the part or part diseased." Wells termed the brain "the great electrical reservoir of the physical system" that "furnishes electricity to it." He speculated that the body was a huge compound magnet, with venous blood negative and arterial blood positively charged. Healthy lungs he determined to be positive, repelling arterial blood and attracting blood from the veins. Critical of physicians who "prescribe their gross, ponderable drugs to cure," Wells argued that by applying electrical energy to those parts of the body diagnosed as out of balance, equilibrium and health could be restored. He thought that nerves, not the blood, were the transmitters of health or disease, because they carried "electro-nervous fluid or electricity."[3]

The electrotherapeutic theory seemed to explain not only the origin and treatment of disease, but also the universe, or at least its physical phenomena. It also seemed up-to-date and "scientific" because it employed machines and measurement in an apparently rigorous fashion. As new as it seemed, the electrotherapeutic theory of the postwar era was a derivative of earlier ideas. The magnetic poles Henry Hall Sherwood had identified in *A Manual for Magnetizing* in 1845 were nearly identical to the "grand positive polar centres" (brain, heart, and lungs) that Emma Harding Britten described thirty years later in *The Electric Physician: or Self-Cure Through Electricity* (1875).[4]

Electricity also offered hope that the apparent trend of declining vitality could be reversed. There was a comforting and ancient symmetry to the idea that the body was in a state of equilibrium when healthy, and a self-assured, modern logic to the theory that a man-made machine could correct the body's imbalance and replenish the store of energy depleted by the rigors of a new age. It also seemed to make comprehensible the functions of the brain and nerves, whose actions, like those of electricity itself, were imperceptible. Electricity offered solutions to problems that previous generations had often thought inscrutable. Cholera's visitations, for example, could be explained as "the rapid passage of electricity from the human frame"; and as the "peculiarity of the atmosphere, known to exist during cholera" rather than as divine punishment.[5] But electricity was no threat to religion; rather than offering new explanations for the beginnings of life, it further revealed the order and balance of the world, thus paying homage to the wonders of Creation and the Divine Hand.

The electrical treatment MacDonald received was probably very much like that described by Emma Britten in *The Electric Physician*. Britten and her husband ran an electromedical facility in Brookline, Massachusetts. Treatments were relatively expensive—three dollars for examinations, five dollars for house calls, and three dollars for an "electric vapor bath and treatment."[6]

For a "sick headache" such as MacDonald's, Britten advised home electricians to "apply a [metal] plate, (*positive*), across the loins, and another, (*negative*), across the abdomen, [for] five minutes, then remove the back plate up between the shoulders lengthways . . . and the front across the diaphragm . . . [for] five minutes. Then apply the plate to the nape of the neck . . . and place the feet in a metal foot-tub with about an inch in depth of hot salt and water; into this drop the tin electrode . . . and keep adding hot water to keep up the temperature for ten minutes." The whole apparatus—brass plates, electrodes, and the various cups and sponges of the typical medical electrical kit—would have been wired to a large wet cell. The current was always supposed to be "light," especially in the beginning of treatment, and a "seance" of treatment was not to exceed twenty to thirty minutes, lest the patient be "liable to reactionary fatigue, weariness, and pain."[7]

Like many other authors of medical-electrical books, Britten offered not only advice and testimony for the wonders of electricity but also a chance for readers to buy their own therapeutic device. Advertisements in the back of the book promised to cure "every disease that is curable"; enterprising individuals could purchase the "Home Battery," for twelve dollars (the "extra size and strength model" cost three dollars more). "By the trifling outlay of twelve dollars, together with Mrs. E. H. Britten's admirable Guide to 'Self Cure by Electricity,' any family can possess themselves of an universal and unfailing source of health, and forever dispense with drugs and medical attendance." Additional gear available with the basic battery included a set of five metal plates for three dollars, a sponge-cup and sponge for one dollar, and "eye-cup, ear, throat, and other instruments [vaginal and rectal probes] for special applications . . . at assorted prices."[8] With the battery came a pair of conducting-wire strings and a pair of tin handles, or small cylinders, to serve as electrodes. S. M. Wells, author of *Electropathic Guide: Prepared with the Particular Reference to Home Practice* (1872), also promoted implements similar to Britten's.[9]

There were some general rules for treating diseases with electricity. "Inflammations, fevers, bruises, sprains, expanded muscles, swellings, and extraneous growths should be heated with the positive pole; and debility, chilliness, inaction, tendency to decomposition, and contracted muscles with the negative pole," S. M. Wells wrote. Britten advised wrapping the plates with cotton cloth dipped in hot water, and elaborated in detail how the various connections were to be made.[10]

In 1873, when Henry Lake asked readers "Is Electricity Life?" in *Popular Science Monthly,* his answer was resoundingly positive. "Although we are not continually made sensible to it," he explained, "men and women are electrical machines . . . [and] all parts of the body furnish signs of free

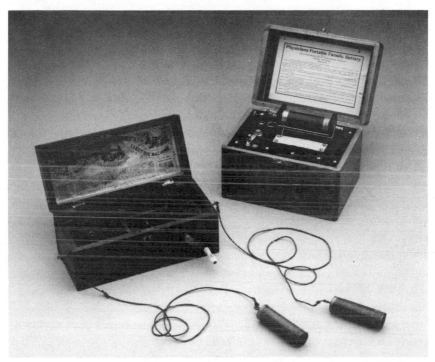

These apparatus consisted essentially of a small wet (galvanic) cell that, when activated, would transmit a modest electrical current (direct) to the patient. Left: magnetic-electric machine, W. H. Burnap, Davis and Kidder, New York, N.Y., bone, brass, mahogany, paper, tin, cotton, ca. 1855. Right: Faradic battery, American, oak, paper, chrome, ca. 1885.

positive electricity, especially when the circulation is excited." According to Lake, illness was caused by a deficiency of this force, and this was to be remedied by an artificial supply of electricity. Lake asserted that electricity was "the very soul of the universe. It permeates all space, surrounds the earth, and is found in every part of it." Lightning could kill a "human body not possessed of its proper quantity of electricity." Further "proof" of his contention that people became ill when they lost electricity was his assertion that "sparks of electricity may be drawn from the body of a patient dying of cholera."[11]

George Beard and Alphonso D. Rockwell's *A Practical Treatise on the Medical and Surgical Uses of Electricity* (1871) was one of a series of books

Beard wrote that concentrated on electrotherapy. Beard thought the nervous system was akin to a galvanic battery, and that in autumn and winter higher positive energy charges existed in the atmosphere and in the earth than in spring and summer. Nervous people would thus be more lively in the two cooler seasons, as well as from nine A.M. to noon and from six to nine P.M., the cooler hours of daylight, when he thought that a higher level of positive electrical force existed. To maintain equilibrium or to boost a patient's energy, appropriate supplements of battery-induced energy were used.

Even some of electrotherapy's supporters were not certain Beard and others had correctly defined the reason for the evident success of the treatment. John J. Caldwell, in *A Review of Recent Theories of Brain and Nerve Action* (1877), agreed that "a knowledge of the brain and of the network of the nervous system should be the aim of every physician who would minister to a body or a 'mind disease.' " He seemed to equate "nerve power" and electricity, but was uncertain about the exact relationship of the two forces. "Precisely how electricity acts as a therapeutic agent," he wrote, "no experimenter has satisfactorily explained."[12]

Some of Beard's medical colleagues questioned his equation of declining vitality and overexertion, either physical, or, more commonly, mental. Dioclesian Lewis had challenged the "fixed amount of vitality" idea in 1862, terming "all this talk about expenditure of vitality" as "full of sophistry." He was joined in his critique by some of the most eminent of the nation's physicians, including Henry Pickering Bowditch (1840–1911). In 1886 Bowditch attacked the first principle of Beard's work on medical electricity —the theory that "nerve force" and electricity were identical. "The important facts which forbid the identification of nerve force with electricity," Bowditch wrote, were "the absence of an insulating sheath on the nerve fibre, the slow rate with which nerve force is transmitted, and the effect of ligature on a nerve in preventing the passage of nerve force while not interfering with that of electricity." J. H. Kellogg was similarly unconvinced in 1882. He allowed that "when rightly used, [electricity's] curative value is immense; but it has fallen, unfortunately, almost entirely into the hands of quacks."[13]

Britten, S. M. Wells, and W. R. Wells—all of whom promoted their inventive procedures and therapies to the lay public—may well have been the "quacks" to whom Kellogg was referring. W. R. Wells stated, "We are frequently asked whether we expect to take people without medical education, and in one or two courses of lectures qualify them to treat diseases safely. We answer, not only with safety, but success, too." The considerable success of home electrotherapy devices in the marketplace indicates that the public did not agree with Kellogg or Bowditch; the academically trained medical profession was not yet seen to be the only true aid to the ill.[14]

Comments by patients about how electric treatments actually felt are nearly impossible to find. But it can be inferred from the educational and cautionary tone of many of electrotherapy's advocates that the experience was at times painful. George M. Schweig urged practitioners to start slowly, maintaining the treatment for only ten or fifteen minutes with a "current not sufficient in intensity . . . to cause any but *slight* muscular contractions." Britten warned that the electrical charge administered "should never cause pain or discomfort," and that "the hap-hazard administration of what used to be vulgarly denominated 'shocks' " were intolerable to the responsible electrotherapist. Patients probably experienced mild shocks when first connected and finally disconnected from the circuit even under the most carefully controlled conditions, as Doctor Moritz Meyer explained in his highly technical *Electricity in Its Relation to Practical Medicine* (1869). Meyer pointed out that in the most careful treatments the aftereffects of "electrization" included an inclination to sleep, earlier and fuller menstruation for women, and relief of pain for many hours afterward.[15]

The broad cultural enthusiasm for and confusion about electricity helped generate a variety of related but tangential theories about health and therapy. The idea that the human body was a large compound electromagnet gave rise to the conviction that electricity was continually escaping from the extremities—in particular, the feet and especially, according to S. M. Wells, during sleep. This, Wells maintained, would explain feelings of "languor and exhaustion on rising in the morning." With characteristic commercialism, Wells asserted that this surreptitious draining of vital force—which, like the effects of unventilated bedrooms, took place when people were most unaware and therefore most vulnerable—could be averted. "We would recommend Hall's Glass Castors, for Insulating Bedsteads" to stop the "circuit" that connected the person with the earth. "Made of pressed glass, about three and one-half inches in diameter, and one and one-half inches thick, with a cavity to allow the feet of the bedstead to rest in," these devices were also advertised as a "protection for lightning."[16]

Wells also advised "sleeping with the head toward the north and the feet toward the south, in order "that the strong currents of Electricity, which are constantly flowing from the poles to the equator, may pass in the same direction as those in the body, which flow from the brain downward and outward." He warned that to sleep in other configurations would lead to "wakefulness, restlessness, and even great nervous derangement in persons of delicate, sensitive organizations."[17] Like others of the decades immediately following the Civil War, Wells was trading on common fears among the populace—declining energy, the symptoms of inability to cope with a changed world as manifested in the various forms of neurasthenia, the vulnerability of humans to unseen but omnipresent forces of great power (electricity and electromagnetism), and madness, which seemed to result from no single identifiable cause.

Inspired entrepreneurs soon developed a series of foot-related electrical products, including "Electripatent Socks." These innersole devices were to "prevent the abstraction of electricity by [the] cold earth," while they simultaneously generated "on the feet those electric currents on which warmth depends." American firms such as "Dr. Bridgman's Electro-Magnetic . . . Appliances" produced innersoles for fifty cents a pair, promising a "quick cure" for rheumatism and gout. Electric slippers, each connected to a small cell, were also widely available,[18] as were electric brushes for other parts of the body. These devices usually had hard rubber handles with inset bristles that allegedly brushed electricity onto the skin. Advertised as good for the relief of "nervous affections, paralysis, rheumatism, kidney and liver complaints," and just about everything else, the brushes probably did cause some electrical sensation because their use could create static electricity.[19]

The afflicted could even get electricity in a bottle. For fifty cents anyone could avail themselves of "Brewster's Medicated Electricity, an infallible remedy for headache, neuralgia, hay fever, catarrh and cold in the head." E. E. Brewster of Holly, Michigan, claimed to produce an inhaler with a "perfect electric battery in every bottle." This "battery" was a small metallic coil submerged in a solution of, among other things, "vegetable compounds." It was advertised as producing a "permanent cure in one to two weeks" through powers described as "truly magical."[20]

Those needing more "vital force" could also get their electric treatment from chains and belts that could be worn about the waist or other ailing parts of the body. The Pulvermacher Company, an English firm that had

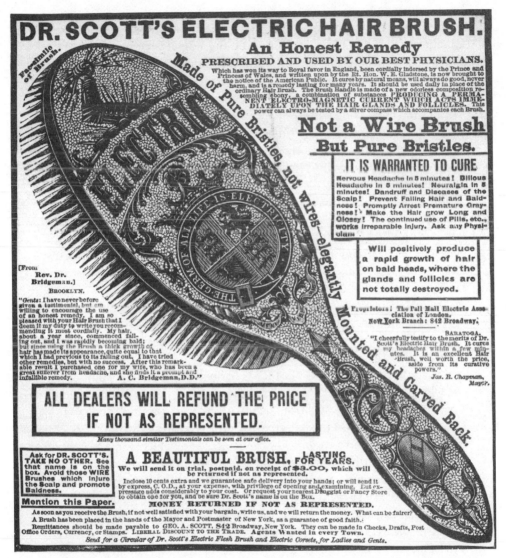

One of the most popular of all expressions of the nineteenth-century craze for electricity was the electric brush, which probably gained its credibility because of the static electricity produced when hair was brushed with thermoplastic materials. On the brush back is emblazoned what for many was an incontrovertible truth: "The Germ of Life is Electricity." Advertisement from Harper's Weekly, June 3, 1882, p. 350.

been producing these devices since before the Civil War, had such success exporting the chains to the United States that a factory was established in Cincinnati soon after the conclusion of the war. They were popular for thirty years. Available in a variety of lengths from six to thirty-six inches and in two widths, the chains were a series of brass-encased zinc cylinders with tapes attached to each end for securing the device to the limbs, the abdomen, or the chest. The battery effect was activated by soaking the chain in a three-parts-water and one-part-vinegar solution, with weaker acid concentrations producing a weaker charge. The usual panoply of afflictions from gout to "female complaints" to cholera were rendered curable by proper use of these apparatus.[21]

The blue-light enthusiasm of the mid 1870s and early 1880s was one of the more creative applications of electromagnetic theory. In 1876 Augustus James Pleasonton had published a rather quixotic book entitled *The Influence of the Blue Ray of Sunlight and of the Blue Color of the Sky in Developing Animal and Vegetable Life, in Arresting Disease, and Restoring Health in Acute and Chronic Disorders to Human and Domestic Animals.* Appropriately printed in blue ink, Pleasonton's work was a combination of his experimentation with and knowledge of light's effect on plants, and a somewhat bizarre set of theories about heat, light, the laws of motion, and the nature of the earth.[22]

Born in Washington, D.C., in 1808, Pleasonton was a West Point graduate who became adjutant general for the state of Pennsylvania in 1838. There he served during "political disturbances at Harrisburg," and later, in 1844, was wounded "in the left groin" during a skirmish "with rioters." In the Civil War, he served as brigadier general of the Pennsylvania Volunteer Militia and came through the conflict unscathed; afterward he spent much of his time developing his theories on light, health, and magnetism.[23]

Pleasonton, like so many other theorists of health and hygiene during the postwar era, began with what was for him a revealed truth. "Without light and heat," he asserted, "life cannot exist, and electricity and magnetism are indispensable to its active vitality." The spinal column, he argued, when exposed to electromagnetic force, conducted it to the brain, from whence the "whole nervous system" carried the force to "all the organs of the body . . . stimulating them into active exercise: hence follows restoration to health."[24]

With some knowledge of the magnetic character of the earth, Pleasonton extended his theories into many more areas than other electrotherapists. He offered explanations for such natural phenomena as the aurora borealis, tropical rainy seasons, and the rotation of the earth on its axis, and theorized that every change in the form of matter—combustion, solidification, liquification, evaporation—produced electricity, "which in turn contributes to form new modifications of the matter which has yielded it."[25] His theories about the sun and earth led him to his discovery about the nature of light and the relationship of blue light to health.

A complicated line of logic convinced Pleasonton that, like the human body, neither the sun nor the moon had atmosphere or heat. He added a more down-to-earth observation as "proof" of his theory—that people became warm while exercising outside in winter, when the snow and ice do not melt.[26] What people perceived to be the great mysterious powers of their time—magnetism and electricity—lent credence to even these flights of fantasy.

His observations about electricity and magnetism pushed Pleasonton to regard Newtonian physics with disdain. "Light, electricity, magnetism, and heat, the vital forces of the universe, all treat gravitation with great contempt," he observed. Failing to comprehend the differences between physical mass and energy were not the only analytical problems Pleasonton had, however. He argued the "gravitation is not universal," and sought to prove it by demonstrating that an iron bar will sink while an iron dish of the same weight can be made to float. He was either unaware of or simply misunderstood that objects that displace a volume of water whose weight is equal to or greater than their weight will float, and instead explained the iron dish's flotation as a "function of magnetism." The iron dish "became magnetic by induction from the water," he thought, which was itself "magnetic," and of the same polarity as the dish. Since opposite poles attract and polarities repel, flotation occurred, according to Pleasonton.[27]

With all this electromagnetic baggage, Pleasonton was nonetheless an astute amateur botanist. In 1871, ten years after he had begun his experiments—first with grapes, then with pigs—he was awarded a patent for an "improvement in accelerating the growth of plants and animals" through the use of blue-tinted glass. Observations revealed that plants grown under blue light fared better, and Pleasonton theorized that, when all the colors of light were filtered out the blue end of the spectrum, the blue, indigo, and violet caused "friction" and in turn produced electricity and magnetism. This "electro-magnetic current . . . imparts to vegetable or animal life subjected to it, an extraordinary impulse to the development of their respective vigour and growth," he wrote. Thus both plants and animals, by virtue of their exposure to electromagnetism, were "strengthened so as to resist disease, and to throw it off in those instances in which it had appeared" already.[28]

Pleasonton figured that the sky's apparent blue color was the key to the health-giving properties of light. "How rapidly might the various races of our domestic animals be multiplied, and how much might their individual proportions be enlarged!" he exclaimed, stopping short of recommending growing conditions for humans like those he found useful for animals. Perhaps because great physical size was not as prized in 1876 as it was in the twentieth century—but more likely because such connections between humans and the flora and fauna were beyond the boundaries of acceptable dialog—Pleasonton recommended that people expose themselves to blue light only as a therapeutic device. The implications were there, however, for those who wished to see them.[29]

Pleasonton first experimented with blue light's effect on the human environment in the servants' sleeping quarters in one of his country houses. "It was observed that large numbers of flies, that had previously infested them, were dead soon after its [blue light's] introduction on the inside sills of the windows," he noted, supposing that because sunlight was negatively charged, and blue glass positively, their attraction generated an electromagnetic current sufficiently strong to destroy the "feeble vitality of the eggs or of the insects themselves." Pleasonton comprehended light and electricity as some sort of energy gun which could vitalize those strong enough to accept it, yet kill those too weak. The roll call of cures was the familiar one —rheumatism, neuralgia, "torpor of the lower extremities," and "cerebral disorders"—for which Pleasonton prescribed "full trials of blue and sunlight baths."[30] Like nearly every other purveyor of a cure-all, Pleasonton had a stock of endorsements and case histories with which to impress the reader.[31]

Pleasonton developed a series of explanations for all sorts of human behavior and human preferences based on his theories of electromagnetism and blue light. Drunkards, he maintained, were always male because men were negatively charged beings, a condition brought about by the "habit of negation or denial of the wants of the females." Women, "from the positive and persistent character of their demands," he wrote, "may be termed positively electrified." Attraction between male and female was thus "electric" or "magnetic"; using an old term, Pleasonton thereby redefined "animal magnetism." He thought alcohol a diabolical force in male-female relations because "it has been shown that the negative or masculine electricity of the man is reversed and becomes positive like that of the woman" when he was drunk. In one of the most hostile characterizations of women written in the 1870s, Pleasonton condemned the drunken male for allowing "his attributes [to] become feminine; he is irritable, irrational, excitable by trivialities, and when opposed in his opinions or conduct, becomes violent and outrageous." Pleasonton warned that men so "feminized" were repelled by their wives, and the couple inevitably became "mutually abusive, [and] engage in conflict and deadly strife."[32]

Healthy, upright, moral persons were, for Pleasonton, in a state of electrical equilibrium. People who for some reason had lost their electromagnetic balance "become sullen, cross, crabbed, quarrelsome, and disagreeable." Children so afflicted, however, were inexplicably best treated with "the rod" rather than with the sun; "the friction produced by the blows evolves electricity of the kind necessary to restore the healthy electric equilibrium of their bodies." His electromagnetic argument appears in fact to have been an after-the-fact rationalization for his traditional ideas about temperance and child rearing: Advocacy of corporal punishment for adults was unacceptable in 1876.[33]

Pleasonton's most bizarre application of his electromagnetic theories was to physical appearance and sexual attraction. He asserted that corpulence prevented the emission of electricity from the body; therefore overweight people were less sexually attractive. They were also, in his estimation, less intelligent. Pleasonton characterized the "Esquimaux, Fins [sic], Laps and all inhabitants of the high northern climates requiring a fatty incarbonaceous food" as both unintelligent and overweight. Pleasonton sarcastically advised people who wished for few or no children to "select for their companions in life the fattest persons of the opposite sex that they can find, and they will be rewarded by an immense reduction in their household and educational expenses when compared with those of their neighbors who chance to be of a lean kind." His advice reflected not so much a concern about declining family size among the "better sorts" of Americans—that would not develop until after the 1880 federal census figures had been analyzed—as it was criticism of those men and women who "resisted the injunction of the Patriarchs of going forth, multiplying and replenishing the earth."[34]

The issue of the sun's relation to health was still highly controversial. Most hygienists and physicians thought the sun health giving; Shirley Murphy, editor and author of one of the standard texts of English reform architecture and furnishings of the postwar era, stated that "pure light is as essential to health as pure food and drink."[35]

J. H. Kellogg summoned the example of the Swiss to demonstrate the healthful effects of the sun. Residents of "the deep valleys" where "the sun shines only a few hours a day . . . suffer terribly from scrofula," he noted. "The women, almost without exception, are deformed by huge goiters, which hang pendant from their necks unless suspended by a sling. A considerable portion of the males are idiots." By contrast, Swiss who lived "higher up on the sides of the mountains . . . are remarkably hardy, and are well-developed, physically and mentally," due solely to increased sunshine. Accordingly, his advice was to "throw open the blinds and draw aside the window curtains . . . never mind if the carpets do fade a little sooner."[36]

As they urged women to expose their skin to the sun, reformers were running headlong into the powerful fashion imperative that identified beautiful skin as white and translucent, a condition that sunburn or suntan would destroy. Women perennially wrote to editors of popular magazines trying to find cures for freckles and spots. They were aware that sunlight darkened freckles and accentuated other imperfections. The fragile, wan look remained fashionable throughout the late nineteenth century in spite of the fulminations of health and moral critics who condemned "phthisical" (tubercular) heroines. Pale skin signified daintiness, and it was not until after 1890 that the "outdoor girl" became a widely accepted cultural ideal.

C H A P T E R · E I G H T

"MUSCULAR CHRISTIANITY" AND THE ATHLETIC REVIVAL

Americans searching for ways to achieve and preserve good health found another series of methods after the Civil War—gymnastics, calisthenics, physical education, and sports—which were actually old movements that had finally found a receptive audience. Charles Follen and Edward Hitchcock had shown enthusiasm for these activities as early as 1830, and the cause had been championed for the next three decades by such reformers as Russell Trall, Catharine Beecher, and, to some extent, by the example of the Turners.

In the Northeast in particular, middle-class and wealthy Americans heeded the advocates of exercise and athletic competition because their environment had changed so radically from that of 1830. By 1860 nearly half the population of the Northeast lived in cities and towns. Many worked in sedentary, "brain work" occupations. The argument that theirs was a position superior to that of people of less developed civilizations appealed to them, as did the idea that physical activity—a positive action—would alleviate the ill effects of this advanced station. The idea that united the advocates and devotees of calisthenics, gymnastics, physical education, and sports was that the body was more than simply a container for the soul that should be kept free from disease; its form could be altered and perfected, and by doing so people could increase their energy and improve their life and, implicitly, their afterlife. Perfection of the body was an essential part of Christian morality in this system of thought and was perhaps the most vivid expression of the prewar millennial spirit, which had promoted the idea that human action could determine individual and social salvation.

The building and success of public gymnasiums was one measure of the new interest. The first efforts of the 1830s failed quickly, but by 1860 more and more Americans had moved to both large and small cities, and entrepreneurs and municipal governments once again began to build gymnasiums to meet the demands of the growing middle-class and wealthy urbanites. In Poughkeepsie, New York, for example, the city gymnasium was incorporated in 1861, its object "to provide for the physical education of youth and citizens."[1] The idea of encouraging physical development dovetailed with increasing cultural worries about mentally overtaxing both the young and the mature in an increasingly urban, bureaucratic, and sedentary society.

Urban gymnasiums were also popular because they were community organizations. As rural, town, and village folk moved to the larger cities, traditional mechanisms of social support and cultural continuity that they had known—community, church, and family—were fragmented or nonexistent. Cities—large, impersonal conglomerations of people, industry, and commerce—had radically different rules of behavior and organization from those that persisted in the small village or town, where nearly everyone knew everyone else. The gymnasium became one urban gathering place where, like the church, groups of like-minded people might both get to know their neighbors and learn ways to combat the health and moral hazards of the big city.

The postwar fitness crusade gained more followers as physical education and body building were linked with the continued strength of evangelical Christianity. Religious revivals of the late 1850s and after were strongest in the cities of the northern states, and Americans seemed especially taken with "Muscular Christianity," a movement that originated in England in the first half of the nineteenth century. Linking moral and physical culture together turned gymnastics, calisthenics, and ultimately sport into a distinctly American pastime—possibly an American obsession.

In early-nineteenth-century England the model of the "muscular Christian" was the popular fictional hero "Tom Brown." Books about the character's life and exploits appeared continuously from at least 1804, but it was Thomas Hughes's rendition of *Tom Brown's Schooldays* that reached a mass audience. Another popular English novelist, Charles Kingsley, coined the phrase itself; his greatest success, *Two Years Ago* (1857), revolved about the assumption that morality was a function of muscularity as well as of piety, and that the best sort of Christians were physically fit. By 1870 "muscular Christianity," according to a book reviewer in *Godey's Lady's Book,* was "so popular with nearly all classes of people" that books on "bodily strength and skill will find abundant favor."[2]

One way to become a muscular Christian was through gymnastics, which in 1857 Russell Trall viewed as "efficient auxiliaries in mental education, by inducing habits of order, exactness, and directness in the mental operations" —skills useful and perhaps essential in an emerging capitalist and bureaucratic society. Trall hinted that mental capabilities might even be improved by exercise. He argued that "people, naturally stupid" may be made "comparatively intelligent, by prevailing on them to take gymnastic exercise." S. D. Kehoe, a popular advocate of exercise with Indian clubs, eloquently refined Trall's ideas of the connections between physical, mental, and moral condition in 1866. "Improve the apparatus, then, and you facilitate and improve the work which the mind performs with it, precisely as you facilitate steam operation, and enhance its product, by improving the machinery with which it is executed." Kehoe's use of the mechanical metaphor was judicious in a culture fascinated with machines and power, and eager for an ideology of positive action to improve life. "The physical education of the human race ought not to be confined to the humble object of preventing disease," Kehoe asserted. "Its aim should be loftier and more in accordance with the destiny and character of its subject—to raise man to the summit of his nature; and such will be its scope in future and more enlightened times."[3]

Nearly all the advocates of gymnastics, calisthenics, and physical education began from a series of deeply critical premises about American culture. Too much "mind work, by the ambitious student, the covetous and careworn merchant, or the adventurer in political life" had hindered Americans, Kehoe wrote. Professor Maurice Kloss, in "The Dumb Bell Instructor for Parlor Gymnasts" (1862), similarly argued that "gymnastics are valuable to all persons, but especially to clerks, students, sedentary artisans, and still more particularly, to those [who] in addition to sedentary habits, perform

exhaustive mental labor. . . . Suffering from indigestion and nervous irritability," Kloss wrote, "such people were threatened with "early failure of the
powers of life" unless they began "a wise system of gymnastic training."
Kloss may well have been referring not only to nervous exhaustion but also
to impotence, given the euphemistic language of publications about sexuality in the mid-nineteenth century.[4]

One of the most popular and enduring advocates of what *Harper's
Weekly* in 1860 called the "Athletic Revival" was Dioclesian Lewis, a
physical education instructor who first integrated girls, women, older people, and very young children into an overall exercise program. An advocate
of temperance, women's rights, health reform, and homeopathy, Lewis
studied German and Swedish gymnastics while in Europe in 1856, and
became convinced that these activities offered Americans their best chance
at improved health.[5] In 1861 Lewis had opened evening calisthenic classes
in Boston and attempted to start two journals to promulgate the new faith,
Lewis' New Gymnastics and Boston Journal of Physical Culture (1861) and
Lewis' Gymnastic Monthly and Journal of Physical Culture (1862). He was
more successful as an author, advocate, and teacher than as a journalist.
Both periodicals survived only one year.

Lewis had published articles on the new gymnastics in the *Atlantic
Monthly* and the *American Journal of Education* in 1861 and had presented
his system to the American Institute of Instruction in 1860. Responses to
both the articles and the lecture were favorable, but mild compared with
the phenomenal success of the book. *New Gymnastics for Men, Women,
and Children,* first published in 1862, went through ten editions and became the standard text for calisthenic exercises in schools, gymnasiums, and
homes for twenty-five years. So pervasive was Lewis's impact that in 1869
tiny Ingham University, in the little upstate New York town of LeRoy,
assured parents of the institution's "earnest attention to the subject of
Physical Culture" by asserting that they adopted "the admirable system of
Dr. Dio Lewis."[6]

Women were encouraged to participate in these activities because, according to educator James Smart, exercise would help produce a "sound
nervous system . . . rendering them normally sensitive, and destroying the
tendency to mental irritability and hysteria." Thomas Wentworth Higginson, the venerable Boston writer, found even more profound reasons for
women to become more athletic, or at least better conditioned. In "The
Health of Our Girls," an article that appeared in 1862 in the *Atlantic*

Monthly, Higginson warned that "unless they are healthy, the whole country is not safe. Nowhere can their physical condition be so important as in a republic. . . . The fate of our institutions may hang on the precise temperament which our next President shall have inherited from his mother." More blunt was physician Edward H. Clarke, who in 1873 asked, "Shall they [the western lands] be populated by our own children or by those of aliens? This is a question that our own women must answer; upon their loins depends the future destiny of the nation."[7]

Dio Lewis claimed his system had been introduced "into female seminaries with comparative satisfaction." In well-ventilated rooms heated to sixty-five to sixty-eight degrees, girls assembled for exercises in loose clothing, with "perfect liberty about the waist and shoulders." The calisthenic crusade that helped undermine the corset in the early 1860s thus owed much of its popularity to Lewis. Fashion in women's clothing had been a source of irritation and concern to both physicians and advocates of women's rights since the 1830s, but the rationale of anticorset enthusiasm changed through the century. Before the Civil War, Beecher, Trall, Shew, and others had condemned "waists," as they were called, because they deformed women's bodies, especially their rib cages, spines, and lungs. In 1857 Trall compared American women unfavorably with "the erect and graceful forms of the hard-working Irish or German servant girls." Their American sisters, by contrast, had "crooked figures and uncouth shapes." Corsets, Trall maintained, caused "the blood to become highly carbonized, thus inducing a dull, dingy, sallow or bilious hue of the skin . . . and . . . a red and carbuncular appearance of the nose."[8]

After the war the cry against the corset and other restrictive garments continued, but its emphasis changed to the deleterious effects of tight-lacing on the abdomen—rather than or in addition to the chest—signaling the growing concern for the reproductive capacities of American women. Corseting was blamed for many cases of collapsed or prolapsed uterus, a condition in which the uterus collapsed, inverted, and sometimes slid into the vagina. Internal supports (pessaries) made of wood, glass, metal, or ceramics were used to combat the condition, as well as hip baths, tonics, medicines, and plasters of different compounds. That a prolapsed uterus might have been a result of advancing years and numerous childbirths was largely overlooked by physicians and other critics; they instead found the fault in an external agent. A cinched waist and pelvis were thought even more dangerous for future generations, since many physicians and most laymen and women of the postwar era believed that acquired characteristics were genetically transferable. Thus many thought that a contracted pelvis (which made birth more difficult) would be passed on to a woman's daughter, whose shape in turn might prevent her from having children at all.[9]

Abba Gould Woolson's *Dress-Reform* (1874) presented women with five lucid anticorset essays. The book criticized the "despotic goddess Fashion," terming its effects a "juggernaut" that was diametrically opposed to the dictates of good health. The "instrument of human torture" was challenged only briefly by the "Bloomer costume," characterized as the "most notable of . . . failures" to reform dress. Woolson thought that "what is needed, then, is not to assail fashion but to teach hygiene . . . to increase the strength, ability, and happiness of themselves and their children."[10]

Corsets and tight, heavy skirts had to be eliminated, according to the reformers. In addition, clothes were to be chosen so as to preserve and evenly distribute body heat in cold weather; fashionable thin sleeves and heavy skirts were unsuitable. But for all the advice and hostility, corsets remained popular. Advertisers even promoted the "electric waist" for women. As Antoinette Brown Blackwell put it in 1874, "with us it is fine clothing *versus* nerves, and the clothes always win."[11]

Dio Lewis's willingness to include women in classes and in his normal school (half of his first class of graduates were women) was one of the building blocks of the system's popularity. Lewis's system allowed women the freedom from corsets and from the "refined" activities that middle-class culture demanded; this, too was a wellspring of its appeal.[12] He advised heads of gymnasiums to stencil their floors at fifty-five-inch intervals with "a large piece of tin, cut out into the shape of a pair of feet," Once aligned, the students began Lewis's system of exercises, to music whenever possible. Lewis maintained that "feeble and apathetic people, who have little courage to undertake gymnastic training, accomplish wonders under the inspiration of music. I believe five times as much muscle can be coaxed out, under this delightful stimulus, as without it."[13]

Lewis's system involved a series of very light stretching exercises, with the aid of a few pieces of simple apparatus he devised. The calisthenics of Catharine Beecher were fine as far as they went but her exercise regimen neglected the hand-eye coordination and the play element he thought essential. Thus he developed an additional series of throwing and catching exercises, first using large rubber balls and then beanbags. "Throwing and catching objects in certain ways, requiring skill and presence of mind,

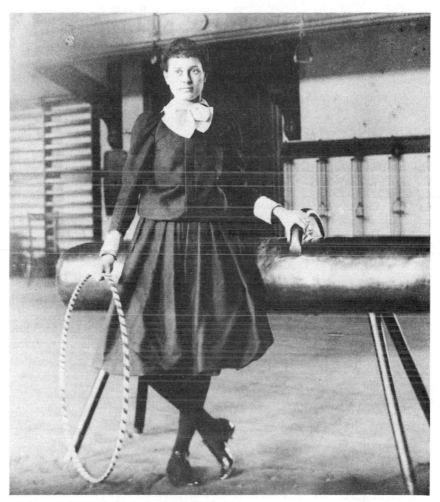

In a properly loose-fitting gym suit, this young woman typified the reformers' ideal of fitness. Photograph, American, ca. 1885.

affords not only good exercise of the muscles of the arms and upper half of the body, but cultivates a quickness of eye and coolness of nerve very desirable." Rubber balls were too difficult to maneuver, Lewis thought. There were thirty beanbag toss exercises, including tossing and catching with both hands or each hand, and more complicated behind-the-back and over-the-shoulder throws for the more advanced. In addition, there were games using a series of hoops lashed together through which gymnasts threw the beanbags to one another. The hoops were "quite high"—and perhaps they planted the seed for basketball in James Naismith's mind.[14]

Lewis also introduced exercise rings, wooden (usually cherry or oak) circles six inches in diameter and one inch thick. In the *American Journal of Education* he recommended that the rings be fashioned of rosewood and carefully polished because in that way "the interest of young ladies is greatly enhanced." Lewis told his readers that "this series of exercises is entirely new, and beyond all comparison, the best ever devised." They were "happily adapted to family, school, and general use." The exercises themselves were fundamentally isometric—an individual or two people held the rings and pulled on them, creating a dynamic tension of the muscles involved. A single person could grasp the ring in both hands and pull outward, working against himself or herself. All these (there were more than fifty variations) were done in time to music.[15]

The "New Gymnastics" also made use of the "wand," a pole four feet long and one inch in diameter, which was employed in a variety of bending and stretching exercises to alleviate the "stiff, inflexible condition of the ligaments and muscles connected with the shoulders," which Lewis thought "the principal obstacle in the way of beginners." *New Gymnastics* detailed sixty-eight different wand exercises, most of them akin to modern barbell lifts. For stronger participants, Lewis recommended a wand with a hollow core, which could be filled with "a pound or two" of lead shot.[16]

Lewis also worked to promote a fundamental change in the way American health seekers used dumbbells, shifting the emphasis from greater weights. Instead of iron, Lewis argued that light dumbbells of wood should be used. There were thirty-four dumbbell exercises in *New Gymnastics,* many of which were very vigorous. Number eleven, for example, began with the participant holding the bells (one in each hand) in front of his or her body with arms extended. From this position, he or she was to "bring them with *great force*" back to the shoulders while leaning backward "forty times."[17]

Lewis included a variety of other games and exercises to increase agility in *The New Gymnastics.* "Pin running" involved setting up a pin fifteen to forty-five feet from a circle in which the athlete began. Upon a signal the individual ran to the pin, picked it up, brought it back to the circle, and stood it upright. Distances could be varied, thought Lewis, to account for differences in strength and speed. He also advocated use of the "Pangymnastikon," or rings suspended from ropes, and "bird's nest" games, in which

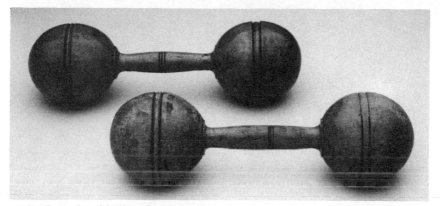

Lighter dumbbells, physical-culture advocates said, increased the flexibility of muscles and joints more than heavier ones. Dumbbells, American, maple, ca. 1870–1900.

a wooden square eight to twenty-four inches on a side, with poles extending one foot diagonally from each corner, was suspended from the ceiling. Participants sought to throw beanbags "weighing three to four pounds" onto the "nests." The "arm pull" consisted of two wooden handles connected to a U-shaped wire form (much like a shovel handle), which in turn were tied to each other with a strong two-foot rope. A variety of isometric exercises for one or two people were also described. The "shoulder pusher" was a wooden rod, thirty inches long and one and a half inches thick with a carved wooden element attached to each end of the rod that could be braced against the shoulder. Two exercisers pushed against each other, placing the carved ends against shoulders or arms.[18]

Lewis advised people to warm up before they undertook any of these exercises. "No machine can suddenly be put in motion at its highest possible speed, and as suddenly stopped, without risk of destroying it," Lewis wrote. He also advised exercisers to avoid workouts "immediately after fatiguing mental labor or just before or after a hearty meal," since the "life force centre" was in the brain in the former case, and in the stomach in the latter. Exercising before a meal prevented this "force" from locating in the stomach, thereby hindering digestion. He also recommended exercises after the morning cleansing of the body, since it produced a "delightful glow." Perspiration—and its attendant smells—were not regarded with the disfavor that twentieth-century Americans attach to them. He thought the slight

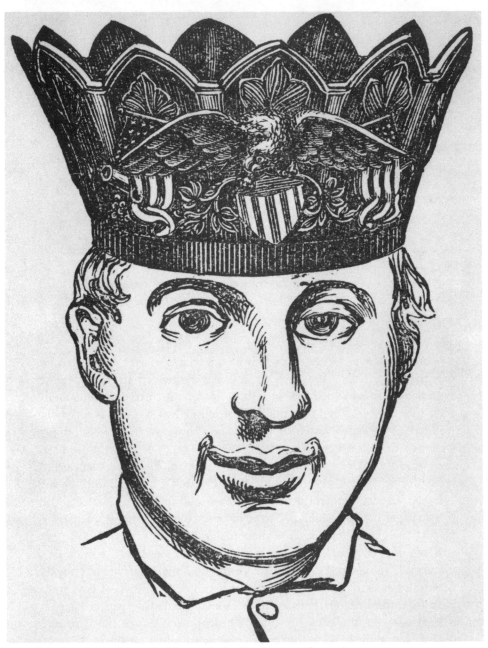

Dio Lewis envisioned this patriotically decorated cast-iron crown as a perfect exercise device to build up leg and back muscles, as well as good posture, but it was heavy, cumbersome, and expensive to use (since many sizes had to be bought for school use). "Gymnastic Crown," illustration from The New Gymnastics *(Boston: Ticknor and Fields, 1862).*

flush of the face that exercise brought was attractive.[19]

Lewis also included exercises with another piece of equipment that became broadly popular after the war. "Indian clubs"—turned wooden devices shaped like bowling pins—were so named because soldiers of the British army in India had adopted and adapted the native exercise and brought it back to England in the middle decades of the nineteenth century. Lewis enumerated twenty-two different exercises using the clubs, nearly all of which involved some manner of swinging them.[20]

Unlike other specific gymnastic or calisthenic exercises and apparatus, Indian clubs had their own literature and became a popular participant and spectator activity. S. D. Kehoe's *The Indian Club Exercise* (1866) described not only the various movements but also acknowledged some of the champions of club swinging. Kehoe advertised his brand of Indian club exercises as beneficial for athletes, both amateur and professional. Baseball teams,

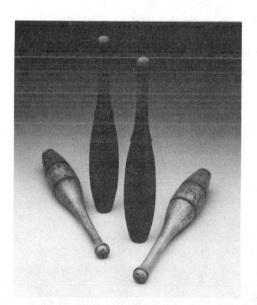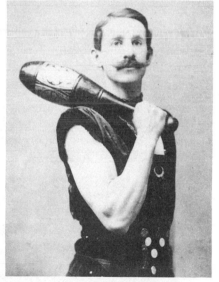

Indian-club exercises were among the attractions of strength, health, and fitness clubs, such as the Turners or native organizations. These groups often adopted uniforms that combined the color of ethnic or folk costume with the formality of dress military garb. Left: Indian clubs, American, maple, walnut, ca. 1880–1910. Right: cabinet photograph, T. D. Jones, West Troy, N.Y., ca. 1885.

such as the Philadelphia Athletics, Brooklyn Atlantics, and New York Mutuals, allegedly practiced with the clubs, as did members of the crew teams at Harvard and Yale. "All are adorned," he wrote, "with Kehoe's Missives on Muscular Christianity." He argued that his exercises would steady the nerves of billiard players and help the coordination of boxers.[21]

In 1866 a male enthusiast could buy the clubs in nine different weights from five to twenty-five pounds each; "ladies and children" were offered four different weights from one to four pounds each. Prices ranged from $1.50 to $15. The true devotee could buy jewelry in the shape of miniature Indian clubs. Sleeve buttons made of ebony or rosewood cost 50 cents for a set of two, and three shirt studs in the shape of Indian clubs were available for 75 cents.[22]

Other advocates of Indian clubs followed close on Kehoe's heels. Samuel T. Wheelwright's *A New System of Instruction in the Indian Club Exercise* (1871) appeared only five years after Kehoe's book, and despite the fact that his regimen was not "new," it was as popular as Kehoe's *Indian Club Exercise.* Wheelwright proclaimed dumbbell exercises "tedious"; in his view, swinging the clubs was more creative and graceful and was better for both men and women. Almira MacDonald's daughter Anne evidently caught the club-swinging fever: on March 24, 1885, she and her friend Daisy went to a "Methodist social where they are to swing clubs"; they went again on April 2. Apparently Anne and Daisy were accomplished performers. They went to "swing clubs" at the "Central Church" on April 10, the Unitarian Church on April 24, and the "Lake Avenue Baptist church" on

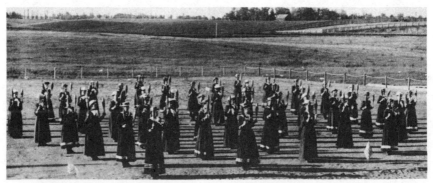

Women Turners participating in a club-swinging drill, State Fair Grounds, Minneapolis, Minn., 1891.

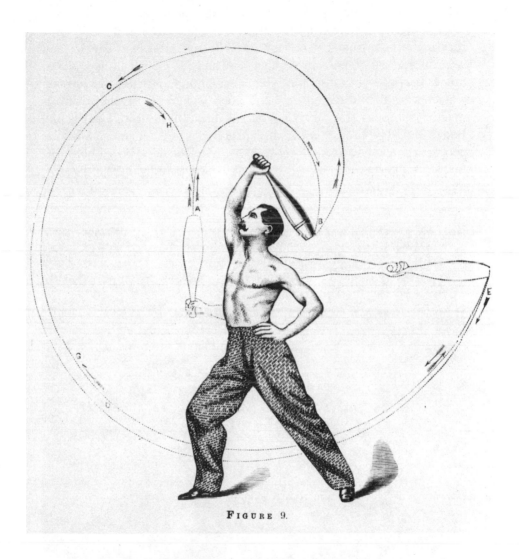

F I G U R E 9.

S. D. Kehoe's book The Indian Club Exercise *was one of the most popular of its kind and was published by the most important sporting goods company of the mid-nineteenth century. Swinging the weighted clubs would allegedly produce the era's ideal male figure, a lean, sinewy muscularity of slight bulk. Illustration from* The Indian Club Exercise *(New York: Peck and Snyder, 1866).*

May 22.[23] The sport was not only popular but evidently ecumenical as well.

Anne seems to have been the athlete of the MacDonald family. She regularly went to the "gymnasium" in 1884 and played lawn tennis and swam at the "natatorium" throughout 1886 and 1887. She may have picked up her interest from her mother, who, in addition to attending lectures on women's health and submitting herself to a wide range of medical treatments, went to hear the fitness luminary William Blaikie lecture on "Sound Bodies and How to Get Them" in January 1885. Like many middle-class people of the late nineteenth century, the MacDonalds enjoyed both participatory and spectator sports, attending many baseball games in the summers between 1885 and 1900.[24]

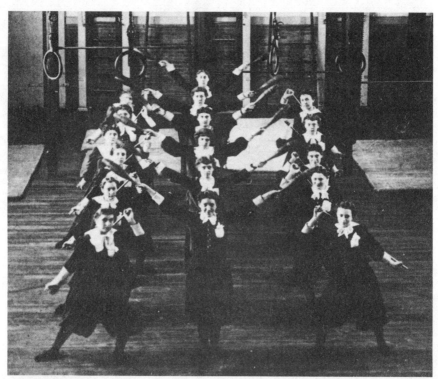

An ideal scene of fitness: young women properly outfitted in loose-fitting gym suits demonstrating their wand and Indian-club exercises, surrounded by the accoutrements of the calisthenic art—rings, ladders, ropes, and horizontal bars. Stereograph, M. H. Zanner, Niagara Falls, N.Y., 1896.

Having a gymnasium in the neighborhood, as Anne MacDonald did, was a convenience. Many—perhaps most—Americans were not so fortunate, especially if they lived in smaller towns or in parts of larger cities distant from such facilities. A few home gymnasiums had been constructed in the early 1860s, but most people settled for various combinations of "parlor gymnasium" gear offered by sporting goods concerns of the late nineteenth century. Most exercise books—Lewis's, Wheelwright's, and the equally popular William B. Dick's *Art of Gymnastics* (1885)—were either promoted as or entitled "family" instruction books for the home, as well as tracts for the gymnasium. Lewis's enthusiasm for the "Pangymnastikon" stemmed in part from his conviction that it was easy to install and use "in a parlor, study, or bed-room." He thought it particularly useful for the "lady done with her morning cares," who could "slip on her Zouave" (a loose-fitting dress like the famous French infantry unit's colorful uniform) and "devote a few minutes to . . . exercises."[25]

Another popular piece of gymnastic equipment—the "parlor gymnasium"—people were urged to use at their desks or sewing machines, placing one hand at each end and pulling outward. "Every business and professional man should have one . . . every teacher, clerk, and seamstress . . . every person whose occupation is sedentary," urged the advertisements. Dr. Barnett first offered this improvement in 1868 and substituted wound cable for the rubber gas tube by the mid 1870s. There were six different sizes ranging from the children's, which cost 30 cents, to the size "for Gentlemen of extra strength," which was available for $1.80. A full set, "for Family or Office use, Two of each size with Hooks," was $13. Barnett's competitors, such as Noyes Brothers of New York, marketed their rubber wand and handles with a pulley rather than hooks. One hook at head level held one handle of the wand. The other handle also had a loop, which was attached to a cable that came through a pulley attached to the floor. The pulley could be hooked either to the floor or the wall so that shoulders, arms, legs, and backs could be exercised.[26]

Barnett also marketed a device to which the rubber wand could be attached to provide rowing exercise. The device consisted of a sliding wooden seat with straps to hold the feet, a shaft that connected the seat with a brace shaped like a swan's head, a mounting ring, and the rubber wand. After attaching two wands—one for each hand—to the swan-shaped hook (attached to the ring, which in turn was screwed into "some convenient solid wood work"), the parlor rower sat on the low seat and began to

DR. BARNETT'S

IMPROVED

Parlor Gymnasium

Adopted by the Boards of Education, and used by the Pupils of the Public and Private Schools in New York and other Cities.

This is a superior and elegant system of exercise, convenient to all in price and other essentials. It is appropriate to the DRAWING-ROOM, the STUDY, the OFFICE, and to the use of both sexes.

Recommended by Drs. MOTT, WOOD, DOREMUS, HAMMOND, DIO LEWIS. Major General WEBB, President of the College of the city of New York, President HUNTER, of the Normal College, City Supt. of Schools HENRY KIDDLE, and numerous other leading professional and business men.

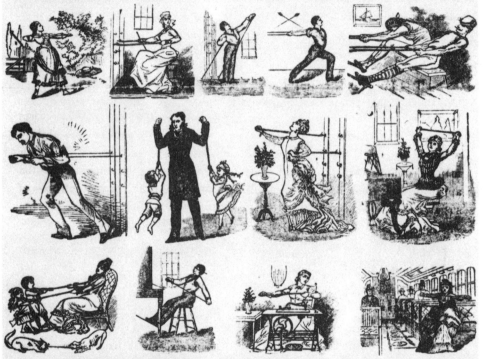

The BARNETT PARLOR GYMNASIUM is the most complete and compact article for health exercise ever invented. It is neither cumbersome nor expensive, and can be used anywhere. BEING LIGHT AND PORTABLE, IT CAN BE CARRIED IN THE POCKET, and is thus always ready for use, without preparation, at any time, and in any place.

IT RESTS THE TIRED BRAIN.   IT RESTS THE TIRED BODY.

Essentially a rubber cord with handles at each end, the "parlor gymnasium" was marketed as the consummately portable and versatile piece of equipment, with endorsements by the most eminent of American fitness advocates. Advertising brochure, American, ca. 1870.

196

"row." This apparatus cost $10 and was made of maple and black walnut. A more expensive parlor rowing machine was the Saunders Pneumatic Parlor Rowing Machine, which utilized a piston and cylinder as a means of generating resistance. Made of brass and hardwoods, the Saunders machine cost $20 in the 1880s, could be easily folded up and stored, and offered women who used it "freshness of complexion and roundness of limb," as well as freedom from "nervousness."[27]

Rowing had become an important spectator and participatory sport after the Civil War, first in colleges, and finally among a broader public by the 1890s. Its earliest practitioners were in the Northeast, and, as historian Donald Mrozek has demonstrated, rowing became a club sport throughout the country by the 1870s. Clubs thrived in Louisiana, Missouri, Pennsyl-

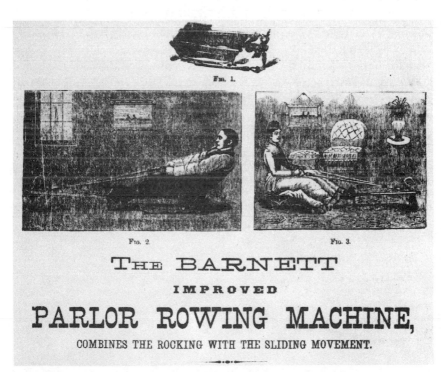

THE BARNETT

IMPROVED

PARLOR ROWING MACHINE,

COMBINES THE ROCKING WITH THE SLIDING MOVEMENT.

The Barnett was a simple device that traded on the American public's interest in rowing, a fascination that began after the Civil War and extended beyond the activities of college teams. Advertising brochure, American, ca. 1885.

vania, Texas, Minnesota, Virginia, Utah, and Washington State, and regional and state rowing associations were in operation by the mid 1880s. Vagaries in weather and water conditions (and the expense and inconvenience of transporting the shells) perhaps prevented rowing from ever gaining a greater foothold in America than it did. Its clubby atmosphere, the expense, and the relatively elite status the sport gained by virtue of its earliest upper-class college associations probably also limited its popularity. In addition, as a sport it had strong competition from baseball, and ultimately football, which could be played anywhere and with minimal equipment.[28]

Barnett also offered his wound rubber wand as part of a "health lift." This popular piece of equipment was essentially a platform of some sort to which the wand was hooked and on which the exerciser stood. With a wand on each side and knees bent, the individual straightened knees, thereby exercising his or her legs. Strong individuals could stand and stretch the rubber further by lifting their arms. The variety of "lifts," exercisers, machines, and gear for home exercising increased as the century progressed. Some had stationary weights, some had pulleys, some had bars to manipulate. D. L. Dowd's Health Exerciser, attached with strong bolts to the wall, with a weight and pulleys hooked to the floor, was a permanent device for the serious "brain-working and sedentary people."[29]

Sporting goods dealers provided alternatives for those uninterested in or not partial to machines. In 1866, Peck and Snyder of New York, one of the largest manufacturers and distributors of athletic and gymnastic gear in the nineteenth century, offered a "complete home gymnasium" which included

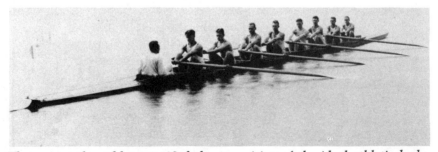

These muscular athletes typified the new vision of the ideal athletic body, a marked contrast from the lean "greyhound look" of the 1860s and 1870s. Photograph, American, ca. 1900.

bars, ropes, rings, and weights. Many of their competitors, such as "Bornstein, King of Clubs," of 24 Ann Street in New York, undercut Peck and Snyder on such items as Indian clubs, dumbbells, and trapezes, selling the latter for a dollar, as opposed to $2.75 for the smallest Peck and Snyder model. Few, however, could match the breadth of the goods offered by the large firms, which were more quickly able to adapt to changing tastes in exercise and athletics.

Lewis and many of his followers were advocates of light exercises, designed to increase stamina and flexibility. While admitting "that no man can be flexible without a good degree of strength," Lewis noted that "it is not . . . that kind of strength involved in great lifting." He thought heavy weights "spoiled" a gymnast's muscles and compared heavy lifters to the "india-rubber men" of the circuses: Each were "mischievous extremes."[30]

Lewis's opinions were difficult to impress upon followers of the great strongmen of the era. Because they were such spectacles—either in the circus or in the gymnasium—body builders attracted attention and admiration. Perhaps the most important of these figures in the 1860s was George Windship, who upon entering Harvard in 1853 was the second smallest member of his class. In a scenario that was to become a classic in the marketing of body building, Windship was allegedly humiliated by a campus bully. He decided to vindicate himself by weight training, which he began in earnest. He entered Harvard Medical School in 1854 and

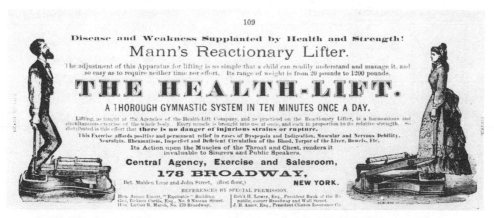

Parlor exercise machines, promoted as a cure for nearly all diseases, were a big business by the 1850s. Advertisement, New York, N.Y., ca. 1860.

Exercise devotees could purchase all the gear they needed to set up a gymnasium in their homes. Advertisement, American, ca. 1900.

soon became known as the "Roxbury Hercules." At five-foot-seven and 143 pounds, he was able to lift a thousand pounds off the ground, gaining notoriety along with his medical degree. An eloquent lecturer, the herculean physician attracted a huge following, and, according to Dudley Sargent, professor of physical education at Harvard, "lifting machines, sprang up in parlors and offices and schools everywhere" as a consequence of Windship's example.[31]

Dio Lewis used Windship as his example of what not to be, stating that "Heenan [a famous boxer] is a very strong man, can strike a blow twice as hard as Windship but cannot lift seven hundred pounds nor put up an eighty-pound dumb bell." But for other commentators, Windship's name was synonymous with body building, health, and great strength. *Harper's Weekly* in 1860 ironically used the same boxer, Heenan, as a starting point for a positive analysis of Windship's significance. "The Homeric combat between Heenan and Sayers set all our youth a-dreaming about physical training," the magazine observed, but it stopped short of approving of boxing by reminding readers of their conviction that "other gymnastic sports are better" for health and strength. They favored the activities of "Dr. Winship [*sic*], the strong New Englander," who could "make any man strong, and in many cases . . . cure him of disease." Many commentators thought Windship's forty-minutes-per-day routine was a good idea for Americans because, according to *Harper's Weekly,* "our race is deteriorating, especially in the large cities. No one who compares the young men of New York or Boston with foreigners of the same age can deny the truth of the statement."[32]

Weight lifting and the body-building examples of Windship and, later, such showmen as Eugene Sandow helped focus attention on the physical condition of American men. Physicians, most of whom were men, spent much of their time criticizing women for their dress and their slavery to "fashion." Men of the working class in particular were chided for their alleged penchant for strong drink, and all smokers were criticized. But men did not wear corsets or tight, high-heeled shoes, and they seemed to dress in ways that would not unduly expose certain parts of their bodies to cold while overheating others. Yet the feats of body builders such as Windship and even boxers such as Heenan helped establish a standard of athletic performance and strength that few men could equal. Whether or not Lewis approved of it, strength was a positive male attribute in American culture. Because it was associated with power and the implicit act of violence, it fit perfectly with a culture that had been in and out of wars and skirmishes since 1607. Moreover, Windship's brand of "physical culture," as advocates called these activities, was something in which women—allegedly because of their constitution and reproductive system—could not participate. More important, they were not allowed to do so. Perhaps men thought that by possessing great strength they would be forever superior—at least in one respect—to women and, perhaps more important, to foreigners.

Windship operated a large gymnasium in Boston, where he situated both his medical practice and his teachings on "Health, Strength, and Development." He also sold gymnastic apparatus, including the "Windship Patent Graduating Dumb-Bell." Though he operated a "separate apartment for ladies," it is clear that Windship's primary concern was for men.[33]

Windship maintained close ties with another pioneer, Dudley A. Sargent (1849–1924), who was altering the methods by which Americans learned about and took their exercise. A native of Maine, Sargent had been an acrobat and weight lifter since he was fourteen and became the director of the Bowdoin College gymnasium in 1869. Two years later he entered the college as a freshman and began to divide his time during the school year between Bowdoin and Yale, where he introduced his methods during winter terms. Upon graduation from Bowdoin in 1875, he assumed the dual role of instructor in gymnastics and first-year medical student at Yale. He received his M.D. in 1878. One year later, after operating his own "Hygienic Institute and School of Physical Culture" in New York City, Sargent became assistant professor of physical training (Harvard's first) and director of the Hemenway gymnasium.[34]

Sargent used pulley and weight machines and "mimetic exercises," which duplicated the activities of certain laborers and sportsmen, to build up students. Hundreds came to Cambridge to his teacher training programs. His ideas and programs were made famous by William Blaikie in his popular books *How to Get Strong and How to Stay So* (1879) and *Sound Bodies for Our Boys and Girls* (1884). Although advocates of physical education had been crusading continually since the 1830s, and although some efforts had been made to train instructors, as Lewis had in the 1860s, it was not until Sargent's school in the 1880s that physical education was truly born. In part Sargent's success was a result of his own ability to define clearly what physical education was and why it was necessary, but it was also a function of his concentration on the entire student body, rather than on a few athletes.

The roots of baseball, cricket, and other organized team and individual sporting activities go back into the early nineteenth century. But baseball, football, track and field, rowing, boxing, tennis, and golf, as well as organized gymnastics, attained broad popularity only after 1860, when demographic, economic, and ideological conditions flowed together in the right proportions.

Football, tennis, golf, rowing, and, to some extent, track and field were originally associated with the well-to-do in the nineteenth century because of the lead colleges and universities had taken in fielding organized teams. The growth of collegiate athletics was itself a result of the efforts of physical education instructors, coaches, and eager alumni who in one way or another envisioned "manly sport" as a way to develop the strength of mind and body that would aid American men as they endeavored to meet the challenges of a new corporate industrial order. Even though baseball, boxing, and football were extremely popular among the working classes soon after their

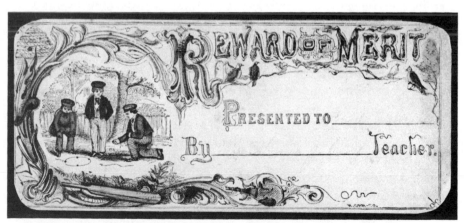

Cricket was a popular game in the middle decades of the nineteenth century. Athletics and hard work were visually linked on this "reward of merit" by the presence of the beehive in the upper left corner and the cricket bat and ball in the lower left border. N. Orr and Company, American, ca. 1850.

introduction to Americans, for the ever-increasing number of collegiate men, the games were considered an ideological statement. In the confines of the university yard, sport was an idea as well as an activity, embracing more than the punches and knockouts, the pitches and hits, or the tackles and touchdowns of the sandlot or the professional arena.

As the dean of American physical educators from the 1880s until his retirement in 1919, Sargent worked hard to develop and maintain an amateur code of sportsmanship as an integral part of collegiate athletics. His counterparts among the coaches and politicians—he trained Harvard undergraduates Theodore Roosevelt and Henry Cabot Lodge—saw in sport desirable values for a nation simultaneously beginning a journey to world prominence while encumbered with a declining physical and mental condition. Sport not only developed teamwork skills and physical toughness, but it promoted the desire and will to win. The genteel values of sportsmanship were never to be forgotten in striving for victory, but winning was a critically important result in the preparation of the social, economic, and political leaders of the new age. Sportsmanship was also thought to be an indicator of class distinction, since the student body at colleges large enough to field teams was composed almost entirely of the children of elites. Thus it became a value that differentiated between collegiate athletes and other participants—the professional and noncollegiate players. Untainted by money, collegiate athletes allegedly played to win within boundaries of fair play they assumed were identical to the parameters of the college grounds. They defined sportmanship as an elite characteristic. Rather than functioning only as an escape from the cares of life or as a chance to "play out" issues of suppressed confrontation and inequality, sport for the collegian—and later for the high school student—was preparation for life.

The will to win and the rise of field sports did not meet with unqualified acceptance in the decades between the war and the 1890s. Dio Lewis was not interested in athletics and field sports, and D.G.M. Schreber, whose "Pangymnastikon" was translated by Lewis and bound with *The New Gymnastics,* regarded field sports as "primitive exercises" with no real use in the effort to maintain health. Sargent continually criticized intercollegiate sports, which he thought were emphasized at the expense of the lesser athletes among the students and chiefly for the fuller development of first-team members. The successful players were too single-minded and were uninterested in a more general athletic training that would make them healthier, if not better, oarsmen, tackles, or hitters. He favored a situation like that at the Fort Edward, New York, Institute, where both faculty and students played together on an almost daily basis. In 1868, for example, Adam Clark Works, a professor of chemistry and natural sciences, played football in the college's "arena" for forty-five to ninety minutes on most days, usually finishing just before tea at five-fifteen P.M. He noted in his diary that he "played too long and too hard." Collegiate sport in the late nineteenth century was a struggle between physical educators and the administration, alumni, and coaches who were hired to win rather than develop all-around, healthy young men. The controversy was lively and vocal throughout the era, but by the 1890s the philosophy of winning began to dominate collegiate sporting activity.[35]

Some of the sports that were ultimately identified with schools and colleges in the late nineteenth century had originally been part of the culture of other groups in America. The German *Turnverein*, freed of their earlier political associations, were the most obvious nonelite source for strenuous gymnastics, which became popular again in the 1880s. Track and field events, as we have come to define them, were originally parts of the highland games that many of the Scottish Caledonian clubs brought with them to the United States. In November 1867 the games held in New York City included three-hundred- and six-hundred-yard races, the "hop, step and jump," and "putting the stone." Earlier in the year the Scottish games at Jones Wood in New York included these events as well as "throwing the heavy hammer," the "running leap," the "running high leap," the "standing high leap," and "the pole vault."[36]

The ideals of sportsmanship and of all-around performance and health urged by such physical educators as Sargent were somewhat compromised by professionalism and the public's obvious love of the contest. Endurance walking was one of the most popular spectacles of the postwar decades, and the exploits of Edward P. Weston, "Weston the Pedestrian," attracted attention as much for his abilities as a walker as for the amount of money wagered on his tests. In 1867 Weston sought to win a ten-thousand-dollar bet on a walk from Portland, Maine, to Chicago. "It is noteworthy," wrote *Harper's Weekly*, "that all along his route crowds of citizens have greeted and encouraged him. . . . No feat of strength or endurance," the magazine rhapsodized, "has ever attracted so much attention in this or any other country."[37]

The same 1867 issue of *Harper's Weekly* that detailed Weston's achievements included another article on competitive sport, in this case a sculling

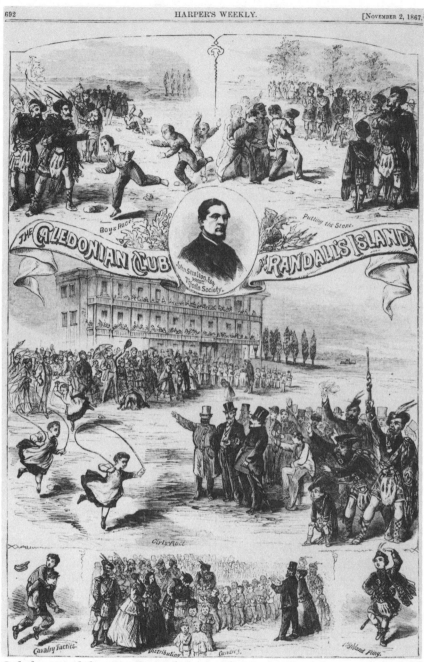

Caledonian clubs were Scottish fraternal organizations that regularly held games very much like modern track and field meets. "Caledonian Club, Randall's Island," illustration from Harper's Weekly, *November 2, 1867, p. 692.*

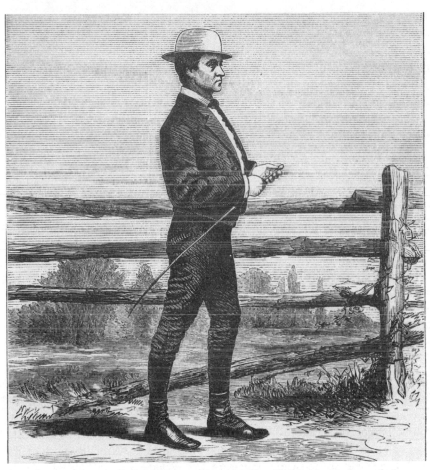

This picture of "Edward Payson Weston, the Pedestrian" showed the nation's foremost race-walker, whose feats of speed and endurance helped make race-walking a popular spectator and participatory sport in the post–Civil War era. Illustration from Harper's Weekly, *November 16, 1867, p. 724.*

race in Pittsburgh. Unlike collegiate rowing, this "five mile sculling contest between Harry Coulter . . . and John Merkel . . . [was] for a purse of two thousand dollars." Coulter took the cash.[38] Playing for pay and wagers was an antithetical philosophy of sport from that of the collegian, and it has been extraordinarily popular from the 1860s to the present day. But the pressure to win ultimately made professionals an important force in the coaching ranks of the colleges, and in this case, elite culture took its cue from popular culture. The professional's concentration not only on one sport but also—in the case of team sports—on one aspect of the game was offensive to physical educators, but it was attractive to both the coaches of collegiate teams and the majority of the American populace.

The relationship between the colleges and the professional—who was most often not of the same socioeconomic background as the college man—was a complex one. Boxing and baseball in particular were working-class sports that were quickly accepted by the colleges. Football began as a college sport, but workers quickly began to play it. Elite acceptance of the substance of boxing and baseball—without the class associations and the money—was made easier by the growing conviction that America's "best" was in need of some sort of renewal. After the Civil War the comparison of the neurasthenic effects of sedentary jobs with the healthy effects of manual work (especially that of the nation's founders) suggested to the elite that some working-class activities might help prepare them better for the future. This sentiment was not in any sense a nostalgia for or a yearning to be workers; it was rooted instead in the conviction that elites could maintain their position in a society as they knew it only through a liberal dose of the perceived vitality of working-class sport and its attitude toward winning. Thus boxing, shorn of the "taint" of professionalism, became the "manly art of self-defense"—with gloves, not bare knuckles—moving literally and figuratively from the public space of the championship ring to a socially restricted arena—the gymnasiums of Harvard, Yale, and other colleges. Baseball likewise became an important collegiate sport, usually shorn of its endless outfield space by the fences of the college playing field or yard.

Theodore Roosevelt was important to this growing acceptance of professionalism and "manly sport." At Harvard, he had overcome asthma and his small size to become an avid boxer, wrestler, tennis player, and all-around athletic participant. He kept up his athletic and sporting endeavors throughout his public life, becoming a symbol for the attitudes that took over sport and society in the 1890s. The foundation for Roosevelt's symbolic popularity, however, was laid in the postwar era, as sport and culture became more and more entwined. Sport was at least as important as the proselytizing of physical educators in developing popular enthusiasm for exercise and health.

The most popular sport of the postwar era was baseball. Amateur teams

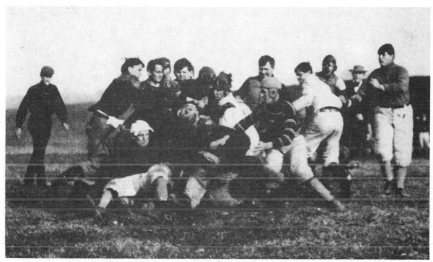

Above: This rare turn-of-the-century action photograph of a football game demonstrates the sport's roots in English rugby football. The "healthy barbarism" that advocates favored is also evident, as are the hazards of getting caught at the bottom of the pile. Stereograph, American, 1880–1910.

Below: A coalyard football game, Pennsylvania, ca. 1900. Football may have begun as an upper class elite sport, played in colleges, but the working class soon adopted the game. The only equipment required was a ball.

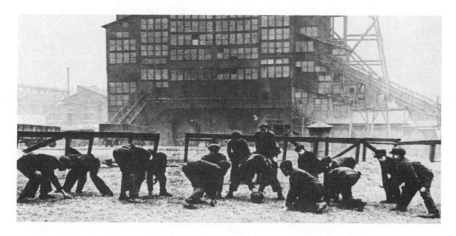

had popped up all over the country by the outbreak of the war, and some soldiers reported playing baseball games during their off hours. In 1865 *Harper's Weekly* had been moved to state, "There is no nobler or manlier game than base-ball, and the more it is cultivated the better the country." By 1867, the game was so popular that even "the little town of Lafayette, Indiana, boasts three clubs, each possessing a championship nine." *Harper's Weekly* observed in August 1868, "The field-sportsmen are in the field in great numbers this year, and thus far several interesting base-ball and cricket matches have taken place." One such contest might have been the baseball "match game back of the Institute between the Institute Club and the Saratoga Club" that Adam C. Works described in his diary entry for May 23, 1868. He proudly noted that the "Institute Club won 21 to 18." (Cricket was popular from the 1850s through 1870, but declined rapidly thereafter, unable to compete with "the national game.")[39]

The Cincinnati Red-Stockings are generally recognized to have been the first professional baseball team in the United States, and they achieved great fame in 1869—the year they were constituted—because of their success while on tour. In July 1869 the team defeated the Brooklyn Mutuals and New York Atlantics on successive days and emerged from its trip as the unofficial but popularly acknowledged national champions.[40]

Some physical educators were troubled by professionalism and spectator sports because the advanced skills of the professional might lead amateurs to attempt feats that led to injuries. In 1868 a columnist in *Harper's Weekly* criticized "something too much of gymnastics," even as he or she admitted that the activity "undoubtedly conduced to a diminution of certain bad habits." The problem seemed to be activities that were "attractive merely because [they were] difficult and dangerous." Professionalism was, for this writer, fine for those trained and proficient, such as the acrobats in one of the nation's most popular spectacles, the circus, but it was not for everyone. Overemphasis on sport was "an evil into which a great many young men of America are running at present with headlong speed and injurious zeal," according to some critics. Horace Greeley had made an impression on the media when he "announced that, if appointed umpire in a base-ball match, he would certainly give the 'champion ball' to the 'nine' who lost the game, as their defective playing at outdoor sports was in some measure proof that they were good husbands, and brothers, and sons, with a commendable love

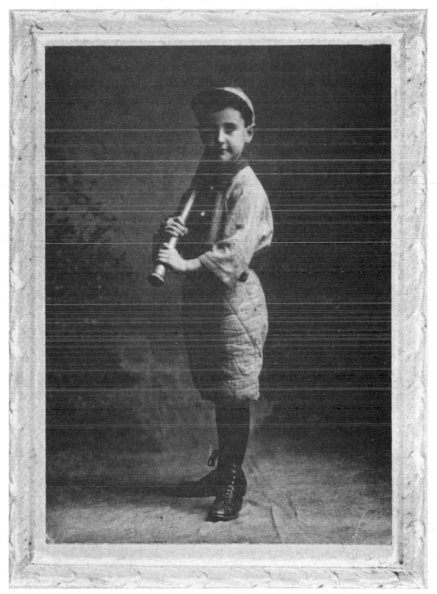

"John L. Parker as a Texas Leaguer": The Texas League was already a famous enough minor league to have entered the language as shorthand for a youngster beginning to play the national game. Photograph, J. E. Beach, Bryan, Ohio, ca. 1900.

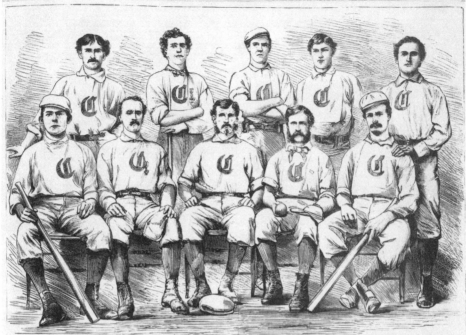

THE PICKED NINE OF THE "RED STOCKING" BASE-BALL CLUB, CINCINNATI, OHIO.—PHOT. BY F. L. HUFF, 244 BROAD STREET, NEWARK, N.J.—[SEE PAGE 422.]

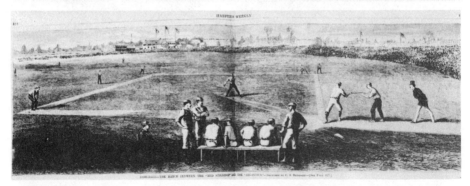

The Red Stockings were the most famous and arguably the best baseball team in 1870. They traveled throughout the country, taking on the best nines in various cities. Above: "The Picked Nine of the 'Red Stocking' Base-Ball Club, Cincinnati, Ohio." Below: "Baseball—The Match Between the 'Red Stockings' and the 'Atlantics.'" Both illustrations from Harper's Weekly, July 3, 1870, p. 425.

of home and home pleasures." The sports "widow" or "widower" is thus as old as the Civil War era.[41]

Advocates of physical training and sports usually warned enthusiasts to stay within their capabilities and cautioned athletes against overtaxing their systems or becoming completely exhausted. But for all their warnings, both the proselytizer and the participant operated from the same fundamental assumption about the human body. The pessimism of the ubiquitous critique of Americans' health was counterbalanced by the conviction that human effort could have a positive impact on the condition of the body and the mind. The optimists shared the conviction that "the physical organism is susceptible of indefinite improvement; that it can be made, by certain hygienic processes, so vigorous and resistant, that amid diseases and dangers it may pass through the fire unscathed."[42]

By 1890 the best example of the individual who had molded his or her body was probably Eugene Sandow, the great showman and physical specimen whom Sargent called "the most wonderful specimen of man I have ever seen." Sandow, a Prussian body builder of great accomplishment, popularized muscle building in ways even the great George Windship never imagined. He marketed photographs of himself (sometimes clad only in a leaf) and wrote or had ghostwritten a number of body-building guides. Sandow's legitimacy as model of the human form was more than simple pinup sexuality: he was the best example of someone who had assumed positive control of his own body. Moreover, he not only performed feats of strength, but he also preached the gospel of health, in his books if not in his prodigious eating and drinking behavior. By 1890 he and boxer John L. Sullivan and wrestlers William Muldoon and George Hackenschmidt were probably the most famous athletes in the United States.[43]

The heroes of exercise seem to have been larger than life in their time, and, by most criteria of measurement they were. Still, Dudley Sargent cast the longest shadow in the development of gymnastics and calisthenics and the rise of sport. Among the students he influenced both at Harvard and beyond its walls were most of the prime movers in the causes of fitness and athleticism from the 1860s to the 1930s. Roosevelt and Lodge grafted his ideas onto politics and social structure in the years after 1890. R. Tait MacKenzie, the director of physical education at the University of Pennsylvania, was a student of Sargent's, and Edward Hartwell, director of physical education at Johns Hopkins University, was a convert to the Sargent system.

Luther Gulick, the man who transformed the Young Men's Christian Association into a sports and fitness organization, had also been one of Sargent's students at Harvard, and used the idea of an inseparable link between a sound mind and sound body from the pagan Greeks; still, he asserted that the spiritual whole to which the YMCA was striving was a Christian notion. (The Greeks were pardoned for their paganism, Gulick said, because there had been no Christ.) The Greek origins of this fusion allowed Gulick and others to praise the nearly nude images of Sandow and other exercise enthusiasts, since they were often posed in classical—if scanty —garb.

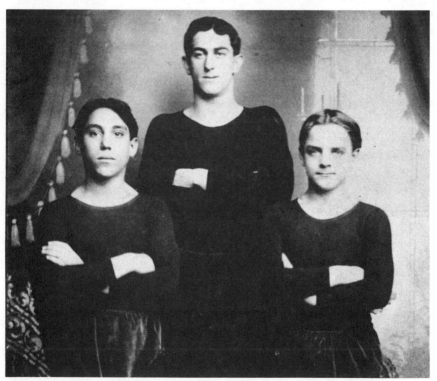

Boxing began as a rough-and-tumble working-class sport and spectacle that quickly attracted a following in colleges and YMCA gymnasiums throughout the country. Young men took up the "manly art of self-defense" to prove both their manhood and their mettle. Photograph, George C. Blakely, Middletown, Conn., ca. 1900.

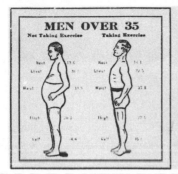
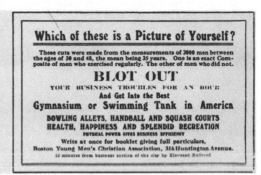

The YMCA promoted itself to a broad spectrum of Americans, from young boys and men who might be kept off the streets and prepared for manhood to businessmen and college men who sought the relief that sports and fitness brought. Advertisement, American, ca. 1900.

Gulick and other devotees of "muscular Christianity" believed that sport and physical training would dissipate or rechannel the energy that could direct young men in particular to crime. In 1861 Thomas Wentworth Higginson had argued that "physical exercises give to energy and daring a legitimate channel, supply the place of war, gambling, licentiousness, highway robbery and office-seeking. . . . It gives an innocent answer to that first demand for evening excitement which perils the soul of the homeless boy in the seductive city." "Muscular Christianity" and sport had taken the place of the frontier, which Frederick Jackson Turner had identified as the outlet through which the pressure of urban populations was eased. In 1893 Turner would formally assert that the frontier had disappeared, and such organizations as the YMCA came to be thought of as critical to the maintenance of order. The YMCA took the responsibility for young urban men that the colleges had assumed for gentlemen of the elite. Yet YMCAs clearly served a broad spectrum of the population, college graduates and the poor alike, and they therefore functioned as purveyors to society as a whole of the collegiate ideology of physical and moral training.[44]

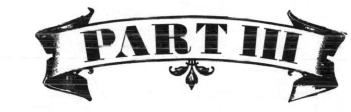

PART III

REGENERATION, 1890~1940

CHAPTER NINE

LIVING THE
STRENUOUS LIFE

I n 1911 Horace Fletcher, who was best known as a nutritionist and health reform activist, was appointed to the National Council of the Boy Scouts of America. In a letter to James West, then the BSA's chief executive, Fletcher expressed his "utmost approval of the aims of the organization" and recounted some of his own experiences with athletics and social policy. "At the time of the Sand Lot Riots in San Francisco," he explained, "I was president of the famous Olympic Gymnastic Athletic Club . . . of that city, and raised a company of athletes and gymnasts within the club which was immediately added to the National Guard of the State."[1]

Fletcher's actions were not exceptional for his time. In many states the National Guard had been formed to combat and control labor unrest and other violence that had been steadily growing from the late 1870s through the turn of the century. The association of gymnastics and athletics with the maintenance of order was no longer a new idea at the turn of the century, but it took on added significance as middle-class and wealthy Americans tried to respond

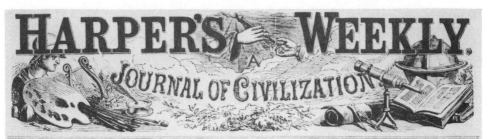

HARPER'S WEEKLY.

A JOURNAL OF CIVILIZATION

Vol. XXI.—No. 1076.]   NEW YORK, SATURDAY, AUGUST 11, 1877.   [WITH A SUPPLEMENT.
PRICE TEN CENTS.

Entered according to Act of Congress, in the Year 1877, by Harper & Brothers, in the Office of the Librarian of Congress, at Washington.

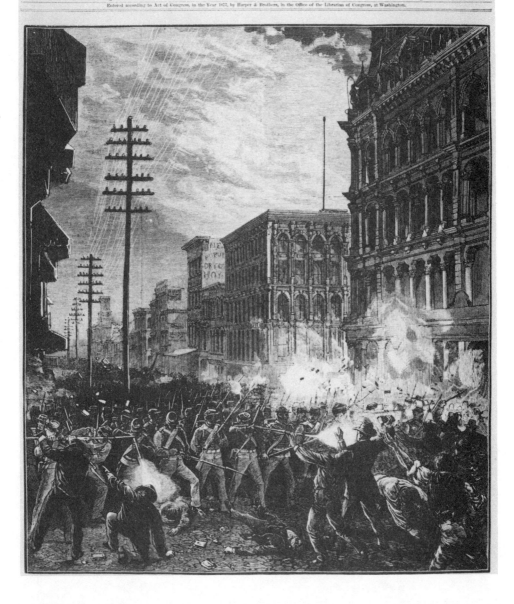

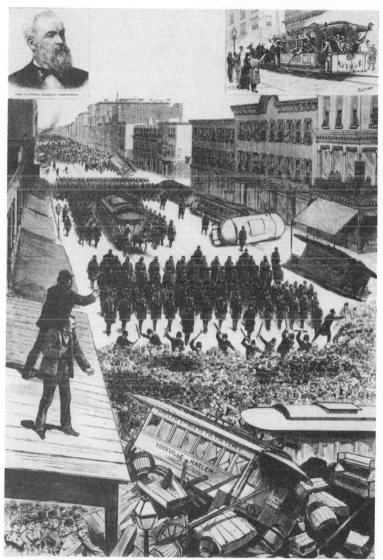

Strikes and riots rocked urban America in 1877 and again in 1886. Left: "The Great Strike—The Sixth Maryland Regiment Fighting Its Way Through Baltimore," Harper's Weekly, *August 11, 1877, front page. Right: "The Great Strike of Street Railway Employees in New York City, March 3–5,"* Frank Leslie's Illustrated Weekly, *March 13, 1886, p. 57.*

to the profound social and cultural crisis that had been in the making for decades but that seemed to have burst upon them in the 1890s.

The genesis of this upheaval was the depression of 1873–1878 and the bitter, often violent confrontations between capital and labor that marked the period. In 1877 violent strikes between railroad workers and management broke out almost simultaneously across the country, a phenomenon that seemed to indicate collusion among the strikers. Sensationalist newspaper accounts of the pitched battles between strikers and state militias were often accompanied by engravings that showed great masses of people marching against less numerous policemen or militiamen while railroad cars and buildings blazed in the background: visions of society run amok, of class war.

The labor strife of the seventies did not recede as the economy improved. Strikes and violence were common occurrences in the Pennsylvania coal fields throughout the 1880s, most of the activity having been initiated by such groups as the Molly Maguires, who allegedly plotted the wholesale assassination of management. At first immigrants were used by the owners to break the strikes, but soon they too organized into unions. Coal workers, many of whom were Hungarian, struck in 1886; their action was labeled the work of foreign radicals. Even more ominous was the strike of street railway workers in New York City in the same year. Europe's riotous disarray had come to America.

Until the 1880s—or so critics of the "new immigration" from southern and eastern Europe liked to think—those who came to America were "the best of the lot," hardy souls who were steeled first by their passage over the Atlantic, and then by the experience of life on the frontier. In his introduction to *The Descent of Man* (1871), Charles Darwin had noted that "the wonderful progress of the United States as well as the character of the people are the results of natural selection; for the more energetic, restless, and courageous men from all parts of Europe have emigrated during the last ten or twelve generations to that great country and have there succeeded best." D. H. Wheeler, in an 1873 *Popular Science Monthly* article entitled "Natural Selection and Politics," expressed a common if simplistic optimism: "History shows us a struggle of races," Wheeler wrote, "and we who survive are ready enough to believe that the strongest survive because they are the best." Anglo-Saxon culture was thought vital enough to absorb the best aspects of foreign cultures, while maintaining its essential character.[2]

The "more energetic, restless, and courageous" men and women Darwin had observed had, by 1899, become "beaten men from beaten races; representing the worst failures in the struggle for existence," as prominent economist Francis A. Walker argued. "They have none of the ideas and aptitudes which . . . belong to those who are descended from the tribes that met under the oak trees of old Germany to make laws and choose chieftains."[3] A generation of American historians who trained in the 1880s had traced the history of American governmental institutions to thirteenth-century England and the struggle between the knights and King John for the Magna Carta, and ultimately to the Black Forest of Germany, where tribes of Germans congregated and produced the "germs" of democracy.[4] By finding the origins of American institutions in England and Germany, historians not only identified their roots but also excluded all others, not just from cultural traditions but, they hoped, from any claim to legitimate governmental power. In his two-volume study, *The Life and Letters of John Hay* (1915), William Roscoe Thayer characterized the settlers of the Old Northwest (the present upper midwestern states) as vastly superior to the "Irish bogtrotter, [who was] as illiterate and bigoted as the Calabrian peasant or the Russian serf . . . the pitiable offscourings from the capitals of Europe who in the late nineteenth century were seeking American shores."[5]

This sense of exclusiveness in part explains the surge in nationalistic fervor and popular interest in American history that occurred in the late nineteenth century. Fueled first in mid 1870s by the Centennial celebration of 1876, the craze for colonial and Revolutionary War relics and information reached an almost fever pitch by the 1890s. Scores of local and regional histories of the ancient towns of the East Coast were published from the mid 1880s through the 1920s. Americans bought new "colonial"-style furnishings by the roomful, as well as foodstuffs, carpet sweepers, and just about everything else that had *Colonial* as a brand name.

They also formed a variety of genealogical organizations, which tied membership to an ability to trace one's lineage back to the Revolutionary armies, specific political groups (such as the Society of Cincinnati), or passage on the *Mayflower*. Americans of Anglo-Saxon descent busily plowed through archives in libraries all over the country, hoping to establish their connection to the proper sort of American described by such popular fiction writers as Winston Churchill, Maurice Thompson, and Paul Leicester Ford, whose novels contained detailed genealogical tracings of the old heroes and heroines and thinly veiled hostility to immigrants.[6]

The Haymarket bombings of 1886 fused together middle-class fears of workers and immigrants, identifying those involved in union activities and violence as somehow not American, whatever their country of birth. In *Public Opinion,* a business-oriented periodical, one writer warned of imminent disaster. "I am no race-worshipper," he stated, "but . . . if the master race of this continent is subordinated to or overrun with the communistic and revolutionary races, it will be in grave danger of social disaster." The stampede image touched one of the great fears of the late nineteenth century: the presence of great numbers—masses—of people who did not comprehend established American values. They were arriving on American shores in greater numbers than ever before, and at a time when changing social, demographic, and even environmental conditions seemed to make immigrants capable of challenging the established American power structure.

In 1886, the same year as the "anarchist" Haymarket bombings, Thomas P. Gill had written an essay for the *North American Review* that was full of foreboding for its readers, who were primarily middle-class and elite Americans. "The public domain in the United States is now exhausted," Gill warned in "Landlordism in America." The significance of Gill's observation—which Frederick Jackson Turner built upon in his paper of 1893, "The Significance of the Frontier in American History"—was that newcomers to the American soil would no longer have the opportunity to experience the rigors of farm and frontier life. Neither would those adversely affected by the overcrowding of cities be able to release this pressure through the "safety valve" of moving west. Moreover, the industrialized economy had resulted in large cities much like the "capitals of Europe" Thayer had decried—dens of filth and crime so intolerable that immigration to the United States seemed to many the only remaining hope. These newcomers, and their allies among the working class and the corrupt city politicians (most of whom were devoted to the Democratic party) could "overrun" the "master race" by the sheer force of their numbers.[7]

The threat to established American institutions was not solely an external one. The 1880 census had revealed a steadily declining birth rate among Anglo-Saxon families throughout the nineteenth century, committing, in the terminology of the day, "race suicide." "It is perfectly clear," wrote the Reverend John Ellis in *The Deterioration of the Puritan Stock and Its Causes* (1884), "that without a radical change in the religious ideas, education, habits, and customs of the natives, the present populations and their descendants will not rule . . . a single generation." In 1901 Edwin A. Ross raised the specter of race suicide as he berated Americans for their neglect of familial duties, their neurasthenic urban lives, and general physical debility. Twenty years later, Irving Fisher, a distinguished professor of political economy at Yale, still worried that white Americans would "quietly lie down and let some other race run over us."[8]

The question revolved not around the identity of those threatening the system, but around how to combat the problem. The notion that the "Puritan stock" was fundamentally superior and inherently good persisted, but it was a dwindling and unhealthy stock. The formulation of the race suicide theory and an increasing emphasis on the study of heredity (in particular, eugenics, or selective breeding) helped focus American concerns for the vitality of the nation on the health of both men and women. Women were a special concern because they bore, nursed, and raised children. "We want to have body as well as mind," wrote T. S. Clouston in *Female Education from a Medical Point of View* (1882), "otherwise degeneration of the race is inevitable." Eight years later, the much more popular *Ladies' Home Calisthenics* (1890) began with the statement, "The health of coming generations and the future of a nation depend in great part upon the girls. They are to be the coming mothers; and, as such, obligations for the formation of a new race are incumbent upon them. These obligations they can by no means fulfill unless they are sound in body and in mind." Mary Wood-Allen, author of many popular advice books for young women, maintained that "each girl's health is a matter of national and racial importance" because "evil traits and tendencies of mind or morals are transmissible."[9]

As schoolgirls, women had been able to participate in calisthenic exercises —sometimes with men—from middle of the nineteenth century. Calisthenic guides written specifically for women abounded in the latter years of the century, in part as a response to the concern for women's health. One writer traded upon turn-of-the-century American admiration for things and designs of the Japanese and expressed the hope that "the science of *jui-jitsu*" would show "the path for the new physical woman to pursue." The "new physical woman" was the reformer's dream—the woman who finally rejected corsets, ate sensibly, worked hard at becoming an athlete, and bore a large family.[10]

In the 1890s athletic opportunities expanded beyond tennis, badminton, and croquet to include basketball (especially at midwestern colleges), golf,

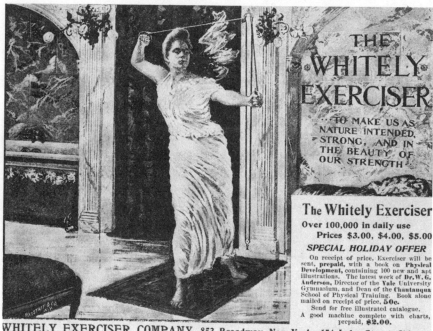

Women had been encouraged to participate in calisthenics since the 1850s, and by the turn of the century, magazines published for women regularly carried advertisements for the health-conscious reader. In the privacy of her dressing room or bath, any woman could be beautiful. Advertisement from The Ladies' Home Journal, *December 1897, p. 43.*

swimming, cycling, and some track and field. The "national game" of baseball, football, and boxing were too strenuous for women, but rowing and canoeing were popular activities. Only those sports which invigorated women's constitutions without endangering their reproductive capacities were considered appropriate. Exercise enthusiasts also asserted that properly supervised sport might help delay a young woman's sexual curiosity and awakening, a situation that many physical educators, physiologists, and parents thought desirable.

The nineteenth-century sportswoman was not encouraged to compete as her male counterparts were, but to strive against herself using her own performance as an index of health. Colleges such as Smith and Mount Holyoke in the East and the Universities of Minnesota and Wisconsin in

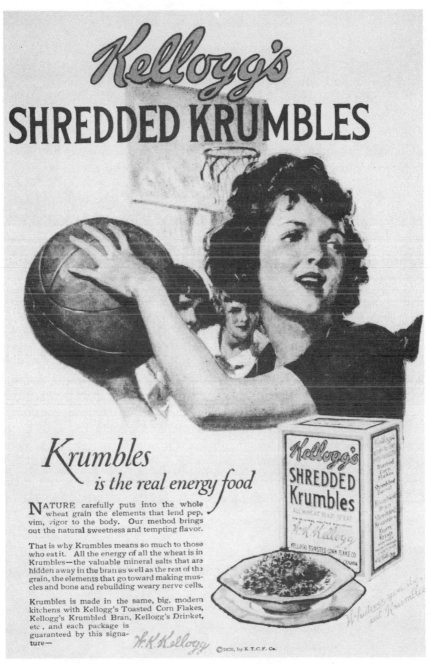

Physical fitness and health food advocates were among the first to support a more equal position for women in American society, even if most saw dietary reform mainly as a vehicle to prepare for their traditional role as mothers. Advertisement, American, ca. 1920.

the Midwest had active teams, but there was no intercollegiate play. High schools established programs for their students but discouraged interscholastic games or rivalries. Even when two schools met, the teams were mixed and divided, the assumption being that competition—playing to win—was unladylike; it might lead to behavior that might be appropriate in the business world, but would certainly be unfit for the home, where women were thought to belong. (That practice continued into the 1970s at some private schools.) Yet for all this aversion to the aggressiveness of the ideology of winning, physical educators justified the need for exercise and sport as a way to better develop women for the struggle for survival. "Life is one long competition, so why not prepare for it in the gymnasium," wrote Bryn Mawr's director of physical culture, Louisa Smith.[11]

Collegiate sports for women were an experience of the few. Marriage was still considered a more important goal than education, and even those with enough money were not necessarily convinced that postsecondary training was important or even proper for a young woman. The popular breakthrough into athleticism for women came not at school, but on the roadway. The "wheel," as the bicycle was called in the 1890s, did more to engage women in health-related exercise than any other single activity or invention.

The bicycle appeared on the American scene in the late 1880s and became a "craze" by the 1890s. "The present and steadily increasing popularity of the 'bipendaliferous wheel,'" wrote a columnist in *Demorest's Monthly* in 1887, "that is to its enthusiastic advocates 'a thing of beauty and a joy forever,' . . . promises to be the universally accepted steed of the

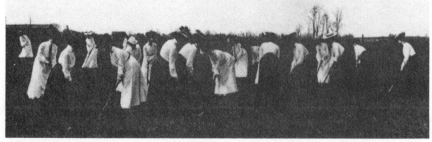

Women learning the basics of field hockey at Hood College. Many women's colleges adopted their male counterparts' enthusiasm for sport, if not for "healthy barbarism." Even in competition decorum was important.

future." The early "celeripedes" of the 1830s—two wheels connected by a bar—had no pedaling or braking mechanisms and were dangerous, if exciting for the thrill seeker. Crank-driven velocipedes were introduced in the 1860s, but like "celeripedes," they were expensive and exhausting. More people—men especially—took up the bicycle with the introduction of the "ordinary" in the 1870s. With its large front wheel and small back wheel, riding an ordinary was popular sport for those who could master it. But it too had no brakes; its large front wheel—sometimes as much as five feet in diameter—made it difficult to control, and a spill was a nasty experience. Few if any women rode them. The "safety" bicycle, with both wheels the same size, was designed and produced in great numbers by 1890s. With the addition of pneumatic tires, mass-produced for the first time in 1889, the bicycle assumed its present form.[12]

For many young men and women, to own a bicycle was to realize a dream. Harriet Baillie of Massachusetts recorded in her diary for 1894 that "Russell [her brother] and I each have a safety. I have dreamed about it ever since they first appeared."[13] Bicycles were not cheap by the standards of the 1890s: a "Crawford" cost $60 to $75 in 1895. Few members of the working class owned one. Still, unlike gymnastics or sports, which were too vigorous or expensive for many people, almost anyone who could find the money— men, women, older, thin, or overweight people—could ride a bicycle, which in part explains its popularity. Bicycles also gave young people mobility. Bicycle posters often subtly promoted this feature, sometimes showing a young man and woman on their bikes without the presence of other people, surely an attraction for courting couples.

The "wheel" was also good for one's health. Bicycle exercise in the open air was considered particularly beneficent, and both advertisers and health advocates seized upon this aspect of the bicycle almost immediately. In 1893 the Columbia Manufacturing Company advertised its purposes in lofty terms of economic realism. "It is our business to do good and make money," their advertisements proclaimed, "to preach the glorious gospel of Outdoors —to supply the vehicle of the healthful happiness—to suggest that everyone join the bicycle army of vigorous health."[14]

Like nearly every other panacea of the nineteenth century—water, calomel, gymnastics, electricity—the wheel was allegedly able to cure everything from neurasthenia to consumption. In the June 1885 issue of *Outing*, Minna Gould Smith endorsed cycling as a great curative for a woman suffering from the ailments variously categorized as "exhaustion," "nervous-

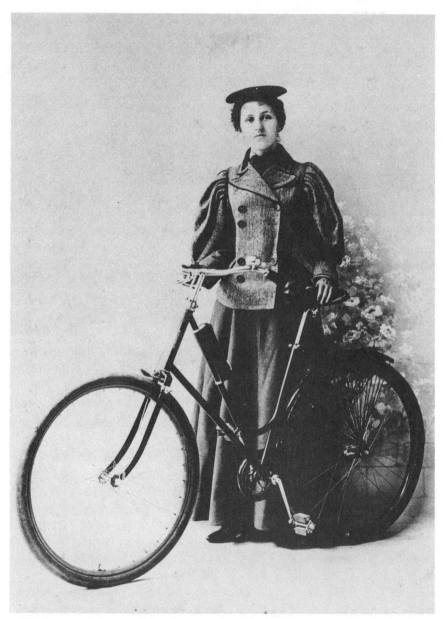

Glorious mobility and freedom made owning a bike the dream of men and women alike and a sign of progress for most advocates of fitness. Cabinet photograph, Jackson, Norwalk, Conn., ca. 1900.

ness," or neurasthenia. Mary Wood-Allen, in *What Every Young Girl Ought to Know* (1905), considered bicycling a capital exercise if done in moderation—and if the cyclist remembered to keep the "gluteal muscles . . . closely held together." The medical and sporting journals of the late 1880s and 1890s are replete with articles applauding the bicycle as a great instrument of health. In the *Medical News* in 1897, one author noted a decrease in cases of phthisis among young women in Massachusetts, a decline that corresponded to an increase in the use of bicycles among the same group.[15]

The bicycle also offered another potential boon to American womanhood, or so its proponents maintained; it helped women carry and bear children —according to one enthusiast, developing the muscles of the uterus, thereby easing childbirth. Such reasoning was usually subtly presented under the general idea that bicycling made women fit for marriage, childbirth, and motherhood. As a practical matter, however, the bicycle enthusiasm of the turn of the century was restricted to the middle class—almost totally white and of Anglo-Saxon or northern European descent. This advocacy may have implicitly addressed the problem of "race suicide," or at least the perceived need to have healthier and larger families.[16]

The bicycle also received support from physicians and health reformers because it made dress reform for women almost a necessity. Corsets did not disappear with the advent of bicycling, but they became less restrictive and omnipresent. Sporting fashions for women, with shorter skirts (though still far below the knee) and even pantaloons or bloomers (for the daring or the political liberal) provoked E. D. Page to warn in 1879 that the bicycle could be a catalyst to immorality because women riders would inevitably hike up their skirts, demonstrating their lack of modesty and provoking lewd comments from male passersby. He also thought the riding position helped shrink a woman's chest cavity, and that for women to overdo the exercise was harmful because it "runs their flesh off."[17]

Critics of bicycling identified its health hazards, in addition to the obvious dangers of falling, as primarily spinal and pelvic for both men and women. *Kyphosis bicyclistarum* was a curvature of the spine that some physicians tried to correlate directly to excessive bicycle riding. Women were also urged to limit their riding because of the potential hazards presented by the bicycle saddle. Until 1895 the saddles on all bicycles and tricycles were molded for the male anatomy, and women were warned that the design might damage their reproductive organs. Cycling was also thought to cause uterine displacements, distorted or bruised pelvic bones, contracted birth canals, and even collapsed uteruses. The advent of the "Komphy," an elaborate pad to be worn by women under their bicycling clothes, helped alleviate this concern somewhat, as did the manufacture of the broader and blunter women's saddles of the late nineties.

Bicycling was also attacked because it allegedly offered women a chance to engage secretly in the "solitary vice" of masturbation while seemingly riding their cycles for health. Shrill critics charged that women might gain sexual gratification by tilting the saddle's front slightly upward. Less scandalous but certainly of equal importance was the conviction noted by Dr. C. A. Vander Beck, in his journal for 1896 that patient Christine McMattie had irregular menses, and that "riding of [the] Bicycle sometimes brought on the flow."[18]

Men were also thought to be placing themselves at risk in their enthusiasm for the wheel. Less inhibited by their clothing, and certainly allowed more variety in sport and exercise than women were, middle-class men found in the bicycle craze a perfect sort of quick exercise for the faster-paced world of the urban industrial era. It was a sport capable of producing great speeds over the land, and it would not occupy as much of the busy businessman's time as calisthenics or gymnastics did.

But bicycling could have its drawbacks for men as well as for women. Physicians warned serious, competitive bicyclists (almost always men) that they could develop a whole series of deformities. "Bicycle face" was characterized by a strained facial expression, a result of continually trying to maintain balance while pedaling hard. "Bicycle throat" was a malady brought on by gasping for air that was dirty, dusty, and full of bacteria. "Bicyclist's heart" was a disorder that supposedly occurred because of the high pulse rates strenuous riding, or "scorching," incurred.

Even the noncompetitive joy-riding cyclist might endanger his pelvic and genital region. Historian James C. Whorton has shown that physicians worried increasingly about the effects of the bicycle saddle horn on men's genitals. They reported treating numerous cases of tenderness of the testicles, constipation, bladder troubles, difficulty in discharging urine, and, most ominously for the late-nineteenth-century man, "shrivelling of the penis." Changes in the saddle design—from a flat seat with a long protruding horn to a curved saddle much like those of the 1980s—helped decrease and nearly eliminate such fears by 1900.[19]

Sport and such activities as bicycling were also important because they helped maintain a "spermatic economy." Most physiologists assumed that each man possessed a finite amount of sperm, and that this had to be conserved for purposes of procreation. For young men, sport was considered a diversion from sexual cravings, masturbation, and other such potential or actual wastes of sperm. "Football," wrote B. W. Mitchell in the *Journal of Hygiene and Herald of Health* in 1895, "has ended a career of debauchery for more than one youth."[20] Even more important for such political and cultural leaders as Henry Cabot Lodge and Theodore Roosevelt, however, were sport's rejuvenating capabilities for young men.

The intellectual balance between athletics as a restorer of energy and athletics as a drain on energy was a tricky one, but in the 1880s and 1890s the idea that action brought regeneration and renewal predominated. Gymnastics and calisthenics had been part of the American enthusiasm for maintaining or regaining health since the 1850s, but they had usually been considered less important than other forms of treatment, such as rest or water. By the 1890s exercise and sport—expending one form of energy (muscular) to maintain another (spermatic) or to renew still another (nervous)—became the preferred activities of the middle-class American male.

Sport—especially team sports, such as football, rowing, and baseball, and strength sports, such as boxing and wrestling—became the most important parts of athletics at the turn of the century. Not only did they require young men to develop physically, but they developed "team spirit" and certain militaristic tendencies thought essential for success in the business community. In 1897 Edward Hitchcock thought that football forced players not only to learn to protect themselves but also to be aggressive while controlling their tempers, thus becoming "better fitted for the stern work of life that assails us all at some time." By experiencing defeat, men would learn to accept life's setbacks while developing the discipline necessary for ultimate triumph. Similar sentiments had been expressed by Walter Camp and Loren F. Deland, whose classic *Football* appeared in 1896. Camp and Deland implied that football was training as essential for life as anything gained in the classroom.[21]

Football caught on quickly among American young men, from the coal yards of Pennsylvania to the playing fields of major universities. But if the enjoyment of the game cut across class, its ideology did not. Lodge and Roosevelt, and their confreres among the military and the health reformers,

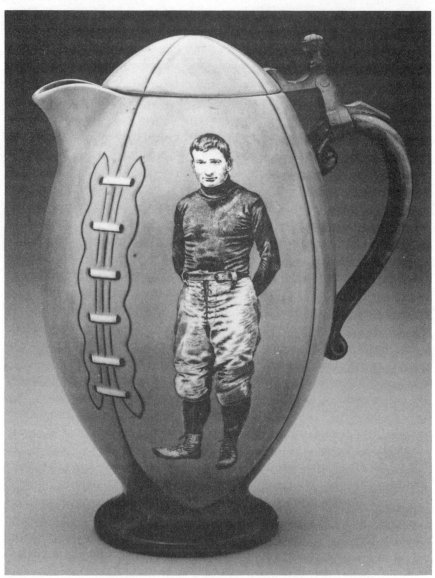

Football was so popular that novelties in a multitude of forms were produced and purchased all over the United States. The young man in his football uniform exemplified the sturdy athlete reformers and cultural critics sought in the younger generation. Pitcher, American, glazed earthenware, ca. 1900.

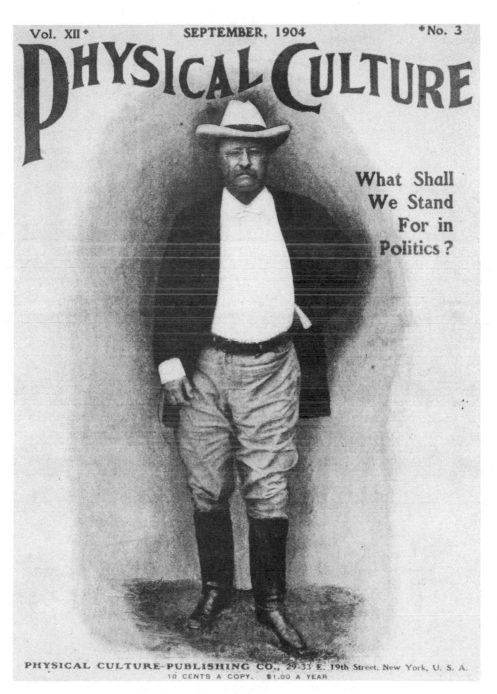

Vol. XII *   SEPTEMBER, 1904   *No. 3

PHYSICAL CULTURE

What Shall
We Stand
For in
Politics?

PHYSICAL CULTURE-PUBLISHING CO., 29-33 E. 19th Street, New York, U. S. A.
10 CENTS A COPY. $1.00 A YEAR

*Teddy Roosevelt's rough-rider "strenuous life" philosophy was compatible
with muscleman and huckster Bernarr Macfadden's ideology of fitness
and health. Illustration,* Physical Culture, *September 1904, front cover.*

perceived athletic training as part of the general preparation of American men for the struggle between the nations and the races of the world.

Roosevelt was the most famous advocate of action and sport as a revitalizing agent for the neurasthenic and dyspeptic American male. His expertise in riding and marksmanship transformed him into a folk hero for both the eastern elite establishment and the common man in the rest of the country, and his exploits on the plains, in the mountains, and ultimately in the Spanish–American War were well documented in his day. Sport was, in effect, Roosevelt's model for life. Though he favored competition, the genteel sportsmanship of his Harvard years turned him against "unfair" advantage, which probably explains why he went after the "bad" trusts

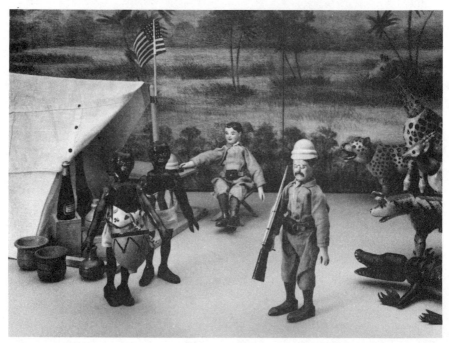

Roosevelt's safari of 1909 was followed in newspapers across the country and inspired all sorts of consumer goods, including these toys, which reveal something of Roosevelt's mythic status and America's racial stereotypes. "Teddy's Adventures in Africa" toy set, Schoenhut Toy Company, Philadelphia, Pa., painted wood, glass, metal, elastic, ca. 1909.

during his presidency: they were not playing by his rules.

Two of Roosevelt's comrades from Harvard had somewhat different views about the role of athletic competition in social renewal. Economist Francis A. Walker worked for the United States Immigration Service in the 1890s, where he made no secret of his distaste for the "new" immigrant populations that he saw rushing into America. Henry Cabot Lodge, the conservative senator from Massachusetts, was one of the most vocal advocates of immigration restriction and was one of the founding members of the Immigration Restriction League in 1894. Lodge thought the English-speaking "race" was the supreme group in the world and owed much of its capacity to triumph in world affairs to the strengths of character and body that sport had taught them. Like his friends Roosevelt, Walker, and historians Henry and Brooks Adams, Lodge worried about the nation's future, should the condition of American men be left untended.[22]

Roosevelt's stress upon action, athleticism, and the "strenuous life" spread outward from the gymnasium and the playing fields to the abundant and seemingly boundless spaces of the outdoors. Roosevelt typified the male-oriented conquest of the wilderness that seemed to be the new "safety valve" or "frontier," which could replace that which Thomas Gill and Frederick Jackson Turner thought had disappeared. This wilderness was a special sort of frontier, however; whereas it may have been "rough," Rooseveltian adventure was not the hardship of subsistence agriculture, conflict with Indians, or threat of wild animals that the frontiersman had experienced. It was, rather, an outing, an opposite and invigorating antidote to the urban experience of most Americans. American thinkers from Henry David Thoreau to John Muir asserted that nature was a replenishing force because of its sublime, serene character, but men of action such as Roosevelt sought renewal by the test of their mettle in the world. Nonetheless, it was a controlled and channeled barbarism. Just as the chaotic qualities of football, boxing, and wrestling existed in the controlled, and officiated, environments of the ring or gridiron, the national parks were wild, yet controlled —bounded, penetrated by roads, and preserved by law.

Nationalism and sport received perhaps their greatest boost from the reinstitution of the Olympic Games in 1896. From the outset the games were seen by citizens, if not by contestants or the games' organizers, as a test of national and even racial strength. "The development and training

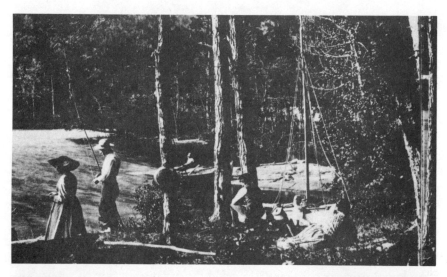

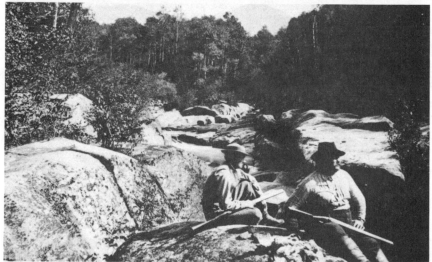

Hunting and fishing were part of the "strenuous" outdoor life that by the 1890s came to be associated with Teddy Roosevelt. Outdoorsmen—and women—such as these were enjoying the beneficence of the woods and streams, unlike their city-bound brothers and sisters, who were subject to "neurasthenia," or nervousness. Above: "Camp Life, Lake George," stereograph, Union View Company, Rochester, N.Y., ca. 1880. Below: "Partridge Shooting," stereograph, American, ca. 1880.

of our college athletes and our gymnasium facilities," wrote the commissioners representing New York State at the Paris Universal Exposition of 1900, "were a revelation to the foreign world." Roosevelt was the honorary president of the 1904 Saint Louis games, bestowing the charisma of his political persona and ideology on the activities. Horace Fletcher, whose own feats of strength and somewhat bizarre nutritional ideas had made him well known, commented on the 1912 competitions with more than a little nationalist fervor. "The importance of organized physical culture is being accentuated by the shame expressed by the English papers at the poor showing they are making in the competition," Fletcher wrote.[23]

In addition to the quadrennial Olympic meets, international expositions and fairs became one of the popular venues for national and international competition. At the Pan-American Exposition of 1901 in Buffalo, New York, commentators remarked that the athletic events and the new stadium would "live in the memory of the many thousands years and years after the electrical display is forgotten." The games at Buffalo not only showcased American athletic superiority, James E. Sullivan wrote in the September 1901 issue of *Cosmopolitan,* but they also gave "thousands an intelligent idea of athletics and of what the brawn and muscle of America represent."

The Buffalo athletic program opened with a baseball game between the Carlisle Indian School and Cornell University. Intercollegiate and American Athletic Union track meets, championship basketball ("which is apparently America's coming indoor game," Sullivan wrote), lacrosse matches, the decathlon, and the marathon completed the summer events (swimming events were held at a nearby lake). Football, bicycling, and auto races dominated fall events. "Nine-tenths of the [athletic] records are held by Americans," Sullivan commented proudly. It was a dramatic change from the situation twenty-five years previous to the exposition, when "all the amateur records [were] . . . held by Englishmen, Irishmen or Scotchmen."[24]

The successes of American athletes in colleges, in the Olympics, and in such professional sports as baseball served notice to the middle class that sluggish, dyspeptic neurasthenics had to mobilize themselves to achieve their potential and assert their claim to leadership. Sporting goods manufacturers were there to help rectify the situation. Late-nineteenth- and early-twentieth-century exercise apparatus for the home changed only slightly from the goods first made available in the three decades following the Civil War. The ideal presented now, though, was one of muscular bulk, a dramatic change from the leaner image depicted in Kehoe's Indian club illustrations thirty years earlier. The marketing campaign for the Whitely Exerciser identified their market. It was billed as "the only practical complete apparatus for travelers," indicating that those whose work required travel or who had enough money to travel for leisure were the prospective consumers. The 1909 A. G. Spalding and Brothers catalog, a thick paperback of approximately two hundred pages of sporting goods and exercise devices, illustrated not only the multiplicity of sporting goods available but also the new American hero. Spalding was big business in 1900, with offices in twenty-two American and four foreign cities, and from them energetic advocates of fitness could get all they needed to train at home.[25]

Gymnastics and calisthenics had changed little from the systems of Lewis or Kehoe. The exercises and the gear—wands, dumbbells, and rings—were the same. The irony of the heightened stress on conditioning for better health was that many of the immigrant groups that such men as Lodge, Walker, and Adams feared and criticized brought with them strong tradi-

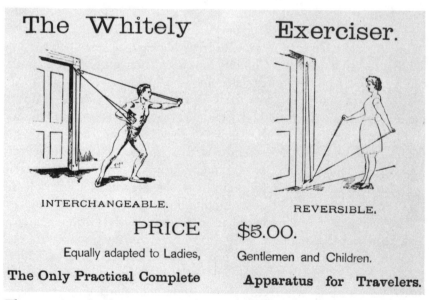

The Whitely   Exerciser.

INTERCHANGEABLE.   REVERSIBLE.

PRICE $5.00.

Equally adapted to Ladies,   Gentlemen and Children.

The Only Practical Complete   Apparatus for Travelers.

The new female ideal form—slender and sleek—and the male model shape—more muscular than before—are evident here, as is the Whitely Company's altered sales pitch to travelers. Advertising brochure, American, ca. 1910.

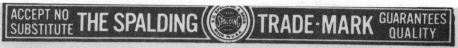
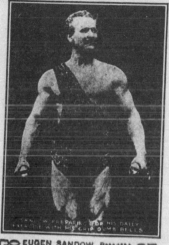
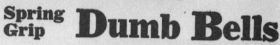
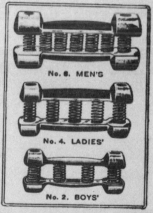
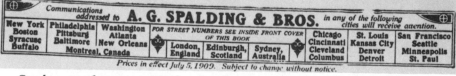
Sandow was by 1909 considered to be the most perfect male specimen in the United States. He parlayed his reputation into endorsements and a comfortable living. A. G. Spalding & Bros. catalog, New York, 1909.

tions of gymnastics. The German Turners revived their activities, holding *Turnfests* throughout the turn of the century, often with military drills accompanying the events. Immigrants from Austria-Hungary brought *Sokols*, or gymnastic and athletic festivals, wherever they settled. At these games, the traditional gymnastic events were combined with precision marching for men and women, and sometimes with American games, such as baseball. In spite of what Lodge and others said about the superiority of the "English-speaking race," critics were forced to admit that the cultures of "new" immigrants from southern and eastern Europe had already integrated the athleticism and action that he and Roosevelt urged upon their own ethnic group.[26]

The Olympian examples of "American muscle and brawn" redefined the image of the well-developed male body. They were not Eugene Sandows, but they were athletes of bulk. The "new" male was large, not like Wilbur Bacon's crew teams of the 1860s, who appeared almost emaciated by comparison. Exercise to build a large, strong body was advertised as a "microbe killer." "Were it possible to find a perfectly healthy individual," wrote Doctor H. C. Stickney in the Whitely advertisements, "that person could walk unharmed amid all contagious diseases. . . . A healthy animal may with impunity eat the tubercule bacilli, drink them, breathe them, sleep among them, and escape tuberculosis." In addition, he argued that sickness was the fault of the stricken.[27]

Among the other endorsements in 1893 advertisements for the Whitely Exerciser were two from a member of the faculty of the Marmaduke Military Academy in Sweet Springs, Missouri. In the early nineties, Bernarr A. Macfadden was just beginning one of the most sensational careers in health and self-help. A ceaseless crusader for fitness, "clean living," and an end to sexual prudery, Macfadden was a consummate businessman and marketing agent for himself and his ideas. In the course of his career he challenged nearly every gospel of American professional health care, amassed and lost a fortune, founded magazines (*True Story* is probably the longest survivor of the Macfadden publications empire), wrote scores of books, and ran up against the law on numerous occasions, usually because of his stand on obscenity. He was, like Sandow, a shrewd publicist for his own cause; he marketed nude photographs of himself as the best promotion for his ideas.

Born in 1868 of an alcoholic father and a tubercular mother, young

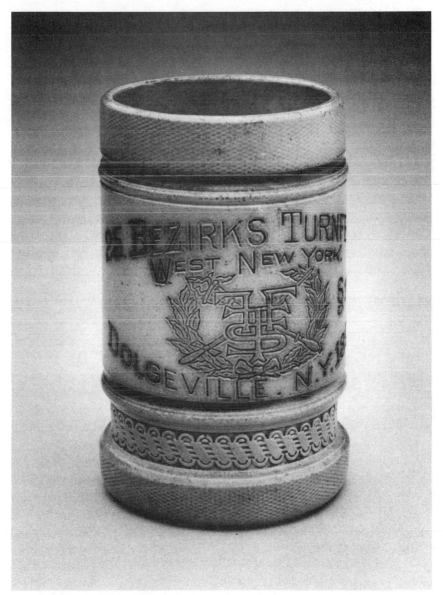

This beer mug commemorates a gathering of Turners in the Adirondack village of Dolgeville, N.Y. The combination of beer and sport irritated those fitness advocates who favored temperance and helped to close saloons. Beer mug from New York State, glazed stoneware, 1894.

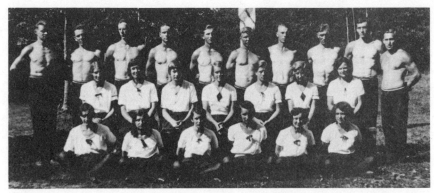

Many eastern European immigrants brought their traditions of gymnastic festivals with them to the United States. Flexing muscles for the camera is a practice that evidently crossed national boundaries with ease. Sokol, Minn., July 5–12, 1931.

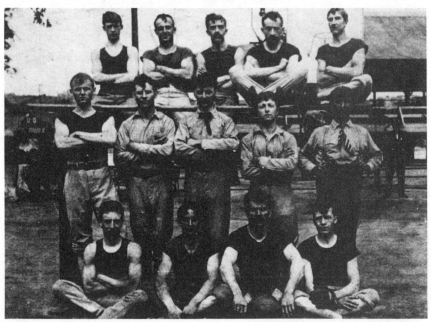

Just as Americans adopted German and other European gymnastics and calisthenics, immigrants took to American sports such as baseball and basketball. "St. Paul, Minnesota, Turnverein on Harriet Island for Sunday Morning Practice," ca. 1920.

Bernard Mcfadden (he changed his name to Bernarr Macfadden in the 1890s) exercised endlessly to build up his weak body. At the 1893 World's Columbian Exposition in Chicago he worked as a roustabout for Florenz Ziegfeld, Jr., who had developed a carefully lighted demonstration of the muscular attributes of the Strongest Man in the World—Eugene Sandow. Here Macfadden learned the tricks of the showman's trade and found a physical specimen whose size and muscle definition he adopted as a model. In his own tour twenty years later, Macfadden would similarly use lighting to give the impression that his five-foot-six-inch frame was actually much bigger.[28]

Macfadden figured a title was a necessity in his quest for credibility, so he manufactured the position of professor of "Kinesitherapy." Macfadden became, in his own mind at least, the guru of "physical culture," a term he claimed to have coined, although it had been in use since the 1830s. In 1899 he took over the management of *Physical Culture* magazine, which, under various titles, had a lineage traceable to Russell Trall's *Water-Cure Journal and Herald of Reforms* (1845–1861). The journal's monthly circulation was approximately three thousand when Macfadden took control; in two years his aggressive marketing, his devotion to displaying women's bodies, and his opinionated stances on a variety of issues increased circulation to more than a hundred thousand.

Macfadden established several "healthatoriums" in the eastern and midwestern states, the most famous across the street from Kellogg's "San." There he initiated the massive amount of printed matter that was to define his theories of "physcultopathy." His aim was to enable people to develop absolute purity of their blood through a regimen of exercise, fresh air, bland diet, and no medicines. Macfadden hated most physicians, particularly "allopathic" doctors, who vaccinated people. *Physical Culture* was full of such articles as "Owning Our Bodies" and "What's Wrong with the Doctors?" Like the rest of the professions Macfadden publications attacked—teachers, writers, and lawyers—physicians were accused of of lying, prescribing unnecessary operations, and being bound by tradition and professional group protection.[29]

Macfadden evidently moved his center of operations from Battle Creek to Chicago in 1909. Horace Fletcher noted his comings and goings with great interest, writing to his friend John Brennan in 1909: "I understand that Mr. Mcfadden [*sic*] has removed from Battle Creek to Chicago and has started a huge physical culture school at the latter place." Macfadden continued to found health-related institutions at various sites around the country—including the ramshackle hotel in Dansville, New York, that had once been Jackson's "Home on the Hillside." Eventually he settled in the "Macfadden Building," at 1926 Broadway in New York.[30]

For all his activity in the real estate market, Macfadden was essentially a showman, on stage and through the printed word. He had been associated with touring shows since at least 1893 and was soon on the road with his own extravaganzas. With an eye for notoriety, he shrewdly calculated that a mixture of sex and body building would certainly draw attention, especially from men.

Macfadden's most ambitious effort to promote physical culture and himself was the Physical Culture Show, which he had scheduled to open in New York's Madison Square Garden on October 9, 1905. The show had taken place in the same arena the year before and had occasioned some notice in the press, but in 1905 MacFadden made headlines in the *New York Times*. On October 5 Anthony Comstock, secretary of the Society for the Suppression of Vice, had Macfadden and two aides arrested for possessing and exhibiting obscene pictures. The pictures were two advertising posters. "One of them shows the women prize winners, ten or twelve young women in white union suits with sashes around their waists standing or reclining in various positions. Another poster shows a man wearing a pair of sandals and a leopard's skin breech-cloth," a *New York Times* reporter who covered the arrest wrote.[31]

MacFadden could not understand Comstock's concern. "All this was done last year," he remarked, referring to the contests and their costumery, "and nobody became indignant." He pleaded that it was too late to call off the event or change the rules, since "over one hundred men and thirty-five young women . . . from all parts of the country" were coming to the show.[32]

The *Times* thought the controversy important enough to devote an editorial to it on October 7. After laying out the boundaries of the dispute, the editors judged, "We are bound to say that Mr. Comstock appears to have the better of it. . . . Let Mr. Macfadden . . . show his culling of the results of Physical Culture in private. . . . But let him not project a money-making show of them, for the express attraction of the 'baser nature,' which will be its effect, if not its purpose." The editors believed that Macfadden intended "to give an indecent exhibition, or else . . . obtain money under false pretenses." By the standards of turn-of-the-century New York, Macfadden's union-suited girls' outfits were too revealing not to be considered

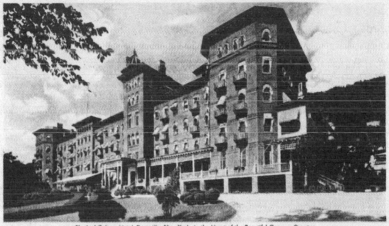

Bernarr Macfadden pitched his institution, which had originally been James C. Jackson's "Our Home on the Hill," to the middle class. Advertisement for Macfadden's "Physical Culture Health Resort," *Physical Culture, July 1939, back cover.*

obscene or at least sexually suggestive. Evidence that the great "professor" knew exactly what he was doing can be found in the response of many businesses that ordinarily might have displayed a pinup or two. The *Times* reported, "Despite the arrest, drug stores, barber shops and many other places are exhibiting the union-suit poster girls bravely on their windows."[33]

Macfadden's British wife, Mary, was described by Macfadden publicists as "Great Britain's Perfect Woman," and no secret was made of the measurements of her figure for those who wished to compare. Mary Macfadden's measurements were "neck, thirteen inches; upper arm, flexed, twelve and three-quarters; forearm, ten; wrist, six; chest, expanded, thirty-eight; small, thirty-four; bust, thirty-eight and a half; waist, twenty-five; hips, thirty-nine; thigh, twenty-four; knee, twelve and a half; calf, fourteen and a half; and ankle, eight inches." In England Macfadden continued to push his show as health-related, but his "physical culture" still carried a strong sexual suggestion. As his somewhat embittered wife recalled forty years later, "The intake from our show had been considerably increased by the sale of glossy postalcard photographs of myself in the flesh tights." The highlight of the show was the 142-pound Mary's leap from "a high table" onto Bernarr's stomach, which he had flexed to show his strength.[34]

In 1914 MacFadden's "International Healthatorium" in Chicago was run by a small army of athletic-looking men and women in white uniforms. In addition to organizing health crusades, the institution was home to various educational operations, such as "The Physical Culture Training School, where, in one year, you could become Doctor of Physcultopathy, Kinesitherapy . . . Hydrotherapeutics . . . [or] Professor of Brain Breathing." It also housed much of Macfadden's publishing empire. In addition to the magazines he controlled, books rolled off the presses in huge numbers, priced from one to three dollars each. Titles suggested self-help on such topics as raising a baby, strengthening eyes and nerves, tobacco's evils, marriage, diabetes, fasting, skin troubles, asthma and hay fever, and "hair culture."[35]

Macfadden found his God in exercise for all parts of the body, including teeth, hair, genitals, and the body's musculature. He hated white bread, although he was not a devotee of Graham or a follower of Kellogg. He did endorse "Kellogg's Krumbles" in the 1920s and briefly marketed "Strengthro," his own body-building cereal; Macfadden complained that he had to develop such foods because he was in danger of being poisoned. He ate flesh food even though he thought it full of impurities, believing, like Doctor Stickney, that a healthy individual's constitution could ward off any problems. He also advocated fasting, often for as long as a week, to cleanse the system.[36]

Macfadden gained his reputation as an apostle of strength and fitness, but he earned his notoriety for his unconventional attitudes toward sex and reproduction. Unlike many of his fitness-minded contemporaries, he did not profess a belief in the "spermatic economy." He viewed intercourse as a healthy, recreative function, not only a procreative one. He recommended large families to readers of *Physical Culture* and practiced his teachings. His wife was in a nearly continual state of pregnancy in the early years of their marriage, and she remembered him as "a Leonardo in his perpetual zest for physical love." She recalled his conviction that "the perfect man should be able to maintain it for an hour's duration." His fascination with sex and identification of power with genitalia led him to invent devices for the care of the male organ. The "peniscope" was a cylindrical glass tube with a rubber hose on one end that was attached to a vacuum pump. Once turned on, the machine would allegedly enlarge a man's penis.[37]

Bernarr Macfadden came of age as a businessman in the high times of the Theodore Roosevelt era, and, like Stickney and others of his bent, he either understood or simply absorbed the idea that the individual was always solely responsible for his or her own condition—economic, social, or medical. If taken by some serious disease, people had only themselves to blame for not being in perfect health. "It lies with you," Macfadden wrote in *Macfadden's Encyclopedia of Physical Culture* (1914), "whether you shall be a strong virile animal . . . or a miserable little crawling worm."[38]

By 1920 *Physical Culture* was crammed with schemes and gimmicks to help readers change themselves. They could perfect their English by spending "15 minutes a day" with books supplied by the Sherwin Cody School of English. They could reshape their noses with the Anita Nose Adjuster, a contraption of straps and bands placed around the head that was also available by mail. In their "spare time" they could "discover" their "unsuspected Self" in the "muddle of wrong thinking, of doubt, and self-distrust" by enrolling (by mail) in the Pelman Institute of America, a "common sense, straightforward course in applied common sense psychology . . . in twelve Little Grey Books." The purpose of the Pelman course was to "give . . . university-trained boys what their college education . . . could never give—

training in original thinking, in initiative." Other aids were marketed to help men develop better memories, speak better in public situations, "read" other men by their eyes and eye movements, improve their eyesight and hearing, improve the tone quality of their voice, build upon their education, eliminate their body odor, and, of course, develop a more muscular body. In December 1933 the magazine appropriately added the subtitle "The Personal Problem Magazine" to its cover, which almost always featured a picture of an attractive young women in some sort of athletic endeavor.[39]

Macfadden's extraordinary success lay in his ability to perceive the needs and evoke the dreams of his readers, nearly all of whom were white middle-class men. The large number of advertisements implicitly offered men aid in their struggle for a place in the bureaucratic and business-oriented world of the American 1920s. There are no images of workers in *Physical Culture*, except for the occasional reference to the man who worked his way up past better-dressed (and perhaps better-educated) colleagues because he studied on his own, either in night or correspondence school. But the most important dream Macfadden promised to make real was the well-muscled body. If Sandow was the apostle of bulk and mass, then MacFadden was the high priest of the flex. He posed nude—in classical poses—from the turn of the century onward. By 1920, *Physical Culture* carried innumerable advertisements promising new ways and new gear designed to build massive arms and chests—not for sport or activity, but to improve health and performance, both in business and between the sheets.

In the July 1920 issue of *Physical Culture*, "Lionel Strongfort" (a perfect moniker for a strong man) asked readers if they were "all in" and promised, "Strongfortism will pull you out." The tall muscular Strongfort clad in trunks and sandals was juxtaposed with a smaller vignette of a haggard businessman at his desk—the dream and the nightmare for American men. Strongfort asked, "Are you a 100% man?" and warned that "no matter how brain-trained and quick a man may be . . . how can he apply his ability if he is weak and sick?" He offered a free book and consultation on forty-four different conditions, both mental and physical. The same issue had advertisements for "Professor" Adrian P. Schmidt's Automatic Exerciser (which promised a "massive chest"); "Professor" H. W. Titus's "Progressive and Automatic Exerciser"; the Whitely Exerciser (now used by a man with a huge chest and arms); Ignatius Neubauer's book on physical culture (accom-

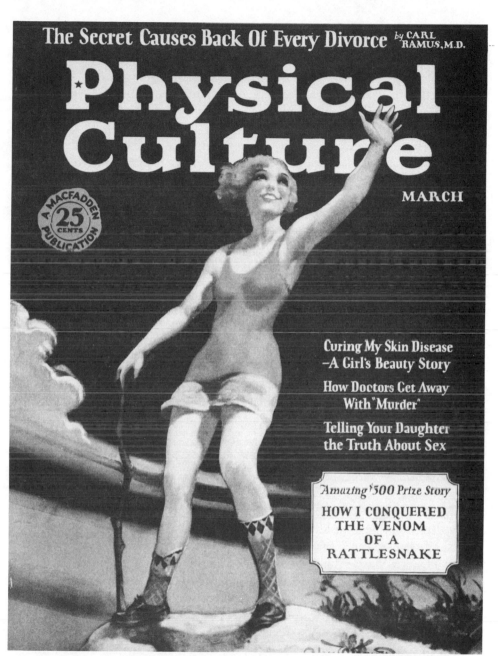

The Secret Causes Back Of Every Divorce *by* CARL RAMUS, M.D.

Physical Culture

MARCH

A MACFADDEN PUBLICATION
25 CENTS

Curing My Skin Disease
—A Girl's Beauty Story

How Doctors Get Away
With "Murder"

Telling Your Daughter
the Truth About Sex

Amazing $500 Prize Story
**HOW I CONQUERED
THE VENOM
OF A
RATTLESNAKE**

Nearly every issue of Physical Culture *had as its cover a painting or a photograph of a healthy, nubile young woman engaged in some sort of athletic activity and clad in a revealing costume. Health and sex were intimately linked for Macfadden and his predominantly male middle-class audience.* Physical Culture, *March 1927, front cover.*

panied by a "handsome halftone picture of the man himself"); and the "physical vitalizer machine" (an electrified pulley-and-rope apparatus with a small battery to supply a mild jolt).[40]

Within six months Strongfort, who regularly took out full-page advertisements in *Physical Culture,* made his approach more bluntly. "Are you Sour on Society?—Is It Your Fault?" his ad asked. "Does it look to you as though every one were against you? Do you feel like rebelling against everything and everybody?" If so, Strongfort declared, "you are bankrupt in health, and lacking in manly vigor and mental courage." Strongfort promised more than body building; he vowed that he could create in his followers a positive attitude, and, perhaps most important for his readers, he promised to "aid in restoring the impotent. . . . I can give you back your dissipated manhood," he proclaimed, "I can give you new courage, increased vigor, more pep."[41]

Other entrepreneurs of muscle culture traded on similar themes and dreams. In the same December issue of *Physical Culture,* "Professor" Matysek offered a "muscle control course" for "but $2.00." Matysek, ironically one of those eastern Europeans about whom Lodge and others fretted, asked his readers the patterned question of the early 1920s: "Why be only half alive?" He promised his readers that he could help them "be a real man!" and cautioned that their "success depends upon health and strength."[42]

By the mid 1920s the verbal message of strength advertisements had begun to change. "Professor" Henry Titus still asked readers whether they wished to be "content to remain a second or third rater all your life, or are you going to be a REAL man?" But Titus's new pitch to sell his exercise machine—two springs joined by a lifting bar which were connected to a platform on which the lifter stood—was to "have big muscles that will make people respect you." Macfadden's advertisement for the "World-Famous Macfadden Muscle-Builder" in 1927 similarly based its appeal on simply building "BIG muscles." For only $1.98 anyone could have the five-cable size, which developed over two hundred pounds of resistance.[43]

Muscles as a key to success in business did not disappear completely from the American advertising consciousness; the idea became a secondary benefit of size and power as the image of the ideal male body had evolved. In 1901 Alois P. Swoboda claimed to be "teaching intelligent men, brain workers, the principles of . . . perfect health"; Swoboda himself was a muscular but by no means bulky individual. The heavily muscled ideal— represented primarily by Sandow—competed with and finally replaced the leaner, sinewy look by the 1920s, and the "brain-worker" model of the physically undeveloped man ceased to have the status that Beard had asserted was his; he was merely the puny ninety-seven-pound weakling that muscleman Charles Atlas made famous.[44]

The idea of building the body to protect the race persisted into the 1920s, with Macfadden as one of its most prominent spokesmen. His business successes fueled his already oversize ego and ultimately led to his caricature. Like Graham, he had an inordinate sense of his own worth and importance, but unlike his religiously inspired counterpart of the 1830s, he got involved in politics. Macfadden thought his crusade should logically take him to the White House, or at least to the governor's mansion in Albany, New York. He actively sought either party's nomination for governor in 1928 and openly tried to discover "what it would cost" him to secure it. Foiled in that attempt, he sought the presidency every four years from 1932 through 1948. His dabbling in politics took him to Italy, where he became enamored of Mussolini. Macfadden thought *il duce* epitomized the action-oriented goals of a "real" man and found the Italian leader's brand of "state socialism" entrancing. It was a curious enthusiasm—he also visited the Pope—because Macfadden had long believed in both eugenics and theories of racial nationalism that favored English and Nordic types. Lodge and others of the Immigration Restriction League mentality fought hard against the United Nations and for the passage of restrictive immigration quotas that effectively kept out southern and eastern Europeans; MacFadden did his part for their cause by publishing articles in favor of selective breeding and racial nationalism.

Macfadden published Albert Edward Wiggam's "Should I Marry a Blond or Brunet?" in *Physical Culture* in July 1921. Wiggam began by asserting that "most people expect to find a difference between a Jap and an Anglo-Saxon, between a Jew and a Gentile," but not between the "Nordic," "Mediterranean," and "Round-head or Square-head Alpine" races. He determined that human progress in government was accomplished by Nordics and recommended that all his readers closely study Madison Grant's *The Passing of the Great Race* (1916). "He [Grant] believes the Great Blond Nordic race which has made nearly all modern civilizations is actually being bred out by the lower types of the brunet races. If so, no greater calamity could possibly happen." Claiming that "the blonds invented democracy," "chivalry," and "the modern high position" of women, Wiggam asserted that democracy will last only "as long as the blond race lasts."[45]

Wiggam carefully defined "blond" and "brunet" so as to not confuse hair color with "race." Body size (Nordics were taller and more muscular) and parentage were his indicators. In a somewhat bizarre turn of logic, he maintained that Nordic blue eyes, fair skin, and light hair were recessive genetically but failed to explain how Nordics were superior if their characteristics could so quickly be subsumed. "All our presidents have been Nordics," Wiggam asserted, even though many were dark in hair, eyes, or complexion. Their national heritage—England—was common; Wiggam's and Grant's great confusion was mixing ethnicity with a strange conglomeration of anthropology and phrenology. Appealing to his readers—primarily white Anglo-Saxon middle-class men and women—Wiggam stated, "It does make an immense difference to your children and the future of America, whether you marry a Nordic or a Mediterranean." Though cautioning that his method of determining a mate could not predict how an individual would behave, Wiggam nonetheless asserted that *"they will not and cannot behave the same"* and *"will emphatically not build the same sort of country to live in."* [46]

The core of the argument in both Grant's *Passing of the Great Race* and in Wiggam's article was the same. Wiggam called World War I "the suicide of the giant white race." The "Nordic who is the backbone of the country, through his recklessly throwing himself on the front line of battle in every war, his drunkenness, his aristocratic love of luxury and his philanthropic, asylum-for-the-oppressed theory of immigration . . . is facing his own extinction," he wrote. Wiggam's language invoked the century-old critique of Americans' love of luxury and drink and added the new twist of suicidal bravery and philanthropy to generate the mixture of pseudoanthropology and racism that in the United States culminated in the immigration acts of 1924—and in Germany led to Dachau, Belsen, Auschwitz, and Buchenwald.[47]

Racial nationalism and eugenics were the dark side of the fitness and body-building crusades of the twentieth century. Macfadden contributed money to Margaret Sanger's contraception campaigns to help prevent conception in the tenements, but he kept his wives pregnant whenever he could. Though insisting that "no wife should have children forced upon her," Macfadden nonetheless maintained that "the imperativeness of motherhood cannot be insisted upon too strongly," but that it should occur only "under favorable conditions." Wiggam agreed in another article in *Physical Culture*, "Can We Make Motherhood Fashionable?" He worried that "lesser" races were outreproducing their "betters" and declared, "The only answer is to make parenthood fashionable among people of brains (meaning yourselves, dear readers) and to encourage birth control among the foolish." He used the fear of numbers to affirm his point. "In our time the lower, more incompetent *one half* produce children *three times as fast* as the other half, which is socially more adequate, [and] the net result is that the lower one-half produces three-fourths of the next generation." Such was one fuel for the conflagration of ethnic hatred and prejudice that burned in the "roaring twenties."[48]

The themes of lost vitality, impotence, and brain-work fatigue permeated the sales pitch for body-building devices until 1924, the year of the immigration acts. Once the "immigrant threat" was under control, when the "bungling horde of dishonesty" that Wiggam characterized as "Mediterranean" and the "millions" of Alpine round-heads (Slavic peoples) who raised big families of "peasants" were effectively shut out, the body-building emphasis began to reveal concern for gender relationships.[49]

The stress on size, which connoted power and perhaps even implied violence, was a product of gender role changes occurring in the twentieth century. Women were gradually gaining some measure of control over their own lives as the 1920s approached. The vote—which they obtained by constitutional amendment in 1920—was certainly the most visible legal sign of change. Suffrage combined with broader cultural changes to alter the way men perceived their own physical needs and ideals, helped shape a new consciousness and definition of health, and helped strengthen the reasons to have it.

In the 1920s, American men and women participated in a sexual revolution. Just as the bicycle gave young couples a chance to get away from parents in the 1890s, the auto gave couples in the 1920s mobility, as well as cushioned furniture for day or nighttime dalliance. Women also found new role models for physical appearance in the twenties. Annette Kellerman, the famous competitive swimmer and movie star, became the new example of the "most perfectly formed woman." As an athletic swimmer, Kellerman was able to challenge older ideas of modesty successfully, transforming women's swimsuits from blousy cumbersome outfits to knitted briefer garb which revealed a woman's contours and bared her legs and arms.

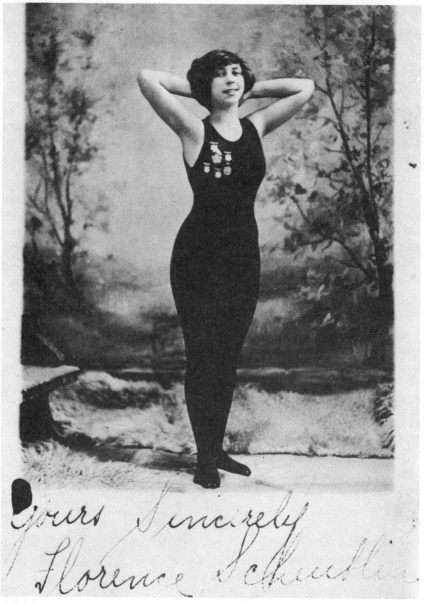

The new twentieth-century silhouette for women is dramatically shown in
this combination of cheesecake and athleticism. Postcard, photograph,
American, ca. 1920.

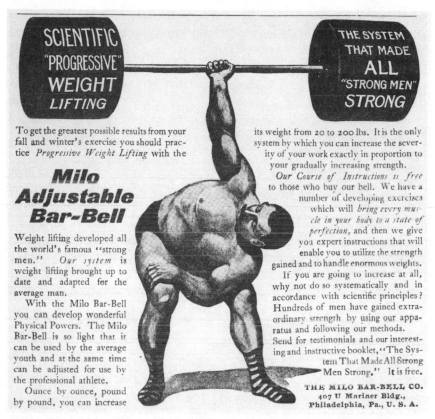

SCIENTIFIC "PROGRESSIVE" WEIGHT LIFTING

THE SYSTEM THAT MADE ALL "STRONG MEN" STRONG

To get the greatest possible results from your fall and winter's exercise you should practice *Progressive Weight Lifting* with the

Milo Adjustable Bar-Bell

Weight lifting developed all the world's famous "strong men." *Our system* is weight lifting brought up to date and adapted for the average man.

With the Milo Bar-Bell you can develop wonderful Physical Powers. The Milo Bar-Bell is so light that it can be used by the average youth and at the same time can be adjusted for use by the professional athlete.

Ounce by ounce, pound by pound, you can increase its weight from 20 to 200 lbs. It is the only system by which you can increase the severity of your work exactly in proportion to your gradually increasing strength.

Our Course of Instructions is free to those who buy our bell. We have a number of developing exercises which will *bring every muscle in your body to a state of perfection*, and then we give you expert instructions that will enable you to utilize the strength gained and to handle enormous weights.

If you are going to increase at all, why not do so systematically and in accordance with scientific principles? Hundreds of men have gained extraordinary strength by using our apparatus and following our methods.

Send for testimonials and our interesting and instructive booklet, "The System That Made All Strong Men Strong." It is free.

THE MILO BAR-BELL CO.
407 U Mariner Bldg.,
Philadelphia, Pa., U. S. A.

Milo was one of the first large-scale barbell manufacturers in the country. Weight lifting, they claimed, would develop a heavily muscled body like that of the century's new hero, the "strong man." Advertisement from Physical Culture, *September 1904, p. 4.*

Kellerman had the typical reformer-athlete's history—invalid at birth and finally a champion swimmer through exercise. *The Body Beautiful,* her life story, was meant to serve as inspiration to her readers and as the come-on for her exercise system, which she organized specifically for women.[50]

The late-nineteenth-century fashionable silhouette of the wasp-waisted, heavily corseted woman was replaced by the unbound figure of the sportswoman whose active life was an indicator of her good health and, implicitly, her ability to bear and nurture a large family. The Victorian woman had been almost a caricature; for if the corset cinched the waist, it also accentuated the bosom and hips, the areas of nurture and generation of children. But as critics continually pointed out, corseting also prevented physical activity, a result that was insignificant for most American women until both men and women accepted the argument that action and strength—the "strenuous life"—were the keys to health. Thus, Mary Macfadden's twenty-five-inch waist was "ideal," as were her thirty-eight-inch bust, and thirty-nine-inch hips. Her body was still a visible message that she could bear and nurse a new generation.

The Olive Company of Clarinda, Iowa, defined more specifically the goal of physical conditioning for women in 1924, with an advertising campaign for its "New National" bust developer. Calling the twenties "the age of beautiful women," the company asserted that "if you are not physically attractive, you lose half of life's joys." "Womanly beauty"—in this instance equated with a full bust—was obviously a sales pitch for a bust-developer manufacturer, but it corresponded with a more general cultural definition of and openness about female sexuality in the 1920s. Macfadden had defined an ample bosom as a mark of a healthy woman two decades before the Olive Company advertisement and had run into trouble with the law when he displayed women's forms in more modest garb in 1905. He encountered similar legal difficulties after he published *The Power and Beauty of Superb Womanhood* in 1901 because the book contained photographs of bare-breasted women exercising to improve their bust size.[51]

The glorification of the bosom had two distinct ideological bases and meanings in the twenties. For Macfadden and his followers, it signaled sexual, procreative, and nurturing functions. For young women, it may have meant similar things, but it also signified sexual freedom and power, which they were beginning to take for themselves. This newly aggressive point of view was manifested in briefer swimsuits and such "roaring twenties" activities as smoking and drinking—activities that challenged traditional female rites of submission and child rearing. They helped generate, by way of counterpoint, the emphasis on great size and musculature that was exclusive to men. While never explicitly stated, invocations to be a "real he-man" embodied a need to assert dominance and power. Size was threatening enough; it made the actual use of force unnecessary.

CHAPTER TEN

OLD-TIME QUIET IN A BREATHLESS AGE

Neurasthenia, or "brain-fag," as Horace Fletcher called it, continued to be identified as an American problem from the late nineteenth century through the 1930s. In 1920 Paul von Boeckmann, who billed himself as a "lecturer and author . . . on mental and physical energy" called Americans "a bundle of nerves" and "the most 'high-strung' people on earth." Neurasthenia had first been defined by George Beard in the 1870s as a sign of advanced civilization—only those societies with sufficient technological and entrepreneurial development produced neurasthenics. But by the turn of the century, it had become a sign of weakness, an American malady just as dyspepsia had been the "American disease" in the middle decades of the nineteenth century. "Jangled nerves," loss of "nerve force," or "nervousness" were obstacles to American businessmen's success and women's happiness in the home.

The radical reversal of Beard's essentially positive attitude toward neurasthenia corresponded with the dramatic alteration of American middle-class culture that had occurred by the 1920s.

Between 1870 and 1920, the American economy—especially in the North-east—had become increasingly bureaucratic, with a continually expanding class of managers enmeshed in the structures of large corporations. Performance and success were evaluated not on the tangible goods produced but on more elusively measured skills such as organizational ability, interpersonal relations, and the ability to "sell" oneself. Success was measured by financial reward and status conferred—and, consistent with American values that had been dominant for at least a century, it was the sole responsibility of the individual. So great was the pressure to succeed and conform that by the mid 1930s Dale Carnegie's *How to Win Friends and Influence People* (1935), which identified "fitting in" as the most important ability a manager could have, was one of the largest-selling books of all time.

Nervous diseases were defined in a manner sufficiently vague that physicians, reformers, entrepreneurs, and hucksters had unlimited opportunities for helping those afflicted with the condition. Physicians were likely to prescribe rest rather than quick cure-alls. In 1900 Dr. W. J. Burnett of New York wrote his recalcitrant patient, D. S. Sanford, he must stop being the "willing ox," always carrying others' burdens. "The best of machinery will wear out in time," he pointed out, and Sanford had "passed the summit" and was "now 'on the down grade,' " he needed to " 'put on the brakes' to avoid an accident." Warning him that he was "on the verge of neurasthenia," Burnett prescribed that Sanford "be taken on a beautiful island in the 'Queen of the Lakes.' "[1]

Sanford's case epitomizes the new provocations for neurasthenia in the twentieth century; "jangled nerves" began to arise from another, perhaps even more ominous, reason than the pressures of success and "fitting in." By the 1920s the American enthusiasm for motion and action that Alexis de Tocqueville had identified in *Democracy in America* in 1835 had itself become a problem. The promised dream of science, technology, and bureaucracy had become a nightmare of anxiety and stress about status, success, and the future—a juggernaut, out of control.

Some responded to this profound sense of discomfiture with a new dedication to strenuous physical activity, others with a variety of external techniques—special clothing, electricity, and motor-driven machines, which provided various types of stimulation. Still others, echoing the inherent criticism of modern culture, turned to the past for examples of lives unaffected by the illnesses of a machine-age civilization, when the labor of head, heart, and hand were seemingly unified.

Personal regeneration through bodily action—sport, body building, or physical labor of some sort—was a response favored by many, and often carried with it strong social and political connotations. As Luther Gulick maintained in *The Efficient Life* (1901), "Bodily vigor is a moral agent, it enables us to live on higher levels, to keep up to the top of our achievement." The ideology of the "efficient life" permeated such organizations as the YMCA and the Boy Scouts of America, both of which devoted their efforts to the young men who were the nation's future—because, as Gulick warned, "We cannot afford to lose grip on ourselves." At the turn of the century young men at the Springfield, Massachusetts, YMCA were given five types of literature ranked in order of "seriousness": "race stories, especially Teutonic myths, legends, and folklore"; nature tales, accounts of individual prowess (such as Samson and Hercules); stories of great leaders and patriots from Moses to George Washington; and finally, tales of love, altruism, family, "beauty, truth, and God." Thus the YMCA sought to order young lives, to prevent the uncontrolled behavior of youth that threatened not only the present social order but also future generations.[2]

The Boy Scouts of America were similarly organized but more directly linked to the military preparedness that was important for a nation flexing its expansionist muscles in the world. Originally a British movement organized by Sir Robert Stephenson Smyth Baden-Powell, the Scouts were a uniformed group of young men who were to learn the ways of life in the woods, an agenda that corresponded in part to Theodore Roosevelt's urgings for the "strenuous life." By teaching the skills of renewal and regeneration —and perhaps those of the battlefield—scouting, like the YMCA, responded to the perception that young men needed to be supervised and controlled in order to prevent what seemed the inevitable evils of male youth. Horace Fletcher, who approved of scouting, wrote James E. West of his concerns regarding this subject in 1911. A vegetarian for much of his life, Fletcher argued that "it is impossible to eat meat without getting an excessive amount of nitrogen into the system. . . . This can be more or less 'worked off' by hard exercise such as boy-scouting involves but it does not prevent the stimulation to sexual yearnings which are the curse and bane of boyhood."[3]

Efficiency—the byword of that diverse group of early-twentieth-century middle-class nature conservationists, political reformers, social activists, and educators known as Progressives—was at the heart of both these organized and supervised youth organizations of the era and broader cultural concerns about the conservation of vital energy. The military model of organization seemed to many Americans the best way to effect the reform goals of Progressivism. As historian Jackson Lears has demonstrated, militarism—in the Scouts or in the proliferation of military schools that were established in the era—was part of a "quest for disciplined vitality." By controlling and disciplining themselves, young men would become better, more dependable citizens.[4]

Between the extremes of exercise—the body acting—and electricity—the application of outside sources of energy to the body—was a whole range of powered machines developed in the mid-1920s. The health and fitness machine industry promoted its goods to both men and women who wished to develop their figures. The Battle Creek Health Builder, for example, promised to help users "oscillate your way to health." Not a muscle builder by any means, the oscillator was designed to stimulate the body and provide "the combined exercise you would get from golf, swimming, tennis, rowing, horseback riding, [and] Indian Club Swinging" in only fifteen minutes a day. It was offered as an "efficient" cure for "Americanitis . . . that physical 'back-sliding' which is caused by the restless rush and hurry of modern life."[5]

The Battle Creek Health Builder typified a new type of exercise machine manufactured in the late 1920s. Users no longer supplied the power, as they had in their "home gyms" with their bar bells, rowing machines, or chest expanders; motor-driven machines vibrated, stretched, or in some way toned the body. The International Health Devices Corporation marketed a "therapeutic couch," which, by means of levers, stretched the patient's spine, rather like a medieval "rack."[6] Zander machines, used in many of the health resorts after World War I, moved and manipulated joints of the infirm or allegedly ill. Vibrating chairs were used at the Battle Creek Health Sanitarium to accomplish much the same end as the "Health Builder" was designed to achieve. These machines were the health-reform counterparts to the body builder's stress on brawn. Implicitly rejecting bulky muscularity in favor of flexibility, they connect the calisthenics of Lewis and the fitness and aerobics practitioners of 1980s America.

Electricity directly applied to the body continued to be a source of curative power from the turn of the century through the 1930s. "Electricity," wrote the advertisers of the Owen Belt and Appliance Company of

Chicago, Illinois, "is the only known force that in any way resembles nervous force, that can take the place of nervous force, or that can correct derangements of nervous force."[7] This equation created an alliance between American physicians, cultural critics, and health-goods manufacturers, a union that had enormous power in an age of widespread cultural concern for the survival of established American society.

The tools of the electrotherapist's trade changed as knowledge about electricity became more sophisticated and pervasive, and as entrepreneurs were able to turn the language of science and medicine to their own ends. After World War I violet rays, ozone, and vibration were invoked, but the 1890s were still the era of "electric" belts, corsets, socks, shoes, and brushes. "Dr. Bridgman's" electric belts were marketed as cure-alls for a variety of familiar diseases. "Dr. Scott's Electric Corsets" probably had small magnets sewn into the waists; advertisements even offered "a beautiful silver-plated compass [with] each corset with which to test their power." Knowledge of its reputed efficiency was assumed to be widespread, but those who did not know or were uncertain about how the corset worked could read a free copy of *The Doctor's Story*, which contained testimonials and diagrams. The smorgasbord of appliances included a nerve and lung invigorator, chest and throat protectors, trusses, knee caps, anklets, wristlets, insoles, office or sleeping caps, hairbrushes, toothbrushes, and suspensories.[8]

Most of the appliances available contained small bimetallic cells that had to be soaked in a weak acid. The Riley Electric Company of Newark, New Jersey, produced an electric brush in the 1890s that carried a small cell in the handle from which current was applied to the hair. "Nature's greatest nerve and voice tonic," Riley's proclaimed, was "the healing power of electricity applied to Head and Hair." Bottled batteries (cells in an acidic solution) that were to be inhaled and battery-powered appliances much like those of earlier decades were still widely used, both at home and in the physician's office.[9]

New electronic devices that flooded the market after World War I promised both renewed vigor and a more beautiful appearance. In the late 1920s the Eko Health Generator, for example, offered four ways to treat illness or debility; it was a modern version of the galvanic and faradic cells of the 1870s but included more attachments and more sophisticated meters and dials. An inhalor, two vibrators (one large, one small), various brushes, and contoured attachments promised relief from a range of maladies from constipation to colds. The Electric Brush, which operated by having the user depress a lever on the back of the brush, generated much noise and a small amount of current, allegedly to help individuals develop more beautiful hair. Although none of these appliances provided any relief, they were purchased in great numbers.[10]

Electric vibrators were popular new gadgets of the twenties and thirties. Vibration therapy operated on the assumption that *"Life* is heat and vibration, *Death* is cessation of heat and vibration." The therapeutic pitch was that vibrators stimulated better circulation, and hence more vitality. Vibration was "practically condensed exercise," perfectly appropriate for modern society. The Star Electric Massage Vibrator was advertised as "Undoubt-

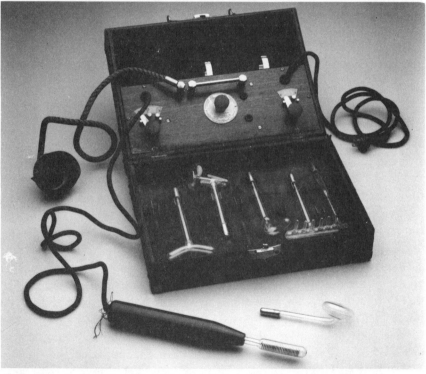

One of a myriad of gadgets that traded on Americans' concerns about decreasing vitality, the Renulife generator was a descendant of the "blue light" enthusiasm of the late nineteenth century. It was ineffective as a revitalizer. Violet Ray Generator, Renulife Manufacturing Co., Detroit, Mich., glass, steel, plastic, copper, wood, paper, ca. 1925.

edly the Greatest of *All* Health Builders!" and invoked one of the dominant metaphors in the culture of the era—sport. "You can't win in business if your muscles are on a strike," the manufacturers warned. "Go after the *big* goal. Play the game hard." Endorsed, its advertisements claimed, by "stage and screen stars . . . athletes, actors, professional men," the vibrator was billed as "an investment that pays *Big* returns." By simply screwing a plug into a light socket, grabbing the handle, and flicking the switch, anyone could win in the business game.[11]

In the 1890s, electricity also began to be promoted as a cure for another important problem, explicitly identified and described in an advertising pamphlet of "Professor" Andrew Chrystal of Marshall, Michigan. In addition to the usual litany of conditions alleviated by electricity, Chrystal emphasized his "electric belts with electric suspensory attachment for all diseases of the urinary organs such as *spermatorrhea, involuntary emissions, weakness of sexual organs, loss of manhood, hanging down of the scrotum, inability to perform the duties pertaining to married life on account of nervous debility caused by early indiscretion, excessive sensuality, or occasioned by having at sometime contracted a loathsome disease."* Chrystal's belts resembled a modern athletic supporter, and consisted "of single and compound magnets" in the form of bimetallic zinc and copper discs that were enclosed in a "band of felt cloth," the outside of which was "covered with a handsome silk band . . . as it is well known that silk is a non conductor of electricity."[12]

Chrystal's catalog of afflictions touched on nearly every late-nineteenth- and early-twentieth-century popular fear about male potency. Nocturnal or other involuntary emissions, for example, "drained" the store of energy in the body. Afflicted men visited their doctors for cures, as H. W. Sweet of Rochester did in 1894. A man of "sedentary habits," Sweet was given a bromide to take four times per day and "iron, arsenic, and strychnine tablets." "Excessive sensuality" worried men, probably for the same reason. John Sheridan, also of Rochester, saw Vander Beck because he "had an erection, which was brought on while 'fooling' with a woman."[13]

Chrystal was convinced that "horrible dreams, restless, fretful spells, blues, gloomy forebodings, loss of memory, loss of energy, etc. etc., are but the outcome of this pernicious evil," masturbation, which nearly inevitably debilitated a man in middle and later years. Other diseases from constipation and paralysis to insanity were also linked to self-abuse, as were "shrunken or undeveloped organs." Although many, and perhaps most, physicians rejected the all-encompassing genital theory of debility (as they had other single causes throughout the century), the power of the argument was sufficient to make "good support" important to most men throughout the twentieth century.[14]

Contrary to late-twentieth-century medical opinion, Americans at the turn of the century were convinced that male potency was enhanced by support of the testicles, believing that if the genital area was kept warm, sperm production increased. Thus suspensories and underwear that supported the genitals became widely popular by 1910. According to a suspensory advertisement, society was "a struggle for existence" that was "getting harder every minute." In this "Survival of the Fittest" environment, they asserted, "health," "strength," and "staying qualities which enable him to withstand any tax upon his system" were necessary for success.[15] The advertisers also suggested that "the consumption of *nerve energy* is a direct strain on the spermatic cord," an idea that had been current in the United States for two decades; men were urged to be concerned because "the testicles are the barometer of a man's physical and mental condition."[16]

This concern for potency and the assumption that it was directly related to genital support endured throughout the twenties and thirties. *Physical Culture* for July 1920 contained four advertisements for suspensories, and the number varied little for the next two decades. Most of the products were sold without overt references to potency and energy; in the two column inches most advertisers bought, comfort was most often emphasized. "The Man Can Come Back," assured an advertisement of the C. C. Lantz Suspensory Company of Atlantic Highlands, New Jersey, in 1920. "Add twenty years to your life enjoying the LANTZ Supporter," men were told, "with freedom of action for mind and muscles." In addition, wearing the Lantz would assure men of the *"refined appearance"* that would be important in business life.[17]

Oblique references to "vitality" and "renewed life" were, by the first decades of the twentieth century, code words for sexual potency. Advertising pieces one might have encountered at a pharmacy or a physician's office were often far more explicit, not only about what any given appliance might cure, but also about how American men had arrived at their debilitated condition. The declining size of middle-class and wealthy American families suggested that men as well as women were responsible. If women bound

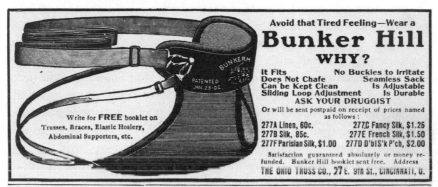

*This suspensory's name invokes nostalgia for the Revolution and its
generation of supposedly healthy men, and links it with the genital theory
of energy. Advertisement from* Physical Culture, *September 1904, p. 4.*

themselves too tightly in corsets and high-heeled shoes, ultimately weakening the muscles used to support the uterus, men, conversely, failed to dress
in a manner that constricted them enough, thereby weakening their vital
centers and in the end, their constitutions.

The ideology of the spermatic economy and its connection to overall
strength encouraged channeling of sexuality toward procreative purposes
and undercut the old idea that young men needed to "sow their wild oats."
As early as 1857, the Sixth Annual Report of the Young Men's Christian
Association had attacked the notion that "young men . . . must go through
fermentation before they could *afford* to be good." Nearly fifty years later,
Mary Wood-Allen, director of the Purity Department of the Women's
Christian Temperance Union, warned women about men who were wanton
in their youth, asserting that such blemished pasts reappear in children and
cause "race degeneracy." Popular writer Emma F. Drake broadened the
argument for forbearance in 1908: sperm would be reabsorbed into the
bloodstream, and the energy redirected to the thought process, increasing
intelligence.[18]

By the time they reached the marrying age (usually the mid-twenties),
men and women were ideally supposed to know how to control their passions. From the 1890s through the 1930s, twin beds were recommended to
make self-control easier to realize. Marriage manuals argued for twin beds
and separate bedrooms, and even Bernarr Macfadden, in *Marriage a Life-*

Long Honeymoon (1903), wanted "no married lovers [to] think of habitually occupying one bed . . . separate beds will in a great measure help overcome sexual excess," he wrote. "Close bodily contact under the same bedclothes is a constant provocation to amorous ideas and suggestions." Although Macfadden, according to his wife, evidently excepted himself from the need to refrain from sexual intercourse, he nonetheless linked "sexual excesses" to failures of memory and eyesight, neuralgia, paralysis, prolapsed uterus, cancer, and evil temperament. While many Americans still clung to the double bed in spite of this advice, the disposition to twin beds that triumphed in the 1940s and 1950s had begun to infiltrate American culture at the turn of the century.[19]

Even those men who had remained pure during their youth and who had practiced restraint when married were not guaranteed good health and abundant energy. In addition to the temptations of drink, tobacco, unhealthy diet, and lack of exercise, the pressure to succeed—and the ideology of individual responsibility for failure—and what seemed to be the quickened pace of life threatened to exhaust American vitality. In the advertisements in the early 1920s for his brief book *Nerve Force*, Paul von Boeckmann identified three stages leading to "nerve exhaustion"—and promised to cure all of them by a variety of self-help and confidence-building procedures. Eleven years later, Richard Blackstone continued to trade on the fear of nervous exhaustion to sell his book, *New Nerves for Old*. "The mad pace at which we are traveling," Blackstone wrote, "is wrecking the entire Nervous Organization." Not one to miss a chance for profit, Bernarr Macfadden added to the list of such self-help guides for relieving tension with *More Power to Your Nerves* (1939).[20]

Underlying nearly every therapeutic promotion was a profound critique of twentieth-century society. Vibration, for example, was unnecessary "in olden times . . . [when] there was no dyspepsia abroad in the land, no prostrated nerves, no headaches, no neuralgia."[21] For many, the invocation of the past was a cue to think romantically and lovingly of the seventeenth- and eighteenth-century yeomanry and patriots that settled the United States. The ambivalence toward modernity took material form in the enthusiasm for reproductions of things "colonial" that were produced in great profusion after 1890 and in the formation of large numbers of hereditary societies, of which the Sons and Daughters of the American Revolution (founded in 1889 and 1890) were but two.

The "colonial" style maintained a firm grasp on American taste throughout the period. In 1904 Frederick Coburn commented on this in an article on the Ellsworth mansion (restored by the D.A.R.) in an arts-and-crafts periodical, *The Craftsman.* The house dated from "an era when, if we may draw conclusions from the high character of the popular arts, life was better ordered than it is to-day, when people were happier. . . . Every stick of timber in the Ellsworth house bears witness to a period of honest, enthusiastic craftsmanship, free from undue commercialism."[22]

Gustav Stickley, a furniture manufacturer and publisher of *The Craftsman,* continued the theme of nostalgic veneration for the colonial past in "From Ugliness to Beauty," inveighing against "fashion," and praising "our forefathers of the Colonial and early Federal periods." He thought them more understanding of the virtues of permanence and praised the work of colonial artisans, who, like the Revolutionary patriots, had become American heroes. Stickley warmly regarded colonial style or re-created colonial interiors, and thought them a suitable alternative to the "chaos" of "fashionable furniture"; they would provide "old-time quiet . . . in a breathless age."[23]

Throughout the 1920s Henry Ford, who did as much to turn workers in his factory into machines as anyone else in history, continued the enthusiasm for the colonial craftsman by collecting tons of household furnishings and tools. His Greenfield Village commemorated the preindustrial past by means of a bank account enriched by the ultimate in mechanization. The Rockefellers, who made their fortune in oil, set about to recapture a slightly different sort of idea—tied more closely to their nostalgic vision of colonial government—when they bankrolled the Colonial Williamsburg project, which formally opened in 1935. So popular was the project that consumers immediately began clamoring for house plans that reflected the "colonial" style. *House and Garden* and *House Beautiful* ran articles on the village in 1937, and Richardson Wright's forty-three-page essay in the November 1937 issue of *House and Garden* presented plans for three houses designed in "the Williamsburg manner."[24]

Colonial America, it seemed, was a society in which good, sturdy citizens contended with neither neurasthenia nor strange peoples with different customs. "Colonial," then, was a form of therapy for middle-class and

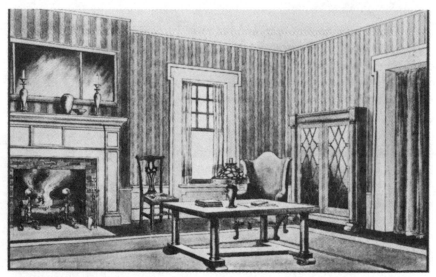

Old-fashioned furniture and decorating forms and designs took on the character of therapy for the modern American troubled by the present. Illustration from The Craftsman, *December 1904, p. 315.*

wealthy, "nervous" Americans: it was a style of life and material goods that both suggested their noble Anglo-Saxon roots and offered them an environmental reprieve from the rigors of the world gone mad with commerce. Many Americans decorated rooms in their homes with accents suggesting both the "strenuous life" (a bearskin rug) and some decorative elements or furniture either of the colonial period or of its style (Windsor or ladder-back chairs, for example). To surround a fireplace—a sign of good ventilation and homey hearthside family relationships—with such furnishings was to construct an almost ideal space.

"Olden times" could and did have other connotations, one of the strongest being a reference to an idealized conception of the medieval craftsman. The intellectual groundwork for this form of historicist therapy was laid in England by Augustus Welby Pugin (1812–1852), John Ruskin (1819–1900), and William Morris (1834–1896). In *The Stones of Venice* (1853), Ruskin had located the strength and vitality of medieval culture in the Gothic cathedral, which he thought realized the interrelationship of craftsmen and the ideal of a society in which individual expression was not only tolerated but encouraged. Ruskin and Morris both sought to alter radically the lives of workers in late Victorian England, hoping to eliminate the tedium and alienation of mass production by encouraging a revival of individual craftwork.

In the United States "craftsman" efforts took a variety of forms, including pottery making at the Rookwood Pottery of Cincinnati, at Newcomb College in New Orleans, and at the Mechanics Institute in Rochester, New

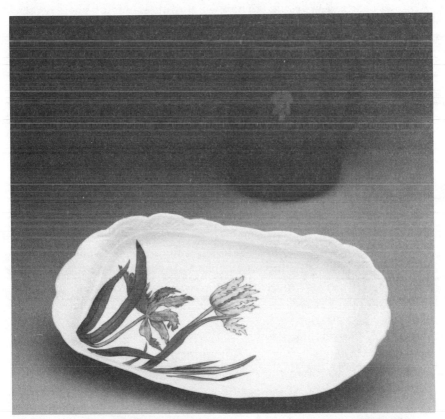

Many women took up china painting, some to calm their nerves. They were part of a large scale "arts and crafts" movement led by professional artists like Frederick Walrath, who produced "art pottery." Plate, Haviland, Charles Field & Co., Limoges, France, porcelain with overglaze painting, 1886. Pitcher, Frederick Walrath, Rochester, N.Y., glazed earthenware, ca. 1912.

York, to cite a few. Here predominantly middle-class women (and a few men) made pottery by hand and signed it. China painting was more broadly based; middle-class and wealthy women all over the country, such as Alice Motley Woodbury, bought blanks from pottery manufacturers and took formal and informal courses to learn how to decorate them at arts societies that were springing up throughout the country.

More thoroughly committed souls to what Jackson Lears has termed "the Arts and Crafts ideal" turned to building furniture, binding books, working metal, or throwing pots as a full-time activity. As in England, colonies of workers were formed to pursue arts and crafts explicitly antithetical or antidotal to modern society. Gustav Stickley's Craftsman Workshops from their founding in the 1890s were established to counteract what he called "nervous prostration . . . the disease of the age." Other, smaller colonies, such as Byrdclyff and Elverhöj in upstate New York, were similarly anchored in an ideology of therapeutic handwork. Here individuals busily worked creating a whole piece, to be sold in the marketplace. The arts-and-crafts ideology of simplicity—in form, design, and construction—was a statement, in part, against modernization and in favor of the "old days."

The ideologues of the arts and crafts movement—primarily Stickley and Elbert Hubbard, the soap-manufacturing company heir who organized the Roycroft community in East Aurora, New York—were also successful promoters of their wares and themselves, and careful not to offend the American corporate power structure. In fact, Hubbard asserted in his journal, *The Philistine* (1895–1915), that he did not favor less big business, but "more of it"; one of his heroes was Henry Ford, the champion of the moving assembly line.

After his initial enthusiastic ideology about the "things wrought by the Craftsman Workshops," Stickley and his magazine, *The Craftsman* (1901–1916), turned sharply to the political right. Occasionally the publication stooped to criticize new immigrant groups, as in an article about John Ruskin in which author Irene Sargent described the "vicious yet cowardly Sicilian with his ever-ready knife."[25] By 1904 Stickley had jettisoned his concern for workers and had begun to identify their work habits and unions as one of the major causes of economic and cultural decline. He soon moved to New York, where he ran the business from the new Craftsman Building, and, like other conservative businessmen, voted Republican.[26]

The arts-and-crafts movement, at least as manifested by the efforts of

Hubbard and Stickley, was ultimately a middle-class and wealthy American activity, even if "mission" or "Craftsman" furniture was rapidly mass-produced and bought by workers. When Horace Fletcher visited the Roycroft shops and stayed at the Roycroft Inn in East Aurora, New York, he was ebullient about Hubbard and his activities, calling the Roycroft colony "the healthiest community I know." "It would do you a world of good to put your auto on the boat once a month," Fletcher advised a friend, "and come up here for three days to mix some sense with business."[27]

Evidently, middle-class and wealthy businessmen and women did just that. "Buffalo folk are driving out in their autos," Fletcher observed in the same letter, "and many are taking houses here for the summer so as to attend the Hubbard meetings." Though Hubbard did not turn against labor as rapidly or as completely as Stickley, his audience was not composed of the folk Morris had in mind—those working in the mills.[28]

Regeneration through work was akin to Roosevelt's concept of action as the critical component to combating the pitfalls of urban industrial life. Working with one's hands was an act of molding or shaping the materials of nature; though it was certainly not electricity, magnetism, or violet light, it was a form of therapy designed for the middle classes suffering from the maladies and malaise wrought by modernity.

A smaller group of Americans than those attracted to medieval or colonial American society found relief and invigoration in Japanese culture. American fascination with the island empire began from almost the moment Matthew Perry sailed into Tokyo Bay in 1854, "opening" the nation to Western trade. When the Japanese Pavilion was erected at Philadelphia's Centennial Exhibition in 1876, newspapers and magazines described with wonder and awe the efficient, quiet and content Japanese craftsmen who seldom used modern construction tools and accessories.[29]

It was the architecture and design of the building, however, that seemed to hold solutions to Americans seeking relief from nervous exhaustion. The serene, flat, planar surfaces and carefully sectioned space in the pavilion impressed observers, and by the turn of the century some wealthier Americans began to have elements of Japanese architecture incorporated into their own houses. Greene and Greene, architects of the Los Angeles and Pasadena area, for example, built a series of expensive homes that employed

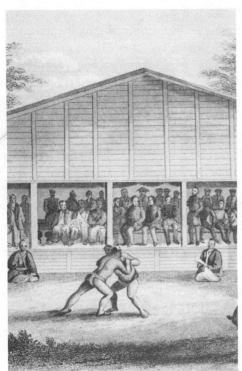
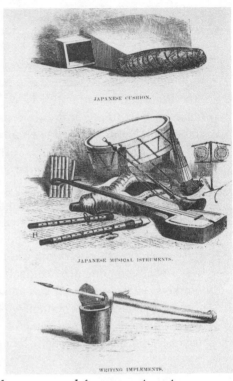

Japanese customs—and artifacts—had great appeal for many Americans, who viewed the island empire as somehow simpler and healthier than American society. Illustrations from Colonel Matthew Perry, Narrative of the Expedition . . . to the China Seas and Japan . . . *(New York: D. Appleton & Co., 1856). Left: p. 431. Right: p. 509.*

not only elements of Japanese design but also Japanese construction techniques as well as Japanese craftsmen. The exterior of many of the Greene and Greene houses in Pasadena resemble Japanese temples, and many had Japanese gardens.[30] Visible evidence of elaborate joinery is everywhere, from the revealed tenons of stairways to the metal strapping of beams used to support the building's mass. The central hearth, with its open fireplace, demonstrates both a turn-of-the-century concern for ventilation and an acceptance of the fireplace as a center for family and important social events; the Gamble family of Pasadena—heirs to the Proctor and Gamble fortune—held church group meetings in the parlor. The ventilation that reformers insisted on was provided by small windows between rooms and halls, some of which were handmade stained glass. Evidence of expensive handwork—ironically available only to those whose money had often been made in industry—was everywhere. Large, handmade doors, stained-glass windows, and hand-worked metal lamps adorn the public and private family

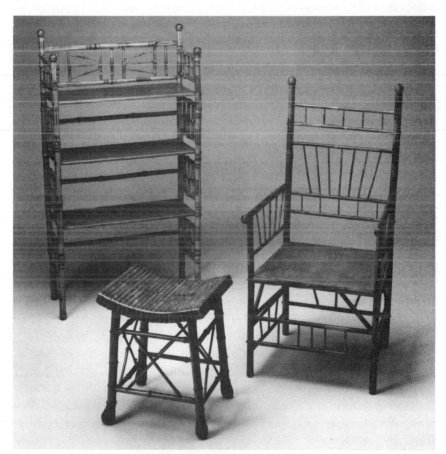

Asian designs and motifs became popular among Americans in the late nineteenth century, in part as a result of a growing conviction that Eastern societies were somehow more serene and less stressful than those of advanced Western civilizations such as those of the United States and England. Bookcase, chair, stool, United States, bamboo, cane, painted oak, pine, 1880–1920.

rooms, while the servants' areas—kitchen and living quarters—are appointed with the goods of a mass-production economy. The kitchen, for example, is a studied attempt at specialization and efficiency.

For a few wealthy Americans, as Jackson Lears has demonstrated, immediate experience of Japanese culture provided direct relief from anxiety. In 1901 and 1905 John Woodbury, who made a fortune first in buggy whips and later in the Eastman Kodak Company, journeyed with his family to the East, where he and his wife began to collect all types of Asian cultural materials. Horace Fletcher also built a large collection of Japanese materials, including a sword stand with several swords, a yellow vase decorated with black and white storks, a brass and paper temple lantern, several drums and gongs, and some suits of armor.[31]

The wealthy patronage of architecture and fascination with Japanese culture extended beyond collecting curios. Manufacturers of household goods parlayed "Japanism" into lucrative sales by producing furniture carved to look like bamboo or decorated with cranes, fans, and chrysanthemums, designs associated with the Far East.

The message Americans might receive from Japanese culture was twofold. Some people were attracted to the serenity and almost fairy-tale quality of the land. Others, like Fletcher, valued the more aggressive aspects of Japanese military discipline. In a 1914 letter to James E. West, director of the Boy Scouts of America, Fletcher revealed this enthusiasm: "My fifty years of acquaintance with Japan and the Japanese and my appreciation of the splendid influence of Fushido (Military-Knight-Ways) makes me keen to notice if similar high ideals held up for acceptance and emulation are not similarly effective in all other countries as well as in Japan."[32]

This enthusiasm for Japanese culture was tempered in the first decade of the twentieth century, after Japan had defeated China (1895) and Russia (1905) in brief but significant wars. Although they gained little territory from their victory in the Russo-Japanese War, the image of the country changed from a serene, peaceful land to a viable competitor for world power. Similarly, the character of the compliant Japanese workman was rapidly being replaced in the public's consciousness by the reality of the dedicated soldier who might well control the Far East.

Far safer to emulate was the medieval knight, a symbol of what the American man could and perhaps ought to be. Invariably strong and full of valor, and almost always tested in battle, he was the opposite of the neurasthenic American. Manufacturers quickly seized upon his image to market their products to the vitality-starved culture. Images of knights were popular in advertising and in magazine and book-length fiction. Novels set in the Middle Ages, such as Charles Major's *When Knighthood Was in Flower* (first published in 1898, in its twenty-third printing by 1899), joined Winston Churchill's *Richard Carvel* (1899) and other fiction detailing colonial American patriots among "best sellers."

The medieval knight-as-hero had two American analogs. American Indians were identified as symbols of health by both American advertisers and cultural critics. Like the knight, they were safe heroes because they posed no threat: By 1900, native American tribes had been conquered and assigned to reservations. Thought to be closer to nature—and therefore more healthy—than white people, images of American Indians were used as decoration by a spectrum of individuals.

American Indian artifacts—particularly baskets, pottery, and rugs—were identified as desirable goods for the decoration of up-to-date homes of the turn of the century. *The Craftsman* regularly included articles describing such materials, as well as occasional selections of native American chants and songs. Decorators at the Rookwood Pottery used the geometric designs of Indian materials, and Navaho rugs in particular were prized by collectors and interior designers. Documented in the late nineteenth and early twentieth centuries by such photographers as William Henry Jackson, Adam C. Vroman, and Edward Curtis, American Indians became still another discreetly distant therapeutic model.[33]

The second analogous American example of health was the colonial craftsman, another idealized figure from an idealized culture. He was no threat to the ideology of those who sought relief from their stress-filled lives in nostalgia for an allegedly simpler culture because, unlike his fellow workers of the 1890s or 1920s, he formed no unions, he never went on strike, and he allegedly cared more for his product than he did for his wages. He was also thought to have a more fulfilling life because he created a piece from beginning to end, unlike his counterparts of the age of industry and the assembly line.

The medieval knight, the American Indian, the colonial American patriot and craftsman, and, more obscurely, the Japanese *samurai* were all steeled by war. Some jingoists and cultural critics saw the Spanish–American War as a chance to revitalize an elite softened by genteel culture or harried into

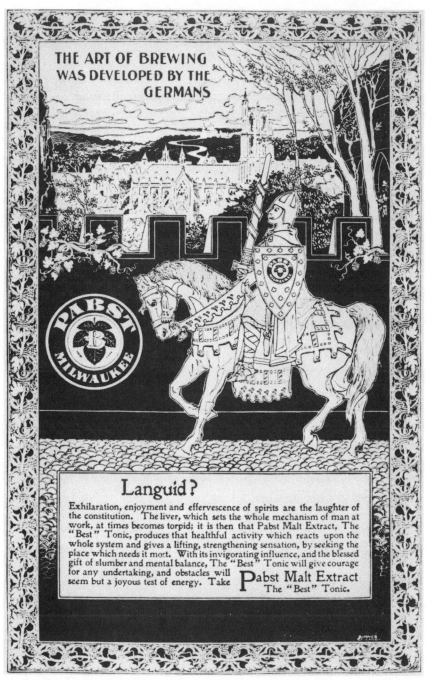

Strong, healthy, brave, and far enough removed in history to be idealized, the medieval knight was a safe hero. Advertisement from McClure's, *ca. 1895.*

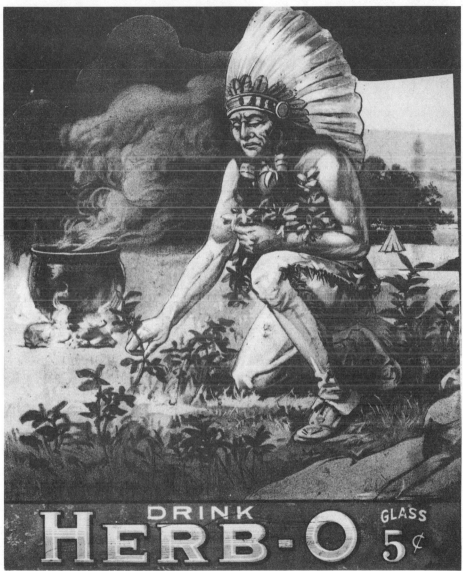

Advertisements of the late nineteenth and early twentieth centuries often evoked the two powerful images combined here—that of natural herbal medicines for health and of the American Indian, who was alleged to be fitter and more in harmony with the natural world than other Americans. Advertising sign, American, lithographed tin, ca. 1900.

nervous exhaustion by the demands of business. But it was preparedness and discipline, not enthusiasm for actual battle that was urged upon American men. Fletcher warmly praised the Boy Scouts' activities, since they taught "preparedness and not beligerency [*sic*]."[34] Physical fitness, efficiency, self-discipline, and elevated moral standards—what Boy Scouting or YMCA activity was supposed to inculcate—were thought to be essential for managing life in the commercial world. Unlike Roosevelt, Lodge, and other patricians of old money and lineage, most Americans trying to gain control of their lives envisioned a mutually reinforcing relationship between fitness and profits. For the middle class, material success was as important a concern as conservation of the environment and support of the flag. Throughout the twentieth century, middle-class Americans have been conscious of their own precarious place in the socioeconomic fabric of the United States. Aware that retreat was as likely as advance, they have continually striven to find the "angle" that would provide them with an advantage in the marketplace. Militarism was therefore a model for security and success in the civilian world.[35]

Women had their stock, albeit smaller, of heroines. Elizabeth Ellet's three-volume study, *The Women of the American Revolution* had first appeared in 1850, but the popular advice writer's work continued to be popular through 1900. Joan of Arc had several biographers during the last decade of the century, and Paul Leicester Ford's *Janice Meredith* (1899) sold 275,000 copies by 1901.

The emphasis on the man or woman alone served to indicate and reaffirm the vital core of American success ideology in the nineteenth and twentieth centuries. To achieve the accoutrements of position and power in America was to be credited with personal qualities that made success happen. To fail was to be personally at fault in some way.

Some flamboyant individuals—Jim Fiske, Jay Gould, and some of the other "robber barons" of the late nineteenth century—drew sneers from such men as Roosevelt, Lodge, and Henry and Brooks Adams because they often illegally manipulated the economy for personal gain. Their fault was not so much that they played unfairly, though Roosevelt would have criticized them for this, but that they did not work. To Roosevelt's way of thinking, J. Pierpont Morgan, Cornelius Vanderbilt, and John D. Rockefeller were individuals in good standing at the helms of their giant firms because they produced; they did not manipulate. Roosevelt went after a few trusts because his sense of "fair play" had been offended, not because he was opposed to great wealth or big business.

Middle- and working-class antipathy to the wealthy was common in the nineteenth and twentieth centuries, but it was always tempered by the gospel of individual success. Horatio Alger's popular heroes made themselves into great men by hard work and fortunate circumstance—luck and pluck. These factors, one force beyond individual control and the other a personality trait, were entwined in the American ideology of individual responsibility. Luck alone would not do it—though hard work might, even with some ill luck. There were just enough true stories of men such as Andrew Carnegie, who rose from nothing to his place as one of the world's richest men, to give general cultural credence to the idea of individual responsibility for one's fate. In this equation, "luck" was akin to the connection between good works on earth and divine grace with which Puritans had wrestled in the seventeenth and eighteenth centuries. For those colonists, to be saved was to be "lucky," since God chose indiscriminately among the fallen because of divine mercy. In the seventeenth and eighteenth centuries, doing good works, the equivalent of Alger's "pluck," did not guarantee salvation but perhaps hinted at the identity of the chosen. So it was with the man who would succeed; hard work was a necessity but not a guarantee.

The solutions to social, economic, and personal problems that advisors, reformers, and manufacturers consistently offered proceeded from an analysis of how individuals had failed. The questions they then addressed would help people redeem themselves and ultimately their society. If American civilization seemed unable to cope with the problems of a changed economy, labor violence, and new and strange groups of immigrants, then the blame lay within. Critics censured the American "mile a minute" society, as writers of the 1920s called it, but there was little suggestion among the middle class that the system should be changed. Most working-class Americans, often identified as a threat to middle-class and elite culture, also questioned the nature of the socioeconomic system but a little; they, too, were victimized by the idea of individual responsibility for their lot. This attitude would ultimately lead to the sense of shame and guilt that many middle- and working-class Americans felt for their plight during the Great Depression, as Studs Terkel, Caroline Bird, and Warren Susman have demonstrated.[36]

Self-help in the form of body building, correspondence-school education, and medicine performed at home with the aid of various gadgets and gizmos all responded to this innate feeling of personal failure when life did not correspond to the ideals propounded in magazines, books, or moving pictures. Macfadden read the pulse of Americans correctly when he cleverly subtitled *Physical Culture* "The Personal Problem Magazine" in 1933. He featured not only physical culture heroes in his magazine but also movie stars and athletes. Here, and in *True Story,* he presented American middle-class readers with optimistic self-help articles to soothe the damaged egos of those victimized by the Great Depression. Implicit in his boosterism and his challenge to established American institutions and professions was the conviction that American men and women had "gone soft."

By having fewer children and by allowing their vigor and potency to decline, middle-class and patrician Americans placed the future of American civilization in doubt. The responsibility for survival rested squarely on each individual's body, mind, and loins. "Race suicide" indicated that a conscious—and disastrous—choice had been made. Mainstream Anglo-Saxon Americans were killing themselves, their culture, and the future of their children's society because they had lost the strength, honor, morals, and grace of their forebears.

CHAPTER ELEVEN

DIETETIC RIGHTEOUSNESS

M ary Wood-Allen, both a physician and an aggressive temperance advocate, echoed a decades-old refrain when in 1905 she stated, "Our bodies are living engines, and use food and air instead of coal and air."[1] Like so many other reformers of the era, she was caught up in the new idea of "efficiency," which promised to make life better for the great bulk of the population by eliminating corruption and waste. Devotees of the arts-and-crafts ideal might cringe at motion studies in the factories and workers might threaten revolt at such overregulation, but, for middle-class and elite reformers, such efforts were heaven made real. Moreover, Henry Ford, one of the early saints of efficiency, paid his workers well, cleverly perceiving them as a market for his basic black Model T. Was that not proof enough that efficiency, despite its negative implications for laborers, might benefit all?

Among health advocates and reformers, efficient management of the body entailed avoiding waste of energy: the "efficient life" was as important as the "strenuous life." But views about the best way to achieve efficiency varied. Roosevelt, Sargent, Macfadden, and others argued that exercise—preferably in the outdoors, and especially in the wilds—built strength and supplemented the body's store of energy, or at least made it possible to realize the body's full potential. Some analysts thought electricity or magnetism could supplement what seemed to be the declining store of energy. Others, seeing the sense of loss or malaise of the middle class as more closely tied to the nature of the economy, argued for a sort of leisured rejection of the world of commerce and industry, advocating handwork as therapy for general debility. Yet whatever their angle of vision, most critics and reformers shared a basic conviction: American dietary habits were closely related to the debilitated condition of American men and women. And just as their principal crusades had taken them in different directions, their approaches to dietary reform encompassed a wide spectrum of solutions.

By the turn of the century the already powerful image of the machine made the clamor for dietary reform insistent: the body needed the proper fuel to run efficiently. Machines, in fact, had an advantage over the human body. The engine seldom ran in ways that would poison itself, and in the event that it did, it could be cleaned and quickly restored to "health."

Public consciousness that the human body was befouling its inner works was raised by the research findings of English physician Alexander Haig (1853–1924), who argued that many of the maladies usually attributed to other causes were in fact the result of one disorder—high levels of uric acid in the bloodstream. This abnormality caused, among other things, migraines, gout, gastritis, eczema, jaundice, and flatulence. Lower uric acid levels would also lead men away from the desire to masturbate as it heightened their procreative interest. Diets high in alkalis forced uric acid out of tissues and into the bloodstream, where the compound could wreak damage.

Haig and his son Kenneth were scorned by many established physicians for advocating this new panacea. In 1912 Horace Fletcher, himself no stranger to faddish solutions to medical problems, seemed to have accepted the importance of "uric acid diathesis" when he wrote that "when fed alone, potatoes dissolve six times their own content of uric acid. . . . Tomatoes are almost equally dissolvent of uric acid, and both . . . will dissolve the uric acid precipitated by meat, cheese, etc."[2]

Like many other thinkers of his day, Fletcher was fascinated with the automobile and thought its operation could be usefully compared with the body's functioning; one of his main goals was "to teach ordinary persons how to become competent chauffeurs of their own corpomobiles . . ." Fletcher was convinced that, like the automobile engine, the body had to be clean internally to operate efficiently. For him, healthy human excretory functions—which depended upon proper diet—were crucial to the maintenance of health.[3]

Fletcher's attention to human excretion bordered on fanaticism and evidently provoked the derision of other professionals. "You will remember," he wrote Professor Irving Fisher of Yale, "that fatty Meltzer of the Rockefeller Institute, who reeked at the time with uric-acid and, I believe, nicotine odoriferousness, condemned me as a crank because I had preserved specimens of absolutely inoffensive feces derived from different sorts of food as proof of the possibility of such inoffensiveness." Fletcher wrote Kellogg in 1910, "I rank it [excretion] as a very enjoyable operation if healthy conditions prevail and it is not accompanied by any rankness of odor. . . . I would like to be doing it all the time."[4]

Fletcher's concern for internal cleanliness was actually shared by many Americans. In 1905 Mary Wood-Allen had cautioned young women to "attend to a daily evacuation" rather than "carry effete or dead matter about in the bowels. . . . It is only politeness and refinement to see that this part of . . . bodily housekeeping is duly attended to." Kellogg agreed that frequent evacuation reduced chances of autointoxication, although he thought that Fletcher stressed roughage too little, thus compounding the allegedly widespread American problem of constipation.[5]

Purgation of the system of dangerous substances took two forms—mechanical and dietary. By 1920, a multiplicity of mechanical solutions were offered to facilitate "internal bathing." In 1921 the manufacturers of the Dupell Internal Bath asked readers (in boldface type), "Do Nine Out of Ten Persons Commit Suicide?" Their advertisement's next question indicated the sinister, unseen nature of the problem: "Why do apparently strong, healthy looking men and women die too young?" The old threat of "premature death" had a new cause: "putrefactive matter from the intestines." The Duprell Internal Bath would prevent loss of "pep" only a few hours after rising in the morning and would save people from feeling "all in."[6]

The "subject" in the Duprell advertisement had learned that "the accumulated waste in the colon . . . causes so much trouble," that the "poisonous" waste accumulates in the large intestine and that the blood flowing "through the walls of the colon . . . absorbs the poisons and carries them through the circulation. That's what causes Auto-intoxication with all its vicious, enervating and weakening results." Internal bathing would enable Americans to "awake in the morning with a feeling of lightness and buoyancy," with an appetite that had "a real edge on it."[7]

Other manufacturers of internal bathing equipment promised "a longer life with tranquility," gains in "physical and mental efficiency," and more specific benefits, such as prevention of appendicitis, high blood pressure, "nervousness, irritability, [and a] tendency to fevers and diseases of numerous kinds." In addition, internal bathing would help bring bodily "weight to what it should be." "Obstinate" conditions, including piles, prostate trouble, rupture, gas pain, and such vaguely defined maladies as "chronic lassitude . . . medicine-taking habits, [and] spells of excitement" would disappear when the internal bath was used.[8]

This new "water cure" was touted as the same sort of cure-all that older forms of water cure had been and continued to be. The differences were of technique (mechanically induced internal use as opposed to external treatment) and in the definition of the problem. Advocates of internal bathing made their sales pitch based on the unwritten and unproven assumption that a healthy human could feel wonderful every day for hours and hours on end. Like the ethic of individual success, which had just enough examples of individuals who struck it rich to seem to be valid, there were few, but enough, examples of what Macfadden called "superb" manhood and womanhood to make the rest of the population doubtful of their own abilities and capabilities, both to stay alive and to hit the "main chance" in business or society.

Internal cleanliness was the watchword of purveyors of other means of regulating digestive and excretory functions. Ingestion of cathartics was, unlike the internal water bath, an old practice. Although it had effectively disappeared by 1900, calomel had been used throughout the nineteenth century, and a variety of other medicines, such as castor oil, were promoted as purgatives. Numerous patent-medicine manufacturers claimed that their products would provide the desired relief, and these combinations of alcohol and, in some cases, vegetable extracts may actually have done so. By the 1920s pharmaceutical companies were manufacturing more "scientific" laxatives to compete with the evil-tasting castor oil and were joined by other firms hoping to cash in on the pervasive concerns about constipation. Standard Oil Company of New Jersey marketed "Nujol" laxative in 1921 and promised "no discomfort while in action." Warning readers that "You May Bathe Daily and Still Not Be Clean," the firm used the rhetoric of the internal bath to sell their "interior cleanser."[9]

Mineral water purveyors also recognized a new market when they saw one. Lithium compounds were promoted as cures for uric acid troubles, especially after British physician Sir Alfred Garrod had shown that lithium

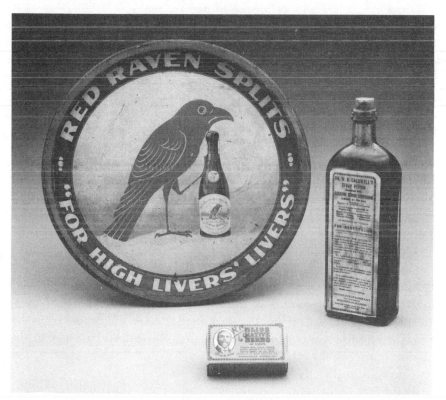

Laxatives became an increasingly important part of Americans' regimen of care for their bodies as they began to worry about "autointoxication" and "internal cleanliness" at the turn of the century. Herbal laxative, Alonzo Bliss Medical Co., Washington, D.C., dried herbs, ca. 1910. Tray, American, painted steel, ca. 1890. Herbal laxative liquid, Pepsin Syrup Co., Monticello, Ill., senna, alcohol, flavorings, ca. 1885–1900.

carbonate dissolved uric acid in a test tube. The Enno Sander Mineral Water Company of Saint Louis advertised its Garrod Spa waters with a rhyme extolling the beneficial effects of lithium bicarbonate:

> *Twinkle, twinkle,* GARROD SPA
> *All the world knows what you are,*
> *Wondrous drink, thy price not high,*
> *So cheap that all the sick may buy.*
> *Thou dost dispel all carking care,*
> *Bring back my youth so debonair,*
> *Make me happy, calm and placid*
> *By chasing out the uric acid.*

Most of the waters marketed as "lithia" spring waters actually had less lithium than some river water. One hundred and fifty thousand gallons of Buffalo Lithia Water, for example, would have had to be ingested to obtain a single dosage that had any therapeutic effect.[10]

Nonetheless, mineral waters continued to be popular among middle-class and wealthy Americans. Railroad lines, such as the Illinois Central and Yazoo or the Mississippi Valley Railways, joined with mineral springs and "health and pleasure resorts" to market the waters to anxious Americans. The juxtaposition of "health" and "pleasure" in the titles of advertising brochures indicated a further broadening of the concept of the spa, which, though it still capitalized on the health angle, more nearly approached the modern "vacation" resort. Real estate entrepreneurs joined railroad and mineral-spring entrepreneurs to push land development. Laurel Springs, outside of Philadelphia on the Atlantic City Rail Line, was promoted in the 1890s as a healthful alternative to urban living, where a working man might buy for himself and his family a grand house whose cost was equal to the rent he paid in the city.[11]

By the turn of the century, connoisseurship of both imported and domestic waters had reached the point that Morris and Schrader, "the only house dealing *exclusively* in mineral waters," published a price list of sixty-three imported and forty-two domestic bottled waters, complete with the geographic source of each and a brief note alerting purchasers to the medicinal and table uses of the liquid. European waters were often two or three times as expensive as native brands were, and drinking imports was a sign of status. One dozen bottles of Viesbaden Gicht Wasser, a muriated, or briny, ther-

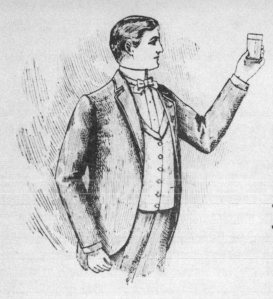

"MINNEHAHA"

MAKES

THE

BEST

HIGH-

BALL

WAGNER'S HUNYADI

Produces a rapid action of the bowels. It never causes cramps and is easily borne by the stomach. It is highly carbonated, thus making it less nauseating than any of the natural Hunyadi waters. In a word, it is

The Best Purgative on the Market.

Mineral and carbonated waters were simultaneously advertised as aids to digestion and as mixers for alcoholic drinks, a combination that horrified most health advocates. Advertisement, "To Defeat Thirst," American, ca. 1910.

mal water from Germany, cost $3.50. The same number of bottles of Saratoga Excelsior Water cost $1.75. Even then, it was a rare working-class home that bought water in bottles when it was free from the tap.[12]

   The crusade for pure, clean tap water, which had begun in the 1840s, became more pressing at the turn of the century as knowledge of the germ theory of disease became almost universal among the American population. Moreover, medical research into the causes of typhoid, typhus, dysentery, cholera, and other virulent diseases had convincingly linked their spread to impure water supplies. The appeal of water filters and stills was heightened by their ability to give the homeowner or renter some sort of control over the water supply. As cities grew throughout the century, individuals accustomed to seeing the source of their water—be it a well, stream, pond, or lake—had to depend on a water supply of unknown origin that simply flowed from a pipe, hydrant, or tap. Country or village people already ambivalent about the urban homes to which they had moved found some assurance in water filters and distilling apparatus in an era when public awareness of health had reached a new height.[13]

   The manufacturers of the "Pasteur Germ Proof Water Filter" warned consumers in 1884 that "clear water, savorless and colorless though it may be, threatens us with the worst of dangers, and the more to be dreaded, as they are hidden, and can escape our best attention." The company offered *"a permanent system of self-protection* which will set our minds at rest and keep away from us all those enemies which may invade our organism and finally destroy our life." These forebodings struck to the marrow of insecurity about the purity of food and drink, a suspicion that was heightened by the spectacular revelations of such "muckrakers" as Upton Sinclair, whose novel *The Jungle* (1906) alerted the public to the filthy conditions of the meat packing industry as well as by the disclosures of the "pure milk" campaigns that pointed out the dangers of raw milk.

   The Chamberland-Pasteur Company warned consumers that the "natural mineral waters," which "in these times of epidemics, people are usually advised to drink," were produced by "dealers, who generally mix them up with ordinary water."[14] In 1894 filters cost between $6.75 and $35 and came in a range of sizes from 6 to 500 gallons. Small, usually globe-shaped filter elements that could be screwed onto a tap were also available for

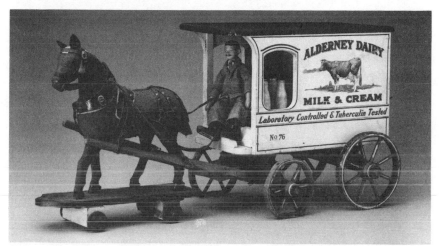

Scientific testing and control of food products became important parts of the marketing strategies of producers and distributors of foodstuffs as Americans became more aware of the work and successes of medical researchers and more trusting of physicians than their ancestors had been. Toy wagon, A. Schoenhut and Company, Philadelphia, Pa., painted wood, 1931.

between twenty-five and fifty cents each. Filled with charcoal or sand, they were designed to remove particulate matter, although grander claims were undoubtedly made.[15] "Water is the greatest distributer [*sic*] of disease germs," as an ad for the McConnell Germ-Proof Filter bluntly stated in 1894.[16]

Still producers were the chief competition for filter manufacturers in the cleansed-water market. These cylindrical oil-, gas-, or kerosene-fired apparatuses were billed as a necessity for those who wished to have absolutely pure water. Dismissing mineral waters as polluted with "earthy matter" and therefore detrimental to health, manufacturers of stills recommended them for cooking, for use during epidemics, and for relief of "nervous prostration," kidney diseases, rheumatism, dyspepsia, and indigestion. Manufacturers also promised that distilled water would "renew youth" by preventing the buildup of mineral deposits in the system. The Cuprigraph Company's advertising pamphlet for the "Sanitary Still" warned readers that mechanical filters could not possibly remove the "500,000 disease germs . . . in a cubic centimeter of water." The company attacked natural spring waters,

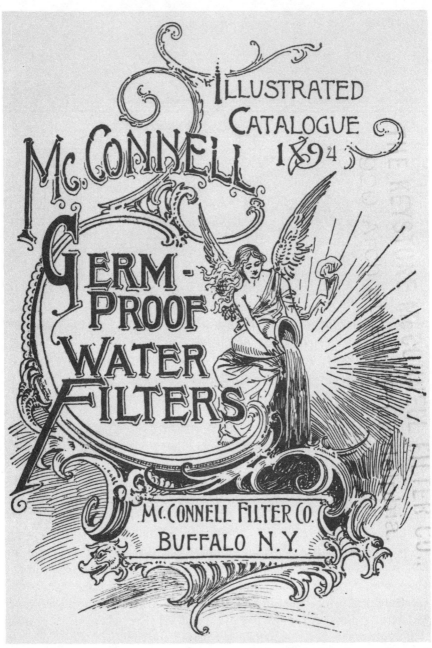

ILLUSTRATED CATALOGUE 1894

Mc.CONNELL

GERM-PROOF WATER FILTERS

McCONNELL FILTER CO.
BUFFALO N.Y.

The McConnell Company vividly portrayed the glories of clean water and the horrors of polluted water. The rococo designs and classically inspired angel attest to the safety of "germ-proof" filters, a characterization that traded on fears of invisible germs. Trade catalog, Buffalo, N.Y., 1894, front cover.

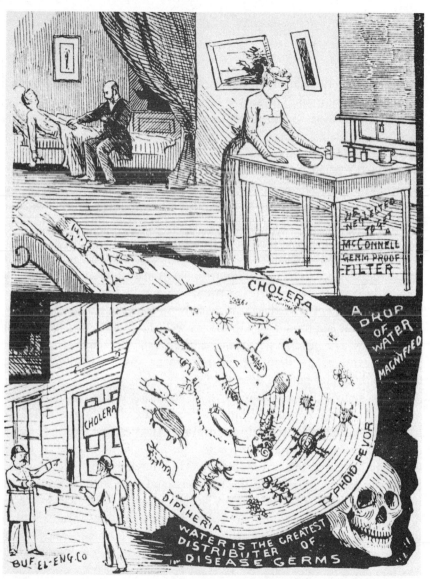

Here are depicted the great fears of Americans regarding their water supply. Fantastic beings allegedly revealed by a microscope brought cholera, typhoid, and diphtheria to a frightened populace that had recently learned of the germ theory of disease. Trade catalog, Buffalo, N.Y., 1894, back cover.

asserting that it was quantity of water consumed, not its mineral content, that brought a cure to the afflicted.[17]

Water was to the body as air was to the engine: it helped remove the foul residue of combustion. The source of the residue—food—had become an even greater concern to Americans between 1890 and 1940 than the purity of water had. Public awareness of nutrition grew as newspapers and magazines reported the findings of scientists and physicians, as well as the often rancorous sectarian arguments between meat eaters and vegetarians. The debates and debacles often turned around the careers and ideas of the "cereal kings"—John Harvey Kellogg, his brother William K. Kellogg, and Charles W. Post—and of the nutrition faddist Horace Fletcher, in addition to more traditional "establishment" physicians and nutritionists.

Horace Fletcher (1849–1919) was one of the most quixotic, dedicated, and sensational characters of the nutrition and hygienic movements of the turn of the century. During the last twenty years of his life, he was as famous as Macfadden or the Kelloggs, in part because of his somewhat obtuse ideology about the proper way to eat (as well the proper food to eat) and with the force of his own personality and exploits. Because he had such a powerful sense of the dramatic, his movement was left without a leader when he died, and faltered accordingly.

Unlike many of his contemporaries or forebears in the hygienic movement, Fletcher did not suffer from any debilitating illnesses from which he had to recover in order to find his salvation. At fifteen he joined the crew of a whaling expedition and discovered for himself the culture of Japan, which he loved for the rest of his life. He attended Dartmouth College briefly, made his way back to the Far East, and then married and settled in San Francisco. An extraordinary athlete, painter, and marksman, he quickly became an important part of Bay Area society, but by the 1890s he was off to New Orleans to manage an opera company. A man of apparently unceasing energy and limitless ego, he was unable to stay at one job or in any one place for very long. By 1898, after sojourns in Paris and Venice, he was back in the United States, conducting experiments at the National Cash Register plant in Dayton, Ohio. He had been around the world four times, and he later maintained that he had practiced at least thirty-eight occupations, not including hygienist.[18]

If Fletcher did not fit the pattern of the weak, sickly youth who fought his way back to health, he did have a skeleton in his closet, albeit a well-padded one. His apparent love of adventure carried over into the culinary arts, not so much into cooking as into eating. In the early 1890s, in his late forties, Fletcher had managed to put 205 pounds on his five-foot, five-and-one-half-inch frame. The athletic body of his younger years was gone, and Fletcher was denied a life insurance policy because of his weight. In an effort to reduce, he became the high priest of chewing.

Fletcher reasoned that by chewing food so thoroughly that all flavor was extracted and the remains involuntarily swallowed, people would eat less, digest their food more easily, and more efficiently use the food they ate. On October 7, 1898, Fletcher wrote his lawyer, Paul Waddell, "I have reduced myself from 205 on June first, when I arrived here, to 169 pounds, today's weight. . . . By a new discovery, which I am explaining in my new book, I am able to regulate nutrition so that I can take on or off a pound of flesh each day as easily as a person can do by putting shot in or taking it out of his pocket." Fletcher weighed 169 pounds or less for the rest of his life and was certain he had made a revolutionary discovery that would dramatically improve the health of the world's people. "I have been experimenting with about a dozen people . . . and [have] prove[n] my discovery to be applicable to any condition. It has not only cured obesity and leanness . . . but I have entirely cured indigestion, bleeding piles, catarrh, pimpled skin and a variety of other ailments."[19]

The ideal fletcherite (a term that, along with *fletcherize,* John Harvey Kellogg coined) was much like a young woman the great masticator encountered in Buffalo in 1909. "Miss Palmer," who was a kindergarten teacher, endeared herself to Fletcher because she "devotes twenty minutes daily to the serving and enjoyment of a single cracker." With perhaps more insight than he recognized at the time, Fletcher compared Palmer's ritual to "a communion service."[20]

Late in 1898 Fletcher attracted the attention of John H. Patterson, president of the National Cash Register (NCR) Company. The firm was one of the most liberal for its time in the treatment of workers, and Fletcher and his system of "efficient" nutrition and mastication appealed to Patterson because the ideas fit in with his beliefs about worker hygiene and welfare. The walls of the company's new factory were almost completely made of glass so that employees could get as much sunlight and fresh air as possible, and the firm's gymnasium and classes in calisthenics were open to all workers. Patterson also hired John C. Olmsted to landscape the plant and design a plan for workers' cottages around it. With classes in gardening organized by educational giant Liberty Hyde Bailey, and with trainloads of plants sold to workers at cost, the NCR experiment became a reality.[21]

Fletcher wrote his sister Abby in November 1898 that he had "the entire facilities of the National Cash Register Company at my disposal." He also told Abby that she would "scarcely know" him, since, on November 11, he weighed "150 pounds, as opposed to the 205 to 210 pounds" he had weighed "for the past fifteen years." Reducing by eating one thoroughly masticated meal had rid him of "catarrh," and returned to him "the strength and activity of twenty-five years ago"—an assertion he was able to support.[22]

For all his boisterous charm and assertive demeanor (shyness was never a problem for him), it was his physical strength that made Fletcher and "fletcherizing" popular phenomena until 1920. In 1903, at the age of fifty-four, he made big news when William G. Anderson, director of the Yale Gymnasium, and Russell H. Chittenden, director of the Sheffield Scientific School at Yale, tested Fletcher's strength and endurance. In a letter to Chittenden, Anderson recounted his findings. "In February, 1903, I gave to Mr. Horace Fletcher the exercises used by the 'Varsity' crew." Fletcher performed them "with ease and showed no ill effects afterwards." Chittenden published the results of these tests in the June 1903 issue of *Popular Science Monthly.* [23]

Four years later, using a leg-exercising machine, Fletcher raised 300 pounds 350 times "and then did not reach the limit of his power." The average number of repetitions by eighteen Yale athletes and gymnasts was 87.4, and the best score 174. His accomplishment seemed all the more remarkable because Fletcher "had done no training" nor had he taken any strenuous exercise since February, 1907, four months before the test. His "two occasions" of "hard work" were typical Fletcher—"climbing a volcanic mountain through a tropical jungle on an island near Mindanao" with Major General Leonard Wood and "wading through deep snow in the Himalayan Mountains, some three miles one day and seven miles the next day, in about as many hours." Fletcher impressed and astonished his testers through five days of stair climbing, three hundred situps, presses, running in place, and exercise with dumbbells, with no apparent soreness, stiffness, or muscular fatigue. "During the thirty-five years of my own experience in physical training and teaching," wrote Anderson, "I have never tested a man who equalled this record."[24]

What most impressed Anderson was that Fletcher's condition seemed to result solely from diet, and an unusual one at that, "with no systematic physical training." Fletcher ate as much as he wanted and whatever he wanted, but he avoided overeating by faithfully following the principle of thorough mastication. Anderson thought there was "pretty good evidence" to support Fletcher's contentions about his chewing practices, since he was so fit and since total mastication left "little or no excess material to be disposed of by bacterial agency," which he thought "might account for the absence of toxic products in the circulation." Anderson endorsed Fletcherism "as not only practical but agreeable."[25]

Fletcher continued to test himself against younger men and his own records, because people evidently did not believe the reports about his feats of strength. "In competition with two husky young New Havenites," he wrote Chittenden, "one of the New Havenites lifted 380 pounds and I followed with 760. Two days later the other did 420 pounds and I followed with 840 pounds." He was sixty years old at the time. On his sixty-third birthday, he "was doing an endurance stunt in the form of a thirty-three mile walk in twenty-four hours." He had bicycled "nearly two hundred miles on [his] fiftieth birthday," with the only negative effects of these endurance trials having been the "chafing of long-continued . . . use" of his feet and posterior.[26] Fletcher's exploits earned him an audience, not only because of the spectacle he presented, but also because he claimed diet and mastication alone produced such positive effects. He offered hope for the sedentary and promise for the overweight without the trials and the pain of training. For the middle class, "fletcherizing" was an easy and effective alternative.[27]

"Fletcherizing" did in fact become a widespread practice in the first two decades of the twentieth century. Fletcher commented in 1910 that "the words 'fletcherism,' 'fletcherizing,' and 'fletcherites' have found their way into the *New International Webster* and *Supplement of the Century* dictionaries since . . . last Spring." In 1905 William James, professor at Harvard and perhaps the most distinguished American psychologist of his day, characterized Fletcher in the Harvard *Crimson* as "one of the most original and 'sympathetic' personalities whom Massachusetts in our day has produced." James's brother Henry was even more enthusiastic. "I Fletcherize," he wrote the champion of chewing in 1906, "and that's my life. I mean it makes my life possible, and it has enormously improved my work. You really ought to have a handsome percentage on every volume I sell." Henry James had evidently been experimenting with fletcherizing in 1905 and had settled on a routine of eating as much as he wanted (rather than a predetermined small amount) and chewing until involuntary swallowing occurred. "My inclination," he wrote Fletcher in 1905, "is to make Fletcherism perhaps a little *excessively* reduce quantity—it does legitimately and triumphantly reduce it when this virtue in it is not made an over-ridden horse. . . . As soon as I prove myself afresh (at any return of malaise), the difference between Fletcherizing on really *enough* (of quantity) and on too little, all my serenity and improvement return." James suffered from "sinister heart-burn" and indigestion, which he blamed on the "abuse of too drastic mouth washes," and credited Fletcher's ideas with ending his troubles. "Be interested (and glad!) to know that I haven't touched listerine since Sunday night, and that thus at the end of three days the abnormal irritation I spoke to you of has most unmistakeably [*sic*] subsided. Glory, glory, Hallelujah!"[28]

Henry James evidently lost his enthusiasm for fletcherizing by 1909. He cabled his brother in February that he had "stopped Fletcherizing. Perfectly Well." William relayed the message to Fletcher, who responded that "a bugbear like your brother's message would set back my work tremendously." William evidently regarded Fletcher with a combination of respect and the derision reserved for those who took themselves and their causes with complete and utter seriousness. He did not wish to "wreak havoc" on Fletcher's cause, but, when he sent Fletcher's letter to his brother, he wrote at the top: "Poor Horace Fletcher! I repeated your cablegram in New York to him the other day. He bore it well, with my explanation, but is evidently afraid of his enemies getting wind of it and exploiting it." Relations between Henry James and Fletcher deteriorated by 1911, when James evidently let it be known that he had "starved" while holding to the regimen. "As for Henry James," wrote Fletcher to Kellogg, "If he has 'starved' as a result of fletcherizing, he has done something else than fletcherize."[29]

While Henry James was vacillating, the Moses of mastication was converting thousands, including other prominent Americans. Elbert Hubbard's Roycrofters became ardent fletcherizers in the first decade of the century. Oil baron John D. Rockefeller endorsed fletcherizing in 1913 in the New York *Evening Mail:* "Don't gobble your food. Fletcherize or chew very slowly while you eat." The previous year Sir Arthur Conan Doyle publicly supported the practice, prompting Fletcher to speak warmly of "Sherlock Holmes" thereafter.[30] Fletcher's frequent correspondents included conservationist Gifford Pinchot, publisher S. S. McClure, *Ladies' Home Journal* publisher Edward Bok, eminent physician Henry P. Bowditch, author and journalist Upton Sinclair, Boy Scouts of America director James E. West, Bernarr Macfadden, Senator Robert L. Owen of Oklahoma, and U.S. Army Chief of Staff General Leonard Wood.[31]

Fletcher was a close friend of Kellogg; he endorsed the "Battle Creek Idea" and visited "the San" several times.[32] He and Kellogg had had a jovial meeting in 1903, prompting Fletcher to compose lyrics "to the old tune of 'Montague Montrose.' "

I choose to chew because I wish to do
The sort of thing that Nature had in view,
Before bad cooks invented sav'ry stew;
When the only way to eat was to chew! chew!! chew!!!

With glands, full up, with juices strong and sweet,
To dextrose lifeless starch from tubers and from wheat,
With buccal muscles furnished for the toughest things to treat,
I choose to munch and chew with every chance to eat.

To cheat the teeth, the muscles and the glands
With artificial muscles is like working without hands;
And hence the exercise that each of these demands
Is lacking, and they wither, as the law of growth commands.

Hark back my friends, to primal times of yore
When instincts reigned supreme and were always to the fore,
And henceforth give allegence [sic] unto them ever more,
With appetite as king to welcome at the door.

Then eat, eat, eat, at will of appetite;
Whenever it permits, you are surely doing right;
But taste, munch, chew, and relish with your might
For nothing in our lives has such importance quite.[33]

Fletcher's composition may never have challenged ragtime, but it reveals an ideological synthesis that was—and perhaps still is—critical to American dietary and other health-restoring movements. In his assertion that thorough mastication meant going back to nature, Fletcher implicitly criticized a civilization he thought had somehow diverted men and women from the purity that was part of life in "primal times." He joined Kellogg and other dietary reformers by criticizing "sav'ry stew," or highly seasoned dishes, and he blamed cookery for people's digestive troubles. Like many enthusiasts of the arts-and-crafts movement and the colonial revival, he wished to go back in time, to allegedly purer days, when "instincts reigned supreme." This primitivism also harmonized with many aspects of Roosevelt's "strenuous life" idea; it was also the sentiment that provoked advocates of such contact sports as football to appreciate "healthy barbarism" in young men.

In addition to the apparent increase in strength the system stimulated, fletcherizing seemed an efficient use of resources—an idea that, by the first decade of the new century, was central to Progressive reformers' ideals; Fletcher thought succeeding generations would actually approach super-manhood and super-womanhood. In a letter to William James in 1908 he figured that "in the ranks of the Christian Endeavor Army alone [Fletcher's name for his followers], it is hoped to attain a true saving of a million and a half dollars a day," an approach to diet that certainly appealed to efficiency-minded businessmen. Fletcher spent "about five weeks" at the Chautauqua colony in the summer of 1908, where he "delivered some fifteen addresses" drumming up support for "Optimum Progressive Human Efficiency as a Result of Dietetic Righteousness and Psychic Righteousness." In the same year he and Irving Fisher, an ardent hygienist and prominent Yale professor of political economy, founded the short-lived Health and Efficiency League of America, which had as one of its goals the establishment of a cabinet-level Department of Health. Other similar groups included the Committee of One Hundred on National Health, which was composed of businessmen, scholars, and physicians.[34]

Fisher lent his considerable intellectual reputation to Fletcher's program because he had come to believe that thorough mastication and decreased protein intake produced greater physical endurance, which he thought prevented disease and therefore increased worker and executive productivity. A more efficient society, Fisher reasoned, would result from more efficient diet. Fletcher summarized the benefits in a four-page brochure produced to promote his lecturing. Under the heading of *Some Possible Profits*, he listed "approximately one-half of the former cost of nourishment," and an "increase of 50% to 200% in physical endurance." He promised "immunity from sickness (at least increased resistance), and 'that tired feeling.'" Fletcherizing reduced desire for alcohol in the "chronically intemperate," as well as suppressing "physical morbidness and immorality" while it restored virility. Fletcherizing, he maintained, would "eliminate from human excreta all offensiveness" and renew "normal confidence and laudable ambition" and "both muscular and mental quality . . . in those already past . . . middle life."[35]

Fletcher directed his appeal at the whole human race, but, like many other reformers of the Progressive era, he found a ready audience in the middle class and a model for organization in big business. "You must always bear in mind," he wrote publisher W. E. Berry, "that fletcherism is [a] system of economics taking tips from all human knowledge and proceeding along the lines of Big Business in cultivating maximum efficiency in all departments." This rang in unison with Hubbard's enthusiastic support of "Big Business and more of it," and the interest among American industrialists in Frederick Taylor's motion-study ideas of the turn of the century. Fletcher worked hard to promote himself among businessmen he thought open-minded. In 1909 he reported to Kellogg that he "was in conference at the Waldorf with three prominent New York bankers, one the president of Bankers Trust Company. . . . The conference was for the purpose of forming a Fletcher Club in the interest especially of bank employees, the object being to induce them to fletcherize . . . so as to get the most efficiency out of themselves."[36]

Fletcher did not neglect the plight of the poor and the working class. When missionary trainees from Tennessee tried fletcherizing for six months while in the field in Appalachia, they reported not only reduced food consumption but also less drinking among the converted. Clearly total social reformation was possible.[37]

Fletcher had been devoted to the cause of bettering the lives of impoverished children since at least 1898. Arguing against the idea that some part of the population must always be poor, he fought for the time when the "last waif" would be saved, thereby ensuring a just society. He dubbed his movement the "Conservation of the Child," a phrase undoubtedly influenced by the Interior Department's natural resource conservation efforts, and once again he began to marshal funds and friends to teach fletcherizing. He wrote Kellogg in 1910 that "they tell me over there also that I am mentioned for one of the Nobel prizes in Economics, and it will not only be a worthy thing to get the prize, but it will give me funds to go on with the good work."[38] He failed to win.

Fletcher believed in the power of environment as the chief determinant of the human condition, thereby setting himself apart from such individualists as Kellogg and Macfadden, as well as from more strident eugenicists, such as Madison Grant and Albert Wiggam. "Heredity," he wrote Kellogg in 1910, "is a factor in condition but it is so insignificant in its strength that it can be counteracted by sufficient purity of environment." But like Kellogg and others of his contemporaries, Fletcher identified the social problems of the nation with immigrants. In 1903 he had written General Leonard Wood that "babies who are born into crime—malarial environment . . . imbibe crime with their mother's poisoned milk . . . [and] become criminal before they ever know that there is any such thing as good in the world. . . . My scheme of Social Quarantine has in view the watching for and wet-nursing of these unfortunate immigrants to our shores by the portal of infected birth, and do for this class of immigrants just what you and [Walter] Reed . . . did in the case of Yellow Jack."[39]

Fletcher's lack of interest in physical training was troublesome, even to those impressed with his dietary system. Army Chief of Staff General Leonard Wood found Fletcher's ideas intriguing but did not compel his troops to adopt them. Like William G. Anderson, the physiologist who tested Fletcher, Wood believed that physical and intellectual vigor were achieved only through rigorous conditioning and proper nutrition. Fletcher was commendable on the latter score but negligent on the former. Moreover, Fletcher's lack of discipline in eating—that is, eating whenever his appetite demanded—probably offended Wood's sense of discipline. Moreover, as a true believer in the efficacy of sport—as Fletcher was not—Wood had other ideas about diet and nutrition.

The growth of intercollegiate sport had been accompanied by a parallel increase of research on nutrition and its relationship to athletic performance. Physician Wilbur Atwater was a leading figure in the development of the "new nutrition" of the turn of the century. Using sophisticated chemical analyses of foodstuffs and compilations of information about eating patterns in the United States, Atwater concluded that protein was the essential element of nutrition. He theorized that only proteins built and repaired tissues, whereas fats and carbohydrates provided energy. Atwater found little use for roughage and consigned bran and such fibers as potato skins to the "refuse" heap. He urged Americans to eat more beans and grain, lean meats, and fewer sweets. In *Dietary Studies of University Boat Crews* (1900), he and coauthor A. P. Bryant found that the standard "training table" (a term and concept invented in the 1890s) for college athletes had two kinds of meat at all three meals, a modest amount of vegetables, and large quantities of carbohydrates.[40]

Atwater's findings were a source of great popular interest because Upton Sinclair's revelations about the meat packing industry had combined with cultural fears of "race suicide" and of autointoxication to cause the debate about vegetarianism to resurface. Vegetarians joined in the argument for another reason—to combat the powerfully persuasive sanction that athletics gave to the eating of meat. The battle lines were drawn: red meat, and lots of it, versus fiber and vegetables.

Atwater's dietary recommendations were supported both by college athletic coaches throughout the nation and by most eminent American physicians. New York City physician Woods Hutchinson, for example, argued in *Instinct and Health* (1909) and in articles in such popular magazines as *Cosmopolitan* and *McClure's* that the configuration and shapes of human teeth indicated that a mixed diet was the natural evolutionary ideal for humans. Civilizations had evolved according to their instincts and that meat eating "races" were inevitably stronger, conquering ones. "White bread, red meat, and blue blood make the tricolor flag of conquest," he crowed, evidently forgetting that the French had been uniformly unsuccessful in the wars and colonial contests of the preceding forty years.[41]

Hutchinson's and Atwater's opponents were a mixed lot. Kellogg was a strict vegetarian; Macfadden, Fletcher, and Russell Chittenden took a less polemical approach. Chittenden's research on eating habits and nutrition led him to conclude that lowering protein intake, not increasing it, as Hutchinson and Atwater advised, helped people improve their health, eased digestive problems, and, he thought, promoted longevity. Fletcher also thought protein-rich diets were unhealthy, and in 1914 he wrote Irving Fisher that Atwater had become "a discredited authority" in America, fallen "from his very high proteid perch."[42]

Vegetarians, as James C. Whorton has pointed out, knew how powerful athletic victory could be in securing public support for their campaign, and vegetarian athletes perhaps had an edge in many sporting events because they were committed to a cause as well as to winning. They were particularly successful in the endurance bicycle, walking, and running races that were widely publicized at the turn of the century. In turn-of-the-century America, cyclist Will Brown (who became a vegetarian in the 1890s) held the record for the two thousand-mile ride, and vegetarian Margarita Gast held the women's thousand-mile record. Vegetarian tennis players, runners, and walkers regularly won matches and races in Europe and America throughout the last decade of the nineteenth and early years of the twentieth centuries, enabling advocates like Kellogg to proclaim the superiority of their nutritional beliefs. Kellogg's Battle Creek College football team, however, lasted only one season in the early twenties, losing more games than it won.[43]

The urge to trust vegetables as curatives and preventives had roots in the American psyche that would have horrified Kellogg or Post. Decades before the "cereal boom" of Battle Creek, American consumers had customarily consumed allegedly vegetable-based compounds as "tonics" and "elixirs."

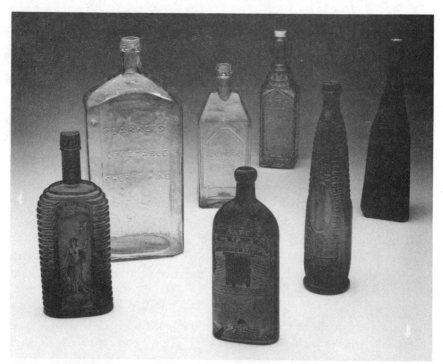

Rather than avoid certain foods, many dyspeptic Americans turned to "bitters" to settle their stomach. This horrified temperance advocates and health critics, since the potions were usually heavily laced with alcohol. Bitters bottles, American, pressed and mold-blown glass, ca. 1860–80.

Lydia Pinkham's famous compound "for all those painful Complaints and Weaknesses so common to our best female population" was a "vegetable compound." Like most others of its ilk, it probably derived its "tonic" effect from the liberal dose of alcohol it contained (as high as 23 percent). Ayer's Sarsaparilla bragged that it too was a product of the vegetable world, in particular sarsaparilla root, "Stillingia, Yellow-Dock, and Mandrake, all celebrated for curative qualities." Americans could even buy "Magnetized Food"—"healthful fruits and cereals vitalized by Magnetism."[44]

The popularity of vegetable and animal extracts indicates that despite Hutchinson's contempt for it, vegetarianism as advocated by Kellogg and Post was not rejected summarily by the American public. Hutchinson had argued that real breakfasts included bacon and eggs or wheatcakes and sausage. He dismissed the cereal kings' products as horse fodder, calling them "shredded doormats," "Gripe nuts," and "Eata-heapa-hay." But while vegetarians were not to succeed as completely with the public as they had hoped, American diet was changing—at least at the breakfast table. From the outset the primary targets for advertisers of breakfast cereals and other health foods were the middle class and the elite. It was a safe and shrewd maneuver, since the working class often shared the same success aspirations implicit in the litany of advertisements warning of the failure to advance because of being "worn out."[45]

According to John Harvey Kellogg, the breakfast food industry was born in about 1878, when he concocted a dough of wheat flour, cornmeal, and oatmeal, fashioned it into biscuits, and baked them. These he had ground into a coarse meal he called "Granula." Jackson's "Our Home on the Hillside" was producing a similar product with the same name, and, threatened with legal action, Kellogg changed the name of his product to Granola.

Breakfast food technology and progress stalled until 1892, when Denver inventor and dyspeptic Henry D. Perky dreamed up shredded wheat. By boiling and steaming the grain, Perky rendered it pliable enough to draw it through rollers—one smooth, the other grooved—to form long strands that were shaped into moist, soft biscuits. Eventually, after he met with Kellogg and moved back east to Boston, Perky began to produce shredded wheat biscuits as contemporary Americans know them.[46]

Shredded wheat was an enormous success in the marketplace, and everything about it was well protected by patents. Kellogg responded quickly to the new rage with a product of his own—"Granose" wheat flakes—in 1895. Competition in the flake market appeared rapidly. In early 1891 Charles W.

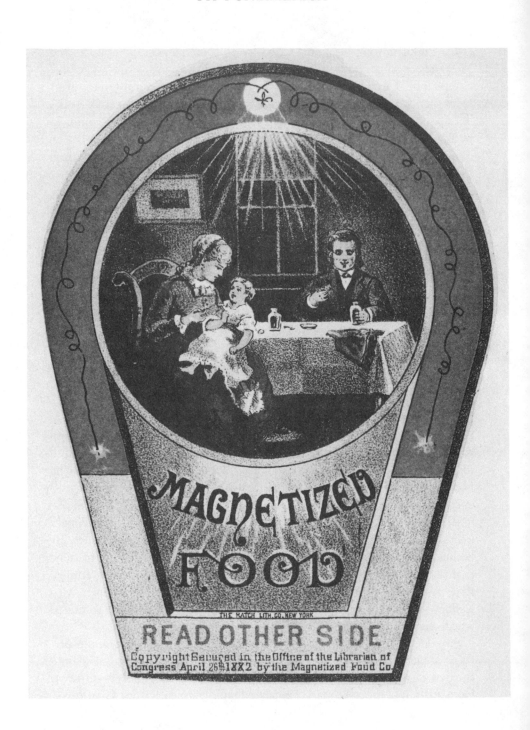

Post, a thirty-six-year-old inventor and engineer, landed at Battle Creek. He had a history of health troubles and had tried nearly every common cure to no avail. He resided at the "San" for nine months but found no relief. He then turned to Christian Science, faith healing, and positive thinking, which seemed to work. In 1892 he established his own health home, LaVita Inn, where he banned tea, coffee, and physicians. Three years later, Post joined the health food industry with the invention of Postum, a cereal "coffee" made from bran, wheat, and molasses. Grape-Nuts (1898) and Post Toasties (1908) soon followed.[47]

Fallout from the "cereal boom" was everywhere. The Battle Creek Pure Food Company made a fortune on Malta Vita (a wheat flake with barley

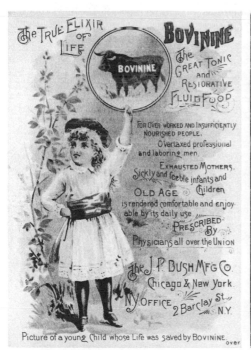 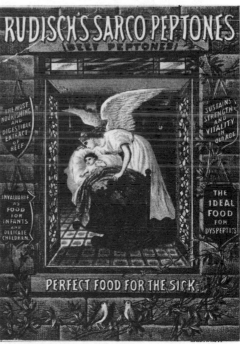

Food products advertised as offering renewed vigor were popular and plentiful in late-nineteenth-century America. Left opposite: trade card, The Match Lithograph Company, New York, N.Y., ca. 1882. Left: trade card, American, chromolithograph, ca. 1890. Right: advertising card, A. Gast and Company, New York, N.Y., ca. 1895.

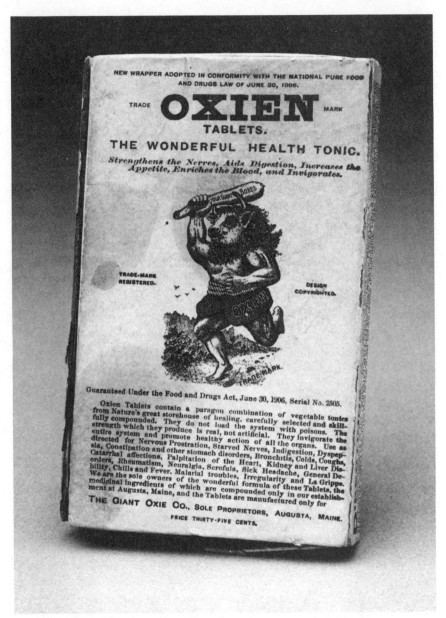

Food-supplement manufacturers appealed to Americans' desire to improve their health without the hard work of exercise. Food-supplement box, the Giant Oxie Co., Augusta, Maine, dried herbs, ca. 1910.

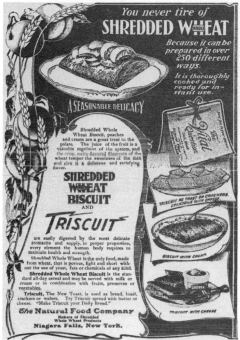
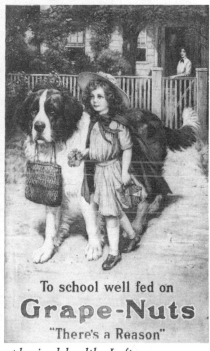

Ad campaigns for new cereal products emphasized health. Left: advertisement from Physical Culture, *September 1904, p. 5. Right: trade sign for Postum Cereal Co. American, chromolithographed tin, ca. 1905.*

malt syrup) and Vim Wheat Flakes. These in turn spawned Force Flakes, Mapl-Flakes, Ceru-Fruto (wheat flakes sprayed with apple jelly), Norka Malted Oats, Golden Manna (a yellow meal product), and Kellogg's Corn Flakes, which John Harvey's brother William K. Kellogg first marketed in 1906.[48]

Alternatives to coffee like Postum had been produced or made at home for most of the nineteenth century. Farm and ranch women in particular had combined various roots or grains with chicory to produce a hot dark drink; cocoa and chocolate had been popular drinks since at least the eighteenth century. Cocoa was marketed by the Van Houten Company in 1893 as a drink for "nervous people who do not know the cause of their ill health . . . [who] would find reason if they'd stop drinking tea and coffee, and substitute an absolutely pure and soluble cocoa."[49] This Van Houten Cocoa advertisement had another message; it featured a line drawing of a

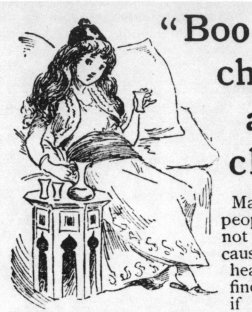

"Boo choke a—ee chere"

Many nervous people who do not know the cause of their ill health would find the reason if they'd stop drinking tea and coffee, and substitute an absolutely pure and soluble cocoa. A trial will show superiority in strength and cheapness of

Van Houten's Cocoa

(BEST AND GOES FARTHEST)

in which the Exquisite Natural Flavor is fully developed. No Vanilla USED

Cocoa was advertised as an alternative to coffee and tea, which some critics argued were "too stimulating," and therefore debilitating. The suggestive pose of the exotic Middle Eastern girl perhaps implied a revitalized sexuality for men worried about their performance. Advertisement from The Ladies' Home Journal, *August 1893, p. 15.*

barely pubescent Middle Eastern girl, surrounded by Moorish-style furniture and with a "come-hither" look. The "look" may possibly be a reference to male sexual longings or concerns in the beginning of the era of male insecurity about potency: cocoa, which calmed the nerves, might also awaken other drives.

Charles Post was a skillful businessman and a vigorous promoter. In 1897 he bought four column inches of advertising space in *The Ladies' Home Journal* in which he proclaimed, "A great popular pure drink and pure food wave is just now passing over the country, and it seems to have come to stay." Post promoted Postum as a "pure natural food such as the Creator intended for man's subsistence," and "a rational method of dismissing sickness."[50] Coffee, he implied, was somehow unnatural and associated with "civilization." Post confused "health foods" with "natural foods," a distinction that was more ideological than biochemical, since many compounds in nature are deleterious to human health. In Post's analysis of civilization, traditional cultures of the past equaled healthier, organic life-styles.

In the serious health-food business's first quarter century, its products were marketed almost exclusively to counter the deleterious effects of industrial civilization, particularly among "brain workers." In 1897 Somatose powder was promoted for "pale, thin, delicate people" who needed to become "vigorous." In 1901, a Post advertisement for Grape-Nuts began with the boldface headline: "Brains are Built by Grape-Nuts." "Brain workers must have different food than day laborers," and Grape-Nuts were appropriate because they contained the "natural phosphate of potash . . . used by the system in rebuilding and repairing the brain and nerve centers."[51]

Bran foods and other "natural" products were also marketed as relief from constipation— and autointoxication. Half the advertisements on one page of the July 1920 issue of *Physical Culture* promised cures for constipation. Great Valley Mills, of Paoli, Pennsylvania, urged consumers to "Use Bran[,] Nature's Cereal Laxative," while the makers of Tyler's Macerated Wheat assured readers they could "eat their way to health" because "its bran content keeps bowels normal" while providing "vitamines and mineral salts." The Yoghurt Company of Bellingham, Washington, warned that "our wrong way of living causes intestinal Auto-Intoxication, which brings about thousands of human miseries, beginning with constipation, and ending with an early death."[52]

The image of the businessman too exhausted to be effective or the woman too tired to be sociable or attractive because of constipation was a dominant theme in thc cereal advertising literature of the 1920s and 1930s. "Half a man on a whole man's job," shouted the headline of a full-page advertisement for Fleischmann's Yeast in the May 1921 *Physical Culture*. One to three cakes eaten daily would "keep your body free of poisons" and help "maintain vigor and zest." Six years later, images of obviously well-to-do men and women—a business executive, a mature socialite or professional woman, and a wealthy young women—replaced those of the young female rower, golfer, and dancer and the male baseball player and fisherman that had adorned a 1926 advertisement in the *Ladies' Home Journal.* Three cakes per day (the required volume steadily increased) would eliminate the "Headache—lassitude—depression . . . digestive troubles, unpleasant breath, skin disorders" that "usually indicate an unhealthy state of the intestinal tract." In an interview conducted in 1985 for National Public Radio, Rudy Vallee remembered that relief of constipation was a new gimmick the marketing people of Fleischmann's had developed in the mid 1920s. He was uncertain of the effectiveness of the product for this malady.[53]

Both the small natural foods concerns and the "heavyweights" of the milling and cereal industries also took advantage of this broad-based cultural concern. In 1924 "at least two tablespoons daily" of W. K. Kellogg's "All-Bran" promised "permanent relief for the most chronic cases of constipation." Three years later the All-Bran advertisement in *Physical Culture* had a somewhat menacing tone, emblematic of the fears of failure that were steadily increasing among white-collar workers in the 1920s.[54]

In 1927 the Pillsbury Flour Mills of Minneapolis took a somewhat different approach in its advertising, mentioning bran's laxative properties only obliquely and providing recipes for a cookie called "bran delights," bran nut bread, and bran, date, and nut muffins. "Pillsbury's Health Bran" was, from the outset, marketed as "a new and delightful appetite experience" that would "do you good." Post similarly began selling Grape-Nuts as a healthful additive to muffins and other baked goods in the mid 1920s, promising better health because it was "crammed with the things the body needs! Dextrins, maltose, and other carbohydrates . . . iron . . . phosphorous . . . proteins . . . and the essential vitamin B."[55]

By the late twenties cereal advertisers were promoting their wares as essential to men who would be strong and women who would be beautiful. Nabisco's Shredded Wheat promised "Strength in Every Shred" in 1931,

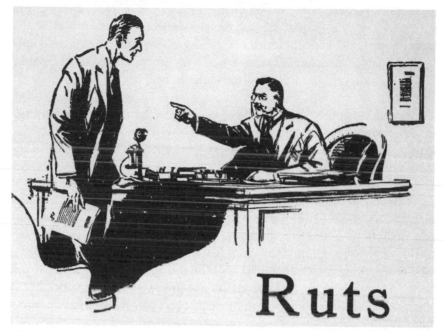

Ruts

This ad portrays one of the great fears of the 1920s man-on-the-make: the severe and dapper executive points an accusing finger at the slouched-over aspirant, who is suffering from listlessness because of his diet. Advertisement for Kellogg's All-Bran, from Physical Culture, *December 1927, p. 51.*

and a typical advertisement showed a father and son exercising with dumbbells while his wife sat on the bed holding an Indian club as she watched proudly. A Post's Bran Flakes advertisement in the August 1927 issue of *The Ladies' Home Journal* sadly noted that the woman pictured *"could* be beautiful," but she was "never quite up to par. . . . There is something almost pitiful about her, the woman who just misses beauty." Her problem was "lack of natural bulk," the Bran Flakes advertisement determined.[56]

Throughout the 1920s and 1930s other foods entered the health and strength marketplace as well. The National Kraut Packers Association of Clyde, Ohio, pushed sauerkraut for breakfast and other meals in 1924, asserting that "its lactic ferments have a hygienic influence." "Parkelp," a concoction of "natural minerals from the sea," was marketed in the 1930s to help "assimilate vitamins." Dedicated health seekers could also obtain garlic juice blended with parsley juice and honey to cure a variety of ailments. By 1939 a "partial list" of merchants who were members of the newly organized National Health Food Association, and therefore sold only "natural foods," took nearly twenty column inches of small print in *Physical Culture*. Thirty states were represented, as well as Hawaii and Great Britain.[57]

Health-food purists—usually vegetarians—never gained a strong foothold in American culture in part because they were never able to counter the claims of great athletes—both amateur and professional—who ate meat-laden meals. Moreover, they were challenging the powerful and ever-growing nostalgia for the idealized people of the colonial American and medieval past—hardly people who refused meat. Breakfast foods succeeded because manufacturers' advertising campaigns promised "cures" for indigestion and constipation without requiring Americans to forgo meat. The "natural" quality of grain foods and drinks appealed to Americans who questioned the effects of civilization in the thirties but who did not necessarily reject all the benefits of machine-age technology. In fact, the American press reveled in the quantity of production and mechanized processes of cereal flake production, and the careers of such barons as Kellogg and Post were the sources of envy and veneration, just as those of Andrew Carnegie and John Jacob Astor had been before. It was, after all, not meat that was problematic for most middle-class Americans; it was civilization. Thus C. W. Post's advertisements could safely state in 1926 that "modern conditions of living and working have banished the Early American breakfast, probably forever!" Besides, one could still eat one's Post Toasties or Kellogg's All-Bran with a colonial-style spoon in an early American kitchen (complete with the latest modern equipment) thereby feeling a unity with both the colonial and the modern world.[58]

The vegetarians also failed to become major forces in the American health movement because the advocates of strength culture—Atlas, Titus, Strongfort, and Macfadden—were effectively competing with them for the position of keeper of the key to health. Though some, like Macfadden, embraced health foods wholeheartedly, many others followed the great Sandow's example of eating meat and lots of it. Athletic training tables overflowed with meats. Vegetarian experiments at these tables often met with opposition; the Cornell crew team went on strike in 1904 when they were denied meat after a tough workout.

Finally, the vegetarian wing of the dietary reform movement fell victim to the ever-increasing power of physicians in the culture of health and fitness. Though Macfadden and a few others continued their vitriolic attacks on the medical community throughout the early twentieth century, the vast majority of Americans had begun to defer to physicians. The gradual alteration in public attitude was in part a result of the increasing professionalization of the occupation, which had begun in 1870. Unstructured and haphazard in the 1830s, medical education was made more rigorous and formal in the 1870s, when Charles Eliot at Harvard and Daniel Coit Gilman at Johns Hopkins undertook its reorganization and stiffened graduation requirements, which now included lab work. The rest of the nation's leading medical schools followed the Harvard example by the 1890s.[59]

Increasingly sophisticated machines and technology augmented physicians' sensory and diagnostic powers and with them, their influence. Stethoscopes, ophthalmoscopes, and laryngoscopes, as sociologist Paul Starr has pointed out, gave the physician powers beyond ordinary human observation. When these tools were joined by the machines of the later nineteenth and early twentieth centuries—microscopes, electronic devices to measure or monitor human functions, and X rays—physicians were able to generate and present data in a fashion that was far beyond the capability of ordinary people. In addition, by the turn of the century, medical researchers had isolated the causes of such ravaging diseases as tuberculosis, diphtheria, and cholera and were able to test for them. Cures for dreaded diseases came with increasing frequency as the century turned. Physicians emerged as the most important guardians of health, a position that led manufacturers of foods to seek their approval and endorsement whenever they could.[60]

Medical research also revealed that nutrition was more complex than Kellogg, Post, Macfadden, or Fletcher had envisioned. Vitamins were first isolated in the early twentieth century (the word *vitamine* was coined in 1911), and the pharmaceutical industry, as well as the food merchants, immediately began trumpeting the powers of these compounds. By 1939 advertisements for packaged vitamins were abundant in all forms of the popular press. Moreover, since most physicians opted for a "balanced" diet of meat, carbohydrates, vegetables, and dairy products, vegetarianism was a hard program to sell.

Yet the urge for health was strong enough and the subject complex enough that physicians of the Harvard-Hopkins model did not exercise complete control over the field. Mineral water advocates and strength proponents had great public appeal by virtue of example and clever marketing, and few physicians ever criticized strong men as unhealthy. Moreover, the health seeker could readily locate, in most urban areas at least, homeopaths and other practitioners who did not conform to the traditional, established medical example. Nearly all of the homeopathic medical schools had disappeared by the mid-1920s (there had been twenty-two in 1900), but the practice of using tiny doses of substances to produce symptoms of a disease

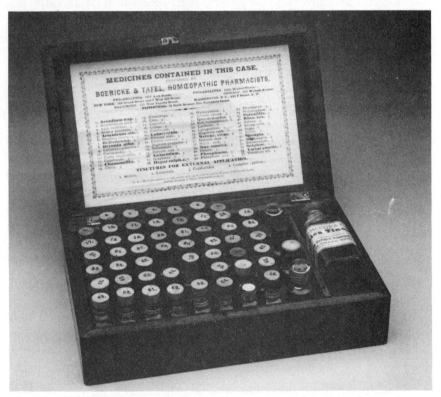

Homeopathy persisted as a minor but important option for Americans seeking medical treatment in the late nineteenth and early twentieth centuries. In a home treatment kit such as this, all the essential compounds were present and could be used with one of the many home-cure and treatment books available at the time. Family Homeopathic Medicine Chest, Boericke and Tafel, Philadelphia, Pa., wood, glass, ca. 1882–1900.

artificially continued to hold some attraction for Americans. Perhaps this was related to the fact that many of the substances were derived from plants, such as belladonna, and this "natural" form of treatment might have seemed more comfortable to those anxious about modern technology. In addition, homeopathic procedure was extremely personal, demanding a thorough reporting by the patient, rather than impersonal diagnostic testing.[61]

The selective way in which Americans responded to dietary and nutritional philosophy and their acceptance of breakfast foods, if not of the entire health-food movement, corresponded to the accommodation that "regularly" trained members of the medical profession made with homeopathic physicians. Resistance to orthodoxy and dogma had been part of the religious tradition of the nation as a whole, and this freewheeling eclecticism characterized American responses to dietary theory and practice. Vegetarianism was too dogmatic, but All-Bran was acceptable. Fletcherism seemed too confining, even though it offered hope to the unhealthy without the pain of exercise. Dietary and health reformers of the pre–Civil War era were often closely connected with religion, either as ministers, or, as in Catharine Beecher's case, as the daughters and sisters of men of the cloth. Religious physicians such as Kellogg bridged the transition between these individuals and the secular scientists of the twentieth century. Though the moral content of health reform has never completely left the good health movement, it, like nearly every other traditional human concern, has responded to the secularization of culture that has characterized the last hundred years.

· EPILOGUE ·

The quest for health in America has been both pursuit and flight. From the very outset of the publication of the *Journal of Health* in late 1829 through the ultimately extremist vantage point of Bernarr Macfadden's *Physical Culture* magazine of the late 1930s, Americans have doggedly searched for fitness even as they have looked nervously over their shoulders. For if the Kelloggs, Sandows, or Alcotts of their times offered a promise, the reality of mortality seemed to take it away. Health was described or classified in ways that changed as social concerns were transformed, but the fear of "early death" was a constant, menacing minor key in the optimism of the reformer's song.

In the three decades preceding the Civil War, Alcott, Graham, Beecher, and others warned Americans of the dangers of their habits, particularly drink and diet, and were convinced that "early death" would befall those who ignored their forebodings. Theirs was a culture steeped in the traditions of evangelical Protestant Christianity. Only a quarter-century from the Second Great Awakening and in the midst of their own "revivals" of religious enthusiasm, most were convinced that the Second Coming of Christ would occur only after they had worked to transform American society to a state of grace that would endure for one thousand years. But they believed it was possible and that human beings could be made perfect if the proper conditions were met. It was, then, an optimistic vision, but one with awesome personal responsibility.

The perfect society most certainly had none of the illness or maladies of American society in the 1830s. To die an "early death," of course, meant "normal" life was much longer, and such a death was perforce one's own fault—not, by implication, God's will. This was a critical intellectual break with the determinism of older theologies. It freed Americans to consider not just the state of their souls but the state of their bodies, as well as the body of their state. As God was relieved of all responsibility for the human body's condition, so too the Divine no longer had run of the state. In fact, the intellectual basis for declaring independence and for forming a new government had already proceeded according to that logic. The transfer of responsibility was nearly complete in the 1830s.

Thus, the religious revivals of the era sought ways to regenerate the fervor of religious experience, with a mind toward the preparation of the good society. They were, at base, individualistic, and they invoked not only a call to arms against sin but also a vision of past generations of greatness, whose presumed noble sense of community responsibility would be necessary for the millennium. Reform was therefore a holistic idea, and ministers to the bodily health of the individual and the republic were often trained in the way of the ministry, or were close to those who were. They flooded the marketplace with mass-produced and inexpensively printed books with advice on everything from courtship to exercise. With death seeming to be ever-present and capricious, they saw as essential nothing less than total reform and regeneration.

Reformers pointed to the sorry state of Americans' physical condition as evidence of decline from the golden age of the nation's founders. They found new cures—water and vegetarianism—for ailments and, in a manner that was to become characteristic, promised to alleviate nearly all forms of human suffering. Those who promised cures and those who preached prevention experienced the same fate. They failed. The millennium did not come.

By the time the Civil War had ended, American society had changed to the extent that older explanations seemed inappropriate. Particularly in the northern states, where fewer and fewer Americans worked on farms or at home, new sorts of diseases seemed to be thwarting the men and women of the nation. Weakened by their new urban lives, spared the rigors of the farm or frontier, vaguely defined illnesses—dyspepsia, neurasthenia, or even uric acid diathesis and autointoxication—seemed to doom Americans. Moreover, the cholera struck again, as it had twice before the war, and consumption appeared to be weakening and carrying away scores of Americans.

Some observers openly longed for the days when (they thought) Americans were sturdier. They were wrong, of course, but they did not know that. And so the lament continued, a persistent jeremiad in the litany of economic boosterism and military braggadocio. Religious enthusiasms grew and declined, but seldom with the consistent social consciousness or broad popularity of the pre–Civil War era. Religion was challenged by a new gospel—that of science and technology. Electricity, with power only suggested by Franklin in the eighteenth century and Faraday in the early nineteenth century, became the new "vital force," as more and more scientists experimented with it and their knowledge was widely circulated. But it, like mineral waters, spas, "wilderness cures," and gymnastics, failed to bring on the millennium.

Neurasthenia was at the core of the crisis in post–Civil War American culture—just as epidemic disease, perceived declension from the noble Revolutionary generation, and (for some) the slave power of the South had been decades before. It was not the only cause for concern, however. Drinking once again became a curse to be fought, and the young seemed out of control (as previous generations had thought the post-Revolutionary generation had been). The millennial content and context were more distant in the zeal of the post–Civil War reformers, as much as they had been immediate for their predecessors. Health had become perhaps as much a way to preserve the present as it had been a blueprint for the future.

Neurasthenia was, after all, a sign of advanced civilization, and Americans were far too pleased with their achievements to reject all of technology's or industry's benefits. Moreover, there was no need to do that. Advanced industrial civilization and health were not mutually exclusive, but complementary. Neurasthenia, dyspepsia, and autointoxication were, after all, one's own fault. This was an amplification, not an alteration, of the earlier idea of personal, individual regeneration. Examples were everywhere. Roosevelt fought and strained his way from effete beginnings to an energetic presidency; Carnegie worked his way to wealth from nothing. With "pluck" and "luck," as Horatio Alger put it, anyone could make it. Action and experience could alleviate the ills of a society "gone soft," and such physical educators as Harvard's Dudley Sargent and Dioclesian Lewis aimed to provide men and women with that chance.

Identifying the problems of the society as a whole with the problems and weaknesses of individuals not only stimulated interest in self-help cures from the turn of the century to the present day but also deflected criticism or questioning from sociopolitical issues in a nation being transformed from a homogeneous agrarian and village society to one of great industrial cities with heterogeneous populations. Moreover, it allowed Americans to explain how others—particularly immigrants not of Anglo-Saxon heritage—could possibly survive, flourish, and even gain power. "Race suicide," "autointoxication," "entropy" (a term used in the late nineteenth century to describe the loss of energy in both people and civilizations), and the rash of unflattering comparisons of men and women to their forebears a century previous all share a criticism of Americans as individuals.

The success of a few athletes made it even more difficult to bear. For if Olympians from the United States could win, as they did from the onset of the games, then why were the rest of the people so weak, so ill developed? This critique was seldom leveled at the working class. They were assumed to be hearty, since they engaged in physical labor, which both exercised them and was allegedly less demanding than "brain work." Brain work offered no exercise, only a drain of the body's vital energy. "The strenuous life" that Roosevelt espoused was not for the workers (who sweated enough), but for the middle and wealthy classes, as were nearly all of the fitness activities related to physical movement and the building of muscles—sport, body building, and gymnastics or calisthenics. This may indicate a fear of the masses of working men and women, an anxiety that crowded urban conditions, crime in the antebellum era, and labor violence in the later decades of the century did nothing to dispel.

But it would be too simple to relegate the various American efforts to heal, preserve, or transform their bodies to fears of death, or of strangers, or of laborers. The persistent American tendency to equate success with individual effort and failure with individual responsibility meant that men and women were constantly looking for an "edge" on the competition, while recognizing that they were always being pursued by those who could pass them on the way to fortune. Death was not the sole pursuer; one's fellow men and women joined the chase. Health increasingly became one of the advantages one might have, like elocution, education, or the ability to "read" character. The millennium was no longer the kingdom of God on earth, but the corporation president's chair. The gates of heaven had become the doors to the boardroom.

In a society such as that of the nineteenth-century United States, to be physically round was to be proof that one had more food than needed. It was a sign of wealth. But by the 1920s, rotundity no longer singled an individual out as endowed in the wallet as well as in the flesh. To have muscles and not work with one's hands had come to mean that one had the leisure time and discipline to train. Leanness in women and muscular bulk in men were new virtues. In the competitive world of business, the intimidation of size as well as the connotation of tireless action were important.

The quest is, of course, unending. Americans periodically turn against technology, only to reintegrate it into their lives. For most of the middle class and wealthy, it is a pattern of selective adaptation. Alfalfa sprouts now form an integral part of many salads that contain ham. Jogging and running have been common practice long enough to have ceased to be fads. Aerobics in the secularized YMCAs are strikingly similar to Beecher's or Lewis's systems. Weight lifting and body building are growing in popularity among both men and women, and the women may yet redefine the ideal of female beauty. Many businesses encourage their executives to exercise, and some even provide such facilities as showers and changing rooms. The entry of women into executive offices and onto playing fields has spread the gospel of health further than ever before, and health clubs have become centers for those looking for friendship, sex, and love.

The characteristic that unites most of these phenomena or activities is that they are individualistic, which should be no surprise. But concomitant with this fitness fascination is the broadening of team sport, not just for children and collegians, and especially for women, but for adults as well. Softball may be the single most popular participatory sport in America, for men, women, and integrated teams. This need to play, as Dutch historian Johan Huizinga identified in his classic book *Homo Ludens* (1950), is both an integral part of many cultural forms and common to nearly all animals. Thus the growth of fitness activity that has characterized the United States since the mid 1970s is not simply a holding action against death or a competitive edge on one's opponents in the workplace but an expression of the desire for community and emotional bonding in a culture of men and women alone.

· NOTES ·

CHAPTER ONE. HEALTH, MEDICINE, AND SOCIETY

1. T. S. Arthur, "The Young Doctor," *Godey's Lady's Book* 23 (July 1841): 7–11.
2. Ibid., pp. 8, 9.
3. Samuel Thomson, *A New Guide to Health* (Boston: E. G. House, 1822), pp. 8–9, 23–25.
4. See Paul Starr, *The Social Transformation of American Medicine* (New York: Basic Books, 1984), pp. 51–54.
5. See James C. Whorton, *Crusaders for Fitness* (Princeton, N.J.: Princeton University Press, 1982).
6. *Boston Medical and Surgical Journal* 19 (1838): 220–21.
7. Whorton, p. 23.
8. Samuel Hahnemann, *Organon of Homeopathic Medicine*, 1st American ed. (Allentown, Pa.: Academical Bookstore, 1836), p. 59.
9. Calvin W. Owen, diary, March 30, 1853.
10. Ibid.
11. Sylvester Graham, *Aesculapian Tablets of the Nineteenth Century* (Providence, R.I.: n.p., 1834) p. 37. Charles G. Finney, quoted in Robert S. Fletcher, *A History of Oberlin College* (Oberlin, Ohio: Oberlin College, 1943) 1: 333.
12. Sylvester Graham, quoted in Whorton, p. 60.

13. *Journal of Health* 1, no. 1 (September 9, 1829): 1; Edward Hitchcock, *Dyspepsy Forestalled and Resisted, or Lectures on Diet, Regimen, and Employment* (Amherst, Mass.: J. S. & C. Adams, 1831), p. 37.
14. *Journal of Health* 1, no. 1 (September 9, 1829): 2.
15. "Popular Medicine," *Journal of Health* 1, no. 5 (November 11, 1829): 65, 67.
16. John Dryden, "Epistle of John Dryden of Chesterton," *The Poetical Works of John Dryden*, ed. George Gilfillion (Edinburgh: D. Appleton & Co., 1855), quoted in Whorton, p. 18.
17. Hitchcock, p. 332.
18. Catharine Beecher, *Physiology and Calisthenics for Schools and Families* (New York: Harper and Brothers, 1856), p. v.
19. Ibid., p. 130.
20. William Alcott, *The Young Man's Guide* (Boston: Samuel Colman 1835), pp. 32–33.
21. David Tappan, *A Discourse . . .* (Boston: Hall, 1798), pp. 18–19; Alexander Hamilton, *The Federalist* 1 (1787).
22. James Monroe, First Inaugural Address, 1817. See Fred Somkin, *Unquiet Eagle: Memory and Desire in the Idea of American Freedom* (Ithaca, N.Y.: Cornell University Press, 1967).
23. Edward Everett, "Principles of the American Constitutions," *Orations and Speeches* (Boston: Cummings, Hilliard & Company, 1826), 1: 129.
24. Timothy Flint, *Recollections of the Last Ten Years* (Boston: Cummings, Hilliard & Company, 1826), pp. 389–90.
25. Lyman Beecher, "The Gospel the Only Security for Eminent and Abiding National Prosperity," *The American National Preacher* 3 (March 1829), 147.
26. Idem, "Propriety and Importance of Efforts to Evangelize the Nation," *The American National Preacher* 3 (March 1829): 154.
27. Hitchcock, p. 328. Owen, diary, sheet inserted between pages for October 11 and October 28, 1855, and dated in his hand "1844."
28. Edward G. Prescott, *An Oration: Delivered before the Citizens of Boston, on the Fifty-eighth Anniversary of American Independence* (Boston: n.p., 1833), p. 17.
29. Andrew Bigelow, *God's Charge unto Israel: A Sermon Preached . . . at the Annual Election, on Wednesday, January 6, 1836* (Boston: Dutton and Wentworth, 1836), p. 22.
30. Charles Caldwell, M.D., *Thoughts on Physical Education* (Boston: Marsh, Capen & Lyon, 1834), pp. 13–14, 15.
31. George W. Burnap, *The Voice of the Times; a Sermon Delivered in the First Independent Church of Baltimore, on Sunday, May 14, 1837* (Balti-

more: n.p., 1837), p. 15. There is a vast literature on reform in antebellum America. See especially John Thomas, "Romantic Reform in America, 1815–1865," *American Quarterly* 17 (Winter 1965): 656–81; David Rothman, *The Discovery of the Asylum* (Boston: Little, Brown and Co., 1971).

32. Kate to Theodosia Dunham, February 13, 1843, Theodosia Dunham Letters, Strong Museum Library, Rochester, N.Y.

33. Kate to Theodosia Dunham, May 31, 1843, Theodosia Dunham Letters, Strong Museum Library, Rochester, N.Y.

34. Caldwell, p. 93; David M. Reese, M.D., *Phrenology Known by Its Fruits* (New York: Howe and Bates, 1836), pp. 73, 73–74, 82, 87.

35. Reese, pp. 124, 129.

36. "Deaths at Different Ages," *Journal of Health* 1, no. 6 (November 25, 1829): 95.

37. "In-Door Exercises," *Journal of Health* 1, no. 10 (January 27, 1830): 151–52.

38. "Diseases of Artisans," *Journal of Health* 1, 9 (January 13, 1830): 142–44.

39. Hitchcock, pp. 333–34.

40. Caldwell, pp. 91–92.

41. Catharine Beecher, p. 147.

42. "Chapter on Females," *The Young People's Mirror and American Family Visitor,* August 1, 1849, p. 87; Catharine Beecher, p. 11.

43. "Chapter on Females," pp. 87–88; Catharine Beecher, p. 147.

44. Catharine Beecher, p. 188.

45. Ibid., p. 147.

46. Benjamin Rush, *Medical Inquiries and Observations,* 3d ed. (Philadelphia: Johnson and Warner, 1809), 4: 409.

47. Unidentified physician's journal, May 28–October 4, 1837, Warshaw Collection of Business Americana, National Museum of American History, Smithsonian Institution, Washington, D.C.

48. Julia to Theodosia Dunham, Philadelphia, November 14, 1842. Theodosia Dunham Letters, Strong Museum Library, Rochester, N.Y.

49. William Alcott, *The Young Husband* (Boston: C.D. Strong, 1851), p. 374.

50. *Journal of Health* 1 (1829–30, *passim*). See also William Alcott, *The House I Live In* (Boston: Light and Stearns, 1837).

CHAPTER TWO. SPICES AND THE SOCIAL ORDER

1. *Southern Review,* August 1829, p. 221, quoted in Edward Hitchcock, *Dyspepsy Forestalled and Resisted, or Lectures on Diet, Regimen, and*

Employment (Amherst, Mass.: J. S. & C. Adams, 1831), 53; Catharine Beecher, *Physiology and Calisthenics for Schools and Families* (New York: Harper and Brothers, 1856), p. 66.

2. Hitchcock, p. 192; R. T. Trall, M.D., *The New Hydropathic Cook-Book* (New York: Fowler and Wells, 1853), pp. 43, 44, 146. Cookbooks of the period are much less specific in their instructions and quantities of supplies than contemporary manuals, but they form a consistent pattern of preparation methods—boiling, roasting, and—most often—frying. See Susan R. Williams, *Savory Suppers and Fashionable Feasts: Victorian Dining* (New York: Pantheon Books, 1985).
3. Beecher, pp. 134–35.
4. Ibid., p. 188. See Karen Halttunen, *Confidence Men and Painted Women: A Study of Middle-Class Culture in America, 1840–1870* (New Haven: Yale University Press, 1983).
5. Beecher, p. 97.
6. Trall, p. 47.
7. Hitchcock, pp. 193–94.
8. Beecher, p. 97.
9. Trall, pp. 101, 98, 100.
10. Beecher, p. 117.
11. Trall, p. 21; Beecher, pp. 93–94, 95.
12. Trall, p. vii; Sarah Josepha Hale, *Modern Cookery* (Philadelphia: Lea and Blanchard, 1845) quoted in Trall, p. viii.
13. Halttunen, chap. 1.
14. Fred Somkin, *Unquiet Eagle: Memory and Desire in the Idea of American Freedom* (Ithaca, N.Y.: Cornell University Press, 1967), chap. 1–5.
15. William J. Rorabaugh, "Estimated U.S. Alcoholic Beverage Consumption, 1790–1860," *Journal of Studies on Alcohol* 37, no. 3 (March 1976): 360–61.
16. Hitchcock, pp. 134–45.
17. "Wines," *Journal of Health* 1, no. 9 (January 13, 1830): 136, 138, 137. See also Hitchcock, pp. 125–26.
18. "Malt Liquors," *Journal of Health* 1, no. 14 (March 24, 1830): 212–13; Hitchcock, p. 171.
19. "Intemperance-Insanity," *Journal of Health* 1, no. 1 (September 29, 1829): 13–14; Beecher, p. 136.
20. Trall, p. ix.
21. "Maxims for Parents," *Journal of Health* 1, no. 7 (December 9, 1829): 110; "Taking Laudanum," *Journal of Health* 1, no. 11 (February 10, 1830): 162.

22. "Panaceas-Mercury," *Journal of Health* 1, no. 6 (November 25, 1829): 93; Beecher, pp. 169, 136, 95; William Alcott, *Forty Years in the Wilderness of Pills and Powders* (Boston: J. P. Jewett, 1859).

23. "Strong Waters," *Journal of Health* 1, no. 7 (December 9, 1829): 99; Hitchcock, p. 176.

24. Hitchcock, pp. 172–73, 178; "Strong Waters," p. 99.

25. Beecher, p. 101.

26. Ibid., pp. 137, 102.

27. "Tobacco," *Journal of Health* 1, no. 3 (October 7, 1829): 36, 37; Hitchcock, pp. 133–34.

28. Beecher, pp. 183, 182.

29. Ibid., p. 182.

30. Ibid., p. 102.

31. Trall, p. 155. Sylvester Graham, *A Treatise on Bread and Bread-Making* (Boston: Light and Stearns, 1837), pp. 43, 46–47; for more on Graham, see Siegfried Giedion, *Mechanization Takes Command* (New York: W. W. Norton Co., 1948), pp. 169–208.

32. Graham, *Lectures on the Science of Human Life* (Boston: Marsh, Capen, Lyon, and Webb, 1839), 2: 448, 455–56.

33. Idem, *Treatise on Bread*, p. 51.

34. Trall, p. 155.

35. Ibid., p. 148.

36. Ibid., p. 150.

37. George Cheyne, *An Essay on Health and Long Life* (New York: Edward Gillespie, 1813), William Lambe, *Additional Reports on the Effects of a Peculiar Regimen* (London: Mawman, 1815); Percy Shelley, *A Vindication of Natural Diet* (London: F. Pitman, 1884) reprint of 1813 edition; see James C. Whorton, *Crusaders for Fitness* (Princeton, N.J.: Princeton University Press, 1982), pp. 68–70.

38. "Animal and Vegetable Foods," *Journal of Health* 1, no. 1 (September 9, 1829): 7; Whorton, p. 89.

39. Beecher, pp. 91–92.

40. Ibid., p. 92.

41. Trall, p. 19.

42. Graham, *Lecture on Epidemic Disease, Generally, and Particularly the Spasmodic Cholera* (New York: n.p., 1833), pp. 6, 11, 31, 66.

43. Idem, *Graham Journal of Health and Longevity* (New York, 1837), 1: 47.

44. Idem, *Treatise on Bread*, p. 48.

45. *Boston Courier*, June 28, 1828, p. 3, *Boston Medical and Surgical Journal*, 14 (1836), 46. Both quoted in Whorton, p. 57.

46. See Steven Nissenbaum, *Sex, Diet, and Debility in Jacksonian America: Sylvester Graham and Health Reform* (Westport, Ct.: Greenwood Press, 1980).
47. *Boston Medical and Surgical Journal,* 14 (1836), p. 25. Graham to Alexander W. Thayer, February 26, 1844, Collection of the Houghton Library, Harvard University, Cambridge, Mass.
48. Graham to Thayer.
49. Ibid.
50. Ibid.
51. James B. Thayer to Justin Winsor, January 3, 1893, Collection of the Houghton Library, Harvard University, Cambridge, Mass.
52. See, for example, *Moral Reformer* 2 (1836): 344ff.

CHAPTER THREE. THE SPRINGS (AND SHOCKS) OF LIFE

1. Siegfried Giedeon, *Mechanization Takes Command* (New York: W. W. Norton Co., 1948), pp. 628–60. See also Fernand Braudel, *The Structures of Everyday Life: Civilization and Capitalism, Fifteenth–Eighteenth Century* (New York: Harper and Row, 1979), pp. 285–86, 310, 329–30.
2. Joel Shew, *Hydropathy, or, the Water-Cure* (New York: Wiley and Putnam, 1844), passim.
3. See, for example, Nicolo Lanzani, *Vera methods di serverse dell' aqua fredda nelli febri* (Naples: Per lo de Bonis, 1723).
4. Edward Hitchcock, *Dyspepsy Forestalled and Resisted, or Lectures on Diet, Regimen, and Employment* (Amherst, Mass.: J. S. & C. Adams, 1831), p. 431.
5. "Watery Regimen," *Journal of Health* 1, no. 9 (January 13, 1830): 129, 130.
6. Hitchcock, p. 243; "Warm Bathing," *Journal of Health* 1, no. 5 (November 11, 1829): 54; see Stow Persons, "The Cyclical View of History," in Cushing Strout, ed., *Intellectual History in America* (New York: Harper and Row, 1968) 1: 46–63; "Warm Bathing," p. 55; Hitchcock, p. 243.
7. "Warm Bathing," p. 55.
8. Ibid., p. 57.
9. Catharine Beecher, *Physiology and Calisthenics for Schools and Families* (New York: Harper and Brothers, 1856), pp. 99, 100.
10. Charles Caldwell, M.D., *Thoughts on Physical Education* (Boston: Marsh, Capen & Lyon, 1834), p. 37; Beecher, p. 138.

11. "Neglect of Personal Experience," *Journal of Health* 1, no. 1 (September 9, 1829): 16; Beecher, p. 190.
12. Shew, p. 5.
13. Beecher, p. 104.
14. Calvin W. Owen, diary, March 30, 1853; January 26, 1854; January 30, 1854; June 2, 1854.
15. Shew, pp. 48, 68–73, 54, 52.
16. Ibid., pp. 117–47.
17. See, for example, Ralph Waldo Emerson, "Nature" (1836); Shew, pp. 270, 271, 272.
18. *The New York Mercantile Union Business Directory* (New York: S. French, L. C. & H. L. Pratt, et al., 1850), p. 397; *Catalogue of the New York Hydropathic and Physiological School for 1854–5* (New York: Fowler and Wells, 1855), p. ii.
19. R. T. Trall, M.D., *The Hydropathic Encyclopedia* (New York: Fowler and Wells, 1852) 2: 4; Idem, *The New Hydropathic Cook-Book* (New York: Fowler and Wells, 1853), p. 144.
20. *Longworth's American Almanac, New York Register, and City Directory* (New York: Thomas Longworth, 1830); *Wilson's Business Directory of New York City* (New York: John F. Trow, 1860), p. 22; *Stimson's Boston Directory* (Boston: Charles Stimson, 1845).
21. "Cautions for the Season," *Journal of Health* 1, no. 14 (March 24, 1830): 209–11.
22. "Strength and Debility," *Journal of Health* 1, no. 1 (September 9, 1829): 3–4; Hitchcock, pp. 2–3.
23. Sylvester Graham, *A Lecture to Young Men, on Chastity, Intended for the Serious Consideration of Parents and Guardians* (Boston: Weeden and Cory 1839), p. 39; Shew, p. 24.
24. J. Stanley Grimes, *Etherology and the Phreno-Philosophy of Mesmerism and Magic Eloquence* (Boston and Cambridge: James Munroe and Company, 1850), p. 46.
25. John Bell, *Animal Magnetism: Past Fictions, Present Science* (Philadelphia: Haswell, Barrington, and Haswell, 1837), p. 2.
26. Kate to Theodosia Dunham, Wilmington, Delaware, January 29, 1844, Theodosia Dunham Letters, Strong Museum Library, Rochester, N.Y.
27. Owen diary, March 4, 1855.
28. H. H. Sherwood, *Manual for Magnetizing, with the Rotary and Vibrating Magnetic Machine* (New York: Wiley and Putnam, 1845), pp. 2, 122.
29. Ibid., pp. 50–56, 29.
30. *Doggett's New York City Directory* (New York: John Doggett, 1846).

31. Sherwood, pp. 26–27.

32. Grimes, p. 11.

33. Bell, p. 2; Kate to Theodosia Dunham, January 29, 1844, Theodosia Dunham Letters, Strong Museum Library, Rochester, N.Y.

34. Sherwood, pp. 18, 119. See also William Leete Stone, *A Letter to Doctor A. Brigham on Animal Magnetism*, 4th ed. (New York: George Dearborn and Co., 1837) for another popular defense of animal magnetism.

35. The 1838 trade catalog of the British scientific instrument makers, Watkins and Hill, devoted 30 of its 112 pages to "electrical," "voltaic," and "electro-dynamical" apparatus. The rest of the goods offered for sale were chemical and other scientific laboratory apparatus, as well as a few toys. Watkins and Hill, *A New and Enlarged Descriptive Catalog of Optical, Mathematical, Philosophical and Chemical Instruments and Apparatus* (London: Richard and John Taylor, 1838). In the United States, instrument makers similarly offered physicians and scientists electrical gear. Daniel Davis of Boston, who listed himself as a "Mathematical Instrument Maker," published at least two books on magnetism and electricity, with specific reference to the medicinal use of the forces.

36. Dr. Moritz Meyer, *Electricity in Its Relations to Practical Medicine*, trans. William A. Hammond, M.D. (New York: D. Appleton and Company, 1869), p. 30.

37. Daniel Davis, Jr., *Manual of Magnetism* (Boston: Daniel Davis, Jr., 1842, 2d ed., 1848) *The Medical Application of Electricity* (Boston: Daniel Davis, Jr., 1846), pp. 3–4.

38. Ibid., pp. 19–20.

39. *Harper's Weekly* 1, no. 16 (April 18, 1857): 255; *Harper's Weekly* 4, no. 167 (March 10, 1860): 158.

40. Advertisement for "Dr. Hankinson's Electro-Chemical Baths, New York, N.Y.," ca. 1860, Warshaw Collection of the Archives of the National Museum of American History, Washington, D.C.

41. Advertisements for Hydropathic and Hygienic Institute and Cleveland Water Cure Establishment, ca. 1855, Warshaw Collection of the Archives of National Museum of American History, Washington, D.C.

42. *New York City Directory for 1845 and 1846* (New York: Groot and Elston, 1845). For an advertisement for "J. V. Pulvermacher's Hydro-Electric Voltaic Chains," see *The Citizen and Strangers' Pictorial and Business Directory for the City of New York and Its Vicinity* (New York: Charles Spalding and Co., 1853), pp. 30–31.

43. Davis, *Medical Application*, p. 18; Grimes, p. 13.

CHAPTER FOUR. "BAD AIR" AND THE "MOVEMENT CURE"

1. Catharine Beecher, *Physiology and Calisthenics for Schools and Families* (New York: Harper and Brothers, 1856), p. 87.
2. *American Journal of Education* 2 (August 1828): 510.
3. "Indelicacy in Breathing Impure Air," *Journal of Health* 1, no. 1 (September 9, 1829): 11; "Impure Air," *Journal of Health* 1, no. 2 (September 23, 1829): 25–26; Edward Hitchcock, *Dyspepsy Forestalled and Resisted, or Lectures on Diet, Regimen, and Employment* (Amherst, Mass.: J. S. & C. Adams, 1831), p. 236.
4. "The Summer Complaint of Children," *Journal of Health* 1, no. 2 (September 23, 1829): 22–24.
5. "Hardiness," *Journal of Health* 1, no. 6 (November 25, 1829): 89.
6. Ibid., p. 89.
7. Beecher, pp. 125, 124.
8. "Rooms Warmed by Heated Air," *Journal of Health* 1, no. 10 (January 27, 1830): 153; Beecher, p. 86.
9. Beecher, p. 86.
10. *Wilson's Business Directory of New York City* (New York: John F. Trow, 1850).
11. Beecher, p. 125.
12. Ibid., pp. 112, 126.
13. Bibliography on education and the nature of children is enormous. See, especially, Bernard Wishy, *The Child and the Republic* (New York: Harper and Row, 1967); M.L.S. Heininger et al., *A Century of Childhood, 1820–1920* (Rochester, N.Y.: The Strong Museum, 1984); Michael Katz, *The Irony of Early School Reform* (Cambridge, Mass.: Harvard University Press, 1968).
14. William A. Alcott, *Essay on the Construction of School-Houses* (Boston: Hilliard, Gray, Little and Wilkins, 1832), pp. 6–16.
15. Beecher, p. 127.
16. "Beds," *Journal of Health* 1, no. 7 (December 9, 1829): 107.
17. Ibid., pp. 107, 108, 109.
18. "Sleeping Apartments," *Journal of Health* 1, no. 6 (November 25, 1829): 84, 85.
19. John Stenhouse, *On the Economic Applications of Charcoal to Sanitary Purposes* (London: Samuel Highley, 1855), pp. 13–15.
20. See John Burnett, *A Social History of Housing, 1815–1870* (Newton Abbot, England: David & Charles, 1978).
21. *Journal of Health*, 1 (September 29, 1829): frontispiece; Hitchcock, p. 205.

22. "Walking," *Journal of Health* 1, no. 8 (December 23, 1829): 118, 119; Hitchcock, p. 226.
23. "Gymnastic Exercises," *Journal of Health* 1, no. 9 (January 13, 1830): 133, 132.
24. Ibid., p. 133.
25. "In-Door Exercises," *Journal of Health* 1, no. 10 (January 27, 1830): 151.
26. Hitchcock, pp. 227–28; Charles Caldwell, M.D., *Thoughts on Physical Education* (Boston: Marsh, Capen & Lyon, 1834), pp. 63–65.
27. "Gymnastic Exercises," p. 132; "Longevity," *Journal of Health* 1, no. 7 (December 9, 1829): 111, 112.
28. "Pulmonary Consumption," *Journal of Health* 1, no. 4 (October 28, 1829): 64.
29. William Alcott, *Forty Years in the Wilderness of Pills and Powders* (Boston: J. P. Jewett, 1859), p. 132.
30. Horace Mann, *Report to the Massachusetts Board of Education* (Boston: Dutton and Wentworth, 1838), p. 47.
31. *Outline of the System of Education at the Round Hill School . . .* (Boston: N. Hale's Steam Power Press, 1831), p. 3.
32. Sarah Josepha Hale, "How to Begin," *Godey's Lady's Book* 23 (August 1841): 41–42.
33. John C. Warren, *Physical Education and the Preservation of Health* (Boston: William D. Ticknor, 1846), p. 5.
34. On the constricting effects of men's ties, see Caldwell, p. 113.
35. "Corsets! Corsets!," *Journal of Health* 1, no. 8 (December 23, 1829): 117–18; Caldwell, pp. 116–19.
36. Beecher, pp. 53, 80, 83, 160.
37. Idem, *Letters to the People on Health and Happiness* (New York: Harper and Brothers, 1855), pp. 93–94.
38. Ibid., pp. 122, 147.
39. Ibid., p. 151.
40. Ibid., pp. 163–64, 11; Augustus Georgii, *The Movement-Cure* (London: T. Harreld, 1853), pp. 5, 6, 8.
41. *Sheldon and Company's Business or Advertising Directory . . .* (New York: John F. Trow, 1845).
42. Beecher, *Physiology and Calisthenics*, p. v. See Barbara Novak, *Nature and Culture* (New York: Oxford University Press, 1980).
43. Beecher, *Physiology and Calisthenics*, p. 9.
44. Ibid., pp. iv, v.
45. Ibid., pp. iv, 9–16, 20–27.
46. Ibid., pp. 39, 177–78.
47. Ibid., pp. 10, 121–22.

48. Ibid., pp. 30, 192.
49. *Wilson's Business Directory for New York City* (New York: John F. Trow, 1855), p. 195; *Wilson's Business Directory for New York City* (New York: John F. Trow, 1860), p. 229.

CHAPTER FIVE. THE SANITATION MOVEMENT AND THE WILDERNESS CURE

1. Almira MacDonald, diaries, September 19, 22, 1871, Strong Museum Library, Rochester, N.Y.
2. Ibid., June 11, 1872; August 29, 1872; September 9, 1872; January 5, 1873; April 17–19, 1873; April 28–29, 1877; December 27, 1879; April 16, 1877–August 20, 1880.
3. "Vaccination at Paris," *Harper's Weekly*, 14, no. 695 (April 23, 1870): 269; MacDonald, diaries, December 16, 1871; January 8, 1872; January 27, 1872.
4. MacDonald, diaries, January 23–30, 1880; November 5, 1883.
5. "New Invention for Surgeons-Collodion," *Rochester Weekly American* 5, no. 19 (May 10, 1849) 2.
6. Elisha Harris, "An Introductory Outline . . ." in David Boswell Reid, *Ventilation in American Dwellings* (New York: Wiley and Halsted, 1858), p. iii.
7. Ibid.
8. Ibid., p. iv.
9. Ibid., p. xi.
10. *Godey's Lady's Book* 61 (August 1860): 175.
11. *The Directory of the City of Boston* (Boston: George Adams, 1850); George E. Waring, "The Sanitary Scare," *American Architect and Building News* 4, no. 153 (November 30, 1878): 180.
12. J. N. Hanaford, "Pure Water," *The Household* 12, no. 4 (April 1879): 81.
13. John Harvey Kellogg, *The Hygienic Cook Book* (Battle Creek, Mich.: The Office of the Health Reformer, 1876), pp. 107–8.
14. Hanaford, p. 81; "The Art of Preserving Health," *The Household* 12, no. 9 (September 1879): 201.
15. Advertising pamphlet for W. L. Ingraham, Rochester, N.Y., ca. 1870, Warshaw Collection of the Archives of the National Museum of American History, Washington, D.C.
16. Advertising brochure for Jewett's Water Filters, Warshaw Collection of the Archives of the National Museum of American History, Washington, D.C.

17. Advertising pamphlet for the Celebrated Cummings Water-Filter, ca. 1890; "Net cash Price List of the Loomis Improved Water Filter," Philadelphia, Pa., ca. 1880; advertising pamphlet for the Stevens Filter Company's Self-Cleaning Upward Water Filters, ca. 1885—all in the Warshaw Collection of the Archives of the National Museum of American History, Washington, D.C.

18. May Stone, "The Plumbing Paradox," *Winterthur Portfolio* 14, no. 3 (Autumn 1979), 283–84; *Godey's Lady's Book* 92, no. 552 (June 1876): 569; Mrs. E. G. Cook, "The Necessity for Ventilation," *Demorest's Monthly Magazine* 23, no. 12 (October 1887): 775–76.

19. Kellogg, *Household Manual of Domestic Hygiene, Food and Diet* (Battle Creek, Mich.: Good Health Publishing Co., 1882), p. 21; "A Lesson about Disinfectants," *Godey's Lady's Book* 94 (April 1877): 370.

20. Kellogg, *Household Manual*, p. 22; billhead, Charles A. Wakefield Co., Pittsfield, Mass., April 29, 1873; Waring, *Earth-Closets: How to Make Them and How to Use Them* (New York: The Tribune Association, 1869); advertising brochure, the Earth Closet Company, Boston, Mass., ca. 1870—all of the above in the Warshaw Collection of the Archives of the National Museum of American History, Washington, D.C.

21. Kellogg, *Household Manual*, pp. 25–26.

22. Ibid., pp. 18, 19; E. G. Cook, p. 774.

23. Shirley F. Murphy, ed., *Our Homes* (London: Cassell 1883), pp. 11, 306, 305.

24. Robert W. Edis, "Internal Decoration," in *Our Homes*, pp. 315–16.

25. Idem, "Floors and Floor Coverings," in *Our Homes*, p. 326.

26. Anna Holyoke, "Wood Carpeting," *The Household* 7, no. 10 (October 1874): 218; Kellogg, *Household Manual*, p. 15.

27. Edis, "Internal Decoration," pp. 313, 314.

28. Ibid., p. 313; Kellogg, *Household Manual*, pp. 35, 36.

29. Edis, "Internal Decoration," pp. 313, 321.

30. Ibid., p. 321.

31. Reid, p. 4.

32. "A French Opinion of Stoves," *Godey's Lady's Book* 86, no. 514 (April 1873): 376; Kellogg, *Household Manual*, pp. 19–20, 11.

33. E. G. Cook, p. 775. See also Dio Lewis, *The New Gymnastics for Men, Women, and Children* (Boston: Ticknor and Fields, 1862), pp. 265–68; Marc Cook, *The Wilderness Cure* (New York: William Wood and Co., 1881), p. 83; "Stoves and Furnaces," *The Household* 7, no. 2 (February 1874): 33; advertisement for the "Sterling Ventilator," *The Jury* 1, no. 1 (November 2, 1889): 13.

34. Kellogg, *Household Manual*, pp. 29, 30; "The Atrocity of Feather Beds," *The Household* 7, no. 10 (October 1874): 221; "Health and Comfort in Sleeping Rooms," *Godey's Lady's Book* 83, no. 495 (September 1871): 275; "Ventilation," *Godey's Lady's Book* 101, no. 604 (October 1880): 391.

35. Kellogg, *Household Manual*, p. 15.

36. Murphy, p. 14; "Sleeping Habits," *The Household* 7, no. 4 (April 1874): 81; P. T. Barnum, *The Story of My Life, with an appendix, The Art of Money-Getting* (San Francisco: A. L. Bancroft, 1886), p. 57.

37. "Bed Rooms and Beds," *The Household* 7, no. 1 (January 1874): 4.

38. Henry I. Bowditch, *Consumption in New England* (Boston: Ticknor and Fields, 1862).

39. Lewis, p. 141.

40. "Consumptions," *The Household* 15, no. 5 (May 1882): 137.

41. Marc Cook, pp. 9–11.

42. Ibid., pp. 12–17.

43. Ibid., pp. 23, 27–30.

44. Ibid., pp. 31, 46

45. Ibid., p. 33

46. Ibid., pp. 38, 106, 43, 44, 51.

47. Ibid., pp. 45–46, 65–66, 81–82.

48. Ibid., p. 142. *Appleton's Illustrated Hand-Book of American Winter Resorts for Tourists and Invalids* (New York: D. Appleton and Co., 1877), p. 136; Marc Cook, pp. 143, 144.

49. For a typical Jackson advertisement, see "How to Treat the Sick Without Medicine," *Hearth and Home* 2, no. 10 (February 26, 1870): 159.

50. See Ronald Numbers, *Prophetess of Health: A Study of Ellen G. White* (New York: Harper and Row 1976).

CHAPTER SIX. THE NEW "AMERICAN NERVOUSNESS"

1. Advertising pamphlet for the "Remedial Institute," Saratoga Springs, New York, ca. 1875; Augustus Georgii, *The Movement-Cure* (London: T. Harreld, 1853), pp. 14–16; Joel Shew, *Hydropathy, or, the Water-Cure* (New York: Wiley and Putnam, 1844), p. 19; Sylvester S. and Sylvester E. Strong, *Remedial Institute*, pamphlet, privately printed, p. 10.

2. Edward Hitchcock, *Dyspepsy Forestalled and Resisted, or Lectures on Diet, Regimen, and Employment* (Amherst, Mass.: J. S. & C. Adams, 1831), 303ff; R. T. Trall, *The Illustrated Family Gymnasium* (New York: Fowler and Wells, 1857), p. 19; "New Diseases," *Godey's Lady's Book* 61 (August 1860): 190; Dio Lewis, *The New Gymnastics for Men,*

Women, and Children (Boston: Ticknor and Fields, 1862), p. 9; "Wear and Tear," advertisement in *Harper's Weekly* 11, no. 561 (September 28, 1867): 623.

3. George M. Beard, "Neurasthenia, or Nervous Exhaustion," *Boston Medical and Surgical Journal* 3 (1869): 217; idem, *American Nervousness, Its Causes and Consequences, a Supplement to Nervous Exhaustion (Neurasthenia)* (New York: G. P. Putnam's Sons 1881); idem, *Eating and Drinking: A Popular Manual of Food Diet in Health and Disease* (New York: G. P. Putnam's Sons, 1871), p. 103.

4. George M. Schweig, "Cerebral Exhaustion with Special Reference to Its Galvano-Balneological Treatment," *The Medical Record,* November 4, 1876, pp. 3, 4, 6–7; "The Rest Needed by Head-Workers," *The Household* 13, no. 12 (December 1880): 270; Schweig, pp. 9–11. See also Edwin Temple, "Overstudy," *The Household* 14, no. 6 (July 1881): 129 for more on brain work and its deleterious effects on its practitioners.

5. Beard, *American Nervousness,* pp. 126, 131. See T. J. Jackson Lears, *No Place of Grace: Anti-Modernism and the Transformation of American Culture, 1880–1920* (New York: Pantheon Books, 1982) for a penetrating study of this dramatic turn of Beard's argument.

6. Beard, *American Nervousness,* pp. 26, 8, 9.

7. Almira D. MacDonald, diaries, sheet inserted, January 31, 1875, Strong Museum Library, Rochester, N.Y.

8. Moses T. Runnels, M.D., "Physical Degeneracy of American Women," *Medical Era* 3 (1886): 302.

9. John Harvey Kellogg, *The Uses of Water in Health and Disease* (Battle Creek, Mich.: The Offices of the Health Reformer, 1876), p. 83.

10. Advertising pamphlet for "Remedial Institute," Saratoga Springs, N.Y. (n.p., ca. 1875), p. 1, Warshaw Collection of Archives of National Museum of American History, Washington, D.C.

11. Ibid., p. 3.

12. Ibid., pp. 3–4.

13. Ibid., pp. 5–8.

14. Ibid., p. 10.

15. Elida Works to Adam C. Works, July 20, 1868, Works Family Papers, University of Rochester, Rochester, N.Y.

16. Elida Works to Adam C. Works, July 23, 1868.

17. Elida Works to Adam C. Works, July 29, 1868.

18. Ibid.

19. Elida Works to Adam C. Works, August 4, 1868; August 24, 1868.

20. Adam C. Works, diary, October 30, 1868, Mrs. C. Works to Adam C. Works, January 5, 1869.

21. Advertising pamphlet for "Remedial Institute," p. 15.
22. Ibid., p. 17.
23. Advertising trade cards for Charles A. Shepard's and Miller's Baths, ca. 1886 and 1885, in the Warshaw Collection of the Archives of the National Museum of American History, Washington, D.C.; *Boston Directory . . . for . . . 1870* (Boston: Simpson, Davenport and Co., 1870), p. 1174; Almira MacDonald, diaries, July 7, 1880; May 24, 1883; February 20, 1900.
24. Advertising pamphlet for the "Remedial Institute," pp. 17–19.
25. Ibid., p. 35.
26. Kellogg, pp. iv, 75, 12–13, 18, 36.
27. Ibid., pp. 49–55, 57, 59.
28. Ibid., pp. 72, 74.
29. Ibid., p. 147.
30. Julia Felton diary, 1880, Houghton Library, Harvard University, Cambridge, Mass.
31. *Appleton's Illustrated Hand-Book of American Resorts for Tourists and Invalids* (New York: D. Appleton and Co., 1877), pp. 135–36, ii.
32. Ibid., pp. 16, 24, 38, 39, 53.
33. Ibid., pp. 71, 71–72, 75, 87; *Harper's Weekly* 34, no. 1749 (June 28, 1890): 496, 499.
34. Kellogg, p. 25.
35. Ibid., pp. 31, 25, 28. For a complete study of concepts of beauty in the United States, see Lois Banner, *American Beauty* (New York: Alfred A. Knopf, 1983).
36. Kellogg, pp. 28–30; "Microscopy," *Godey's Lady's Book,* 82, no. 487 (January 1871): 92.
37. Advertising pamphlet for "Knowlton's Bathing Apparatus," Ann Arbor, Mich., ca. 1876–1880, p. 4, Warshaw Collection of the Archives of the National Museum of American History, Washington, D.C.
38. Advertising circular for "N.Y. Portable Wash Stand Co.," New York, N.Y. ca. 1977, Warshaw Collection of the Archives of the National Museum of American History, Washington, D.C.
39. Advertising flyer for the "Day Mfg. Company," Detroit, Mich., ca. 1890, Warshaw Collection of the Archives of the National Museum of American History, Washington, D.C. For a detailed investigation of portable and collapsible furniture, see Paige Talbott, Rodris Roth, and David Hanks, *Innovative Furniture in America from 1800 to the Present* (New York: Horizon Press, 1981).
40. Advertising flyer for "The Home Vapor Bath and Disinfector Company, New York, N.Y., ca. 1880; advertisement for "The Kelly Bath Shower

Ring," ca. 1890—both in Warshaw Collection of the Archives of the National Museum of American History, Washington, D.C.

41. Advertising pamphlet for "Excelsior" Springs Saratoga Water, 1867, Warshaw Collection of the Archives of the National Museum of American History, Washington, D.C.; *Boston Directory*, 1870, no page number.

42. Ibid., p. 949, for example; *Frank Leslie's Popular Monthly* (December 1888): 765.

43. Advertising pamphlets for the various springs usually had chemical analyses included in them. There are several in the Warshaw Collection of the Archives of the National Museum of American History, Washington, D.C.

44. Advertising pamphlet for White Rock Lithia Water, ca. 1885, Warshaw Collection of the Archives of the National Museum of American History, Washington, D.C.

45. Advertising Pamphlet for Warner and Co. ca. 1880, Warshaw Collection of the Archives of the National Museum of American History, Washington, D.C.

46. Ibid.

47. Kellogg, *The Hygienic Cook Book* (Battle Creek, Mich.: The Office of the Health Reformer, 1876), p. 24; "The Art of Cookery," *Godey's Lady's Book*, 92, no. 547 (January 1876): 91.

48. Kellogg, *Household Manual of Domestic Hygiene, Food and Diet* (Battle Creek, Mich.: Good Health Pub. Co., 1882), pp. 51–52; idem, *Hygienic Cook Book*, p. 86.

49. Idem, *Hygienic Cook Book*, p. 18; idem, *Household Manual*, pp. 64, 65; idem, *Hygienic Cook Book*, p. 96; Robert Tomes, *The Bazar-Book of Decorum* (New York: 1870), p. 11; Kellogg, *Household Manual*, p. 66; Donald Mrozek, *Sport and American Mentality, 1880–1910* (Knoxville, Tenn.: University of Tennessee Press, 1983), pp. 96–97, 217–19.

50. "The Art of Preserving Health," *The Household*, 12, no. 12 (December 1879): 270; Kellogg, *Hygienic Cook Book*, p. 17.

51. Kellogg, *Household Manual*, pp. 66–67; Cook, p. 716. See Barbara Epstein, *The Politics of Domesticity* (Middletown, Conn.: Wesleyan University Press, 1982).

52. James C. Whorton, *Crusaders for Fitness* (Princeton, N.J.: Princeton University Press, 1982), pp. 225–26; Edwin Temple, "Animal Food," *The Household*, 15, no. 7 (July 1882): 201; Dr. C. E. Page, "The Flesh-Food Fallacy," *The Household* 15, no. 10 (October 1882): p. 297;

53. Kellogg, *Household Manual*, pp. 63–64.

54. Anna Holyoke Howard, "An Unseen Enemy: Candy and Its Effects,"

The Household 12, no. 7 (July 1879): 152; "Results of Vivisection: Interesting Experiments," *Godey's Lady's Book* 100, no. 599 (May 1880): 473; Kellogg, *Hygienic Cook Book*, pp. 25, 13, 28–33.

55. Advertisement in *The Youth's Companion* (May 12, 1887), p. 216; advertisement for Imperial Granum, *Ladies Home Journal*, 9, no. 2 (January 1892): 13; "What Shall We Eat?" *The Household* 12, no. 11 (November 1879): 248.
56. "Dr. Hanaford's Replies," *The Household* 12, no. 1 (January 1879): 9.
57. Beard, *Eating and Drinking*, p. 91.
58. "Muscular Education," *Harper's Weekly* 14, no. 710 (August 6, 1870): 510.
59. "Hints to Dyspeptics," *The Household* 14, no. 2 (February 1881): 33.
60. MacDonald, diaries, May 14, 1877.

CHAPTER SEVEN. ELECTRICITY, ENERGY, AND VITALITY

1. Almira D. MacDonald, diaries, April 16–27, 1877. Strong Museum Library, Rochester, N.Y.
2. Ibid., January 22, 26–30, 1875; *City Directory for Rochester, New York* (Rochester, N.Y.: Drew, Allis and Co., 1880); MacDonald, July 7, July 16–August 20, 1880; February 29, 1900.
3. W. R. Wells, *A New Theory of Disease; Based on the Principle That Man Is a Compound Electrical Magnet* (Rochester, N.Y.: C. D. Tracy, 1869), pp. 14, 21–22, 24.
4. E. H. Britten, *The Electric Physician: or Self-Cure Through Electricity* (Boston: Dr. William Britten, 1875), pp. 30–31, 29; H. H. Sherwood, *A Manual for Magnetizing, with the Rotary and Vibrating Magnetic Machine* (New York: Wiley and Putnam, 1845).
5. Henry Lake, "Is Electricity Life?" *Popular Science Monthly* (February 1873): 484; S. M. Wells, *Electropathic Guide: Prepared with the Particular Reference to Home Practice* (New York: American News Co., 1872), pp. 32–35.
6. Britten, p. 63.
7. Ibid., pp. 42–43, 35, 45, 40.
8. Ibid., pp. 63, 61, 19–21, 62.
9. Ibid., p. 17; S. M. Wells, p. 17.
10. Ibid., p. 18; Britten, *Electric Physician*, pp. 31, 21–23; Wells, p. 23.
11. Lake, pp. 483, 477–78, 479.
12. Britten, pp. 12–13, 15; George M. Beard and Alphonso D. Rockwell, *A Practical Treatise on the Medicinal and Surgical Uses of Electricity* (New York: W. Wood, 1871); George M. Beard, *The Medical Use of*

Electricity, with Special Reference to General Electrization as a Tonic in Neuralgia, Rheumatism, Dyspepsia, Chorea, Paralysis and Other Affections Associated with General Debility, with Illustrative Tables (New York: W. Wood, 1867); idem, *Recent Researches on Electrotherapeutics* (New York: D. Appleton and Co., 1872); John Jabez Caldwell, *A Review of Recent Theories of Brain and Nerve Action* (Baltimore: n.p., 1877), p. 13.

13. Dio Lewis, *The New Gymnastics for Men, Women, and Children* (Boston: Ticknor and Fields, 1862), p. 68; Henry Pickering Bowditch, "What is Nerve Force?" *American Association for the Advancement of Science* (Salem, Mass.: Salem Press, 1886), 35: 5; J. H. Kellogg, *Household Manual, of Domestic Hygiene, Food and Diet* (Battle Creek, Mich.: Good Health Pub. Co., 1882), pp. 49–50.

14. W. R. Wells, p. vi. See also Paul Starr, *The Social Transformation of American Medicine* (New York: Harper and Row, 1983), pp. 60–145.

15. George Schweig, "Cerebral Exhaustion," *The Medical Record*, November 4, 1876, p. 14; Britten, pp. 37–38, 8; Moritz Meyer, *Electricity in Its Relations to Practical Medicine* (New York: D. Appleton and Co., 1869), pp. 28–29, 93.

16. S. M. Wells, pp. 29–30.

17. Ibid., p. 30.

18. Advertisement from *The Graphic* (London, ca. 1885), p. 123; advertisement from *Harper's Monthly*, Bakken Library, Minneapolis, ca. 1880. Not everyone agreed as to the efficacy of such treatment. In 1882 J. H. Kellogg thought "electric or galvanic soles are of no use whatsoever" [Kellogg, p. 101].

19. Advertisement from *Frank Leslie's Popular Monthly*, Bakken Library, Minneapolis, ca. 1880.

20. Advertisement for Brewster's Medical Electricity, Bakken Library, Minneapolis.

21. *Instruction Manual for Pulvermacher's Improved Galvanic Chain-Bands* (London: n.p., ca. 1870), Bakken Library, Minneapolis.

22. General Augustus James Pleasonton, *The Influence of the Blue Ray of the Sunlight and of the Blue Color of the Sky in Developing Animal and Vegetable Life, in Arresting Disease, and in Restoring Health in Acute and Chronic Disorders to Human and Domestic Animals* (Philadelphia: Claxton, Remsen, and Haffelfinger, 1876).

23. Ibid., pp. 184–85.

24. Ibid., pp. 27, 117.

25. Ibid., pp. 14–15.

26. Ibid., pp. 14, 15, 41.

27. Ibid., pp. 88–89.
28. Ibid., pp. 5–10, 25, 27, 26.
29. Ibid., pp. 16.
30. Ibid., pp. 3, 24.
31. Ibid., pp. 16–17, 13, 16.
32. Ibid., pp. 118, 118–19, 119–20.
33. Ibid., pp. 128, 28, 128–29.
34. Ibid., p. 170.
35. Shirley Murphy, ed., *Our Homes* (London: Cassell, 1883), p. 18.
36. Kellogg, p. 27.

CHAPTER EIGHT. "MUSCULAR CHRISTIANITY" AND THE
ATHLETIC REVIVAL

1. New York Senate, "An Act to Incorporate the Poughkeepsie Gymnasium," bill 271, March 26, 1861.
2. See Bruce Haley, *The Healthy Body in Victorian Culture* (Cambridge, Mass.: Harvard University Press, 1978), for a solid study of "muscular Christianity." See also Donald R. Mrozek, *Sport and American Mentality, 1880–1910* (Knoxville, Tenn.: University of Tennessee Press, 1983), for a probing analysis of the linkage between mental and physical regeneration. "Literary Notices," *Godey's Lady's Book* 82, no. 488 (February 1871): 193.
3. R. T. Trall, *The Illustrated Family Gymnasium* (New York: Fowler and Wells, 1857), p. 17; S. D. Kehoe, *The Indian Club Exercise, Also General Remarks on Physical Culture* (New York: Peck and Snyder, 1866), pp. 11, 13.
4. Trall, p. ix; Kehoe, p. 19; Maurice Kloss, "The Dumb Bell Instructor for Parlor Gymnasts," in *The New Gymnastics for Men, Women, and Children,* ed. Dio Lewis (Boston: Ticknor and Fields, 1862), 120.
5. The Athletic Revival," *Harper's Weekly* 4, no. 161 (January 28, 1860): 50.
6. *Twenty-Fourth Annual Catalogue . . . of Ingham University* (Rochester, N.Y.: Erastus Darrow, 1869), p. 20.
7. James H. Smart, *A Manual of Free Gymnastic and Dumb-Bell Exercises for the School-Room and Parlor* (Cincinnati, Ohio: Van Antwerp, Bragg and Co., 1864), p. iii; *Ladies' Home Calisthenics* (Boston: Educational Publishing Co., 1890), pp. 10, 8; Thomas Wentworth Higginson, "The Health of Our Girls," *Atlantic Monthly* 9 (1862): 731; Edward H. Clarke, *Sex in Education* (Boston: J. R. Osgood and Co., 1873), p. 63.
8. Lewis, pp. 5, 18; Trall, p. 27
9. Trall, pp. 27, 25; John and Robin Haller, *The Physician and Sexuality*

in Victorian America (Urbana, Ill.: University of Illinois Press, 1974), pp. 171–72, 169.

10. Abba Gould Woolson, ed., *Dress-Reform* (Boston: Roberts Brothers, 1874), pp. 42, 78, 126–28, 54, viii, xiv.

11. F. M. S., "A Possible Improvement," *The Household* 7, no. 9 (September 1874): 197; Antoinette Brown Blackwell, "The Relation of Woman's Work in the Household to the Work Outside," *Papers and Letters Presented at the First Women's Congress of the Association for the Advancement of Women . . . New York, October 1873* (New York: Harper and Brothers, 1874), p. 180. For commentary on warm clothing, see J. H. Kellogg, *Household Manual of Domestic Hygiene, Food and Diet* (Battle Creek Mich.: Good Health Pub. Co., 1882), pp. 43–44.

12. Lewis, p. 5; "The Physical Training of Girls," *Godey's Lady's Book* 81, no. 486 (November 1870): 471.

13. Lewis, pp. 18, 62, 13, 14.

14. Ibid., pp. 18, 19, 20–28, 19.

15. Idem, "New Gymnastics," *American Journal of Education* 11 (1862): 700; idem, *New Gymnastics*, pp. 41, 29–41.

16. Lewis, *New Gymnastics*, pp. 42, 43–67, 58.

17. Ibid., pp. 59, 60, 71–86, 75.

18. Ibid., pp. 94–96, 170, 96–98, 99, 100–101.

19. Ibid., pp. 124–27.

20. Ibid., pp. 87–93.

21. Kehoe, pp. 8, 29.

22. Samuel T. Wheelwright, *A New System of Instruction in the Indian Club Exercise* (New York: E. I. Horsman, 1871).

23. Wheelwright, p. 1; Almira MacDonald, diaries, March 24, April 2, April 10, April 24, May 22, 1885.

24. Almira MacDonald, diaries, October 1, October 14, 1884; August 5, August 20, 1887; September 7, 1885; January 23, 1885; July 27, 1886; August 1, August 6, 1886; July 30, 1887.

25. Lewis, *New Gymnastics*, p. 256.

26. Advertisements for "Dr. Barnett's Improved Parlor Gymnasium," ca. 1875–1885, and "Noyes Brothers Exercising Machine," ca. 1885, both in the Warshaw Collection of the Archives of the National Museum of American History, Washington, D.C.

27. *The Pneumatic Parlor Rowing Machine,* trade catalog in the Warshaw Collection of the Archives of the National Museum of American History, Washington, D.C.

28. Donald R. Mrozek, *Sport and American Mentality, 1880–1910* (Knoxville, Tenn.: University of Tennessee Press, 1983), p. 180.

29. Advertisement for "D. L. Dowd's Health Lift," Warshaw Collection of the Archives of the National Museum of American History, Washington, D.C. See also *Life* 8, no. 196 (September 30, 1886): 203.

30. Lewis, *New Gymnastics*, pp. 62, 59, 10, 123.

31. Dudley Sargent, *An Autobiography* (Philadelphia: Lea and Febiger, 1927), p. 98.

32. Lewis, *New Gymnastics*, p. 61; "Physical Training," *Harper's Weekly* 4, no. 195 (September 22, 1860): 594.

33. Advertising section, *Boston Directory* (Boston: Sampson, Davenport and Co., 1870).

34. Sargent, pp. 145, 149, 202.

35. Lewis, *New Gymnastics* p. 169; Mrozek, pp. 71–73; Adam Clark Works, diary, 1868. University of Rochester, Rochester, N.Y.

36. *Harper's Weekly* 11, no. 566 (November 11, 1867): 689, 692; "Scottish Games," *Harper's Weekly* 11, no. 551 (July 20, 1867): 453

37. *Harper's Weekly* 11, no. 569 (November 23, 1867): 739; 14, no. 702 (June 11, 1870): 380.

38. *Harper's Weekly* 11, no. 569 (November 23, 1867): 737.

39. "Base-Ball," *Harper's Weekly* 9, no. 442 (June 17, 1865): 371; "The Wood-Sawyers' Tournament," *Harper's Weekly* 11, no. 570 (November 30, 1867): 758; Works, diary, April 17, 1868, May 27, 1868; "The Cricketers," *Harper's Weekly* 12, no. 605 (August 1, 1868): 492; Works, diary, May 23, 1868. The best history of baseball is Harold Seymour, *Baseball*, 2 vols. (New York: Oxford University Press, 1960).

40. "The 'Red-Stocking' Base-Ball Club, Cincinnati," *Harper's Weekly* 13, no. 653 (July 3, 1869): 422; "Base-Ball," *Harper's Weekly* 14, no. 705 (July 2, 1870): 427.

41. "The Hygiene of Gymnastics," *Harper's Weekly* 12, no. 580 (February 8, 1868): 83.

42. Ibid., p. 83; Edwin Temple, "Exercise in Relation to Health," *The Household*, 14, no. 4 (April, 1881): 81; Kloss, p. 120.

43. Mrozek, pp. 222–24, 211–14.

44. Higginson, "Gymnastics," p. 296; Quoted in James C. Whorton, *Crusaders for Fitness* (Princeton, N.J.: Princeton University Press, 1982), pp. 284–85; Mrozek, pp. 202–5.

CHAPTER NINE. LIVING THE STRENUOUS LIFE

1. Horace Fletcher to James E. West, January 26, 1911, Fletcher Papers, Houghton Library, Harvard University, Cambridge, Mass.

2. Charles Darwin, *The Descent of Man and Selection in Relation to Sex*

(New York: D. Appleton and Co., 1898); D. H. Wheeler, "Natural Selection and Politics," *Popular Science Monthly,* 3 (1873): 230–32.

3. Francis A. Walker, *Discussions in Economics and Statistics* (New York: H. Holt and Co., 1899) 2: 308–13, 317, 445–47.
4. See Gilman Ostrander, "Turner and the Germ Theory," in *Intellectual History in America,* ed. Cushing Strout (New York: Harper and Row, 1968), 2: 39–46.
5. William Roscoe Thayer, *The Life and Letters of John Hay* (Boston: Houghton Mifflin 1915), 2: 147.
6. For a discussion of these works, see Michael Kammen, *A Season of Youth: The American Revolution and the Historical Imagination* (New York: Alfred A. Knopf, 1978), pp. 161–64.
7. Thomas P. Gill, "Landlordism in America," *North American Review* 142 (1886): 60.
8. Reverend John Ellis, *The Deterioration of the Puritan Stock and Its Causes* (New York: John Ellis, 1884), p. 3; Edwin A. Ross, "The Causes of Racial Superiority," *Annals of the American Academy of Political and Social Sciences,* 18 (1901): 85–86; Irving Fisher, "Impending Problems of Eugenics," *Science Magazine* 13 (1921): 219–20, quoted in James C. Whorton, *Crusaders for Fitness* (Princeton, N.J.: Princeton University Press, 1982), p. 196.
9. T. S. Clouston, *Female Education from a Medical Point of View* (Edinburgh: D. Appleton and Co., 1882), p. 19; *Ladies' Home Calisthenics* (Boston: Educational Publishing Co., 1890), p. 1; Mary Wood-Allen, *What a Young Woman Ought to Know* (Philadelphia: Vir Publishing Co., 1913), p. 220.
10. Harrie Irving Hancock, *Physical Training for Women by Japanese Methods* (New York: G. P. Putnam's Sons, 1904), p. xi.
11. Elizabeth Paine, "Athletics at Women's Colleges—Bryn Mawr," *The Illustrated Sporting News,* 3 (July 9, 1904): 6, quoted in Donald R. Mrozek, *Sport and American Mentality, 1880–1910* (Knoxville, Tenn.: University of Tennessee Press, 1983), p. 156.
12. "Some Forerunners of the Bicycle," *Demorest's Monthly Magazine* 23, no. 8 (June 1887): 488.
13. Harriet T. Baillie, journal, March 8, 1894, Sophia Smith Collection, Smith College, Northampton, Mass.
14. Advertisement for "Columbias," *Ladies' Home Journal* 10, no. 3 (February 1893): back cover.
15. Minna Gould Smith, "Women as Cyclers," *Outing* 2 (June 1885): 318, quoted in Mrozek, p. 141; Wood-Allen, p. 73; "The Bicycle and Phthisis," *Medical News* 71 (1897): 535, quoted in Whorton, p. 308.

16. Henry J. Garrigues, "Women and the Bicycle, *"The Forum* 20 (January 1896): 582–87, quoted in Mrozek, p. 148.
17. E. D. Page, "Women and the Bicycle," *Brooklyn Medical Journal* 11 (1897): 82–83.
18. For a discussion of bicycling and female masturbation, see Whorton, pp. 327–28. C. A. Vander Beck, M.D., journal, 1896, p. 195, Strong Museum Library, Rochester, N.Y.
19. Whorton, pp. 312–26.
20. B. W. Mitchell, "A Defense of Football," *Journal of Hygiene and Herald of Health* 45 (1895): 93.
21. Edward Hitchcock, M.D., "The Gymnastic Era and the Athletic Era of Our Country," *Outlook* 51 (1895): 816–18; Walter Camp and Loren F. Deland, *Football* (Boston: Houghton Mifflin, 1896).
22. For a discussion of Lodge and Roosevelt, see Mrozek, pp. 28–66.
23. *Report of the Commissioners Representing the State of New York at the Universal Exposition at Paris, France, 1900* quoted in James E. Sullivan, "Athletics and the Stadium," *Cosmopolitan,* 31, no. 5 (September 1901) 502. pp. 80–81, Horace Fletcher to J. Brennan, July 11, 1912, Fletcher Papers, Houghton Library, Harvard University, Cambridge, Mass.,
24. James E. Sullivan, "Athletics and the Stadium," *Cosmopolitan* 31, no. 5 (September 1901): 501–8.
25. A. G. Spalding and Brothers catalog for 1909, Warshaw Collection of the Archives of the National Museum of American History, Washington, D.C.
26. Frank L. Bristow, *Calisthenic Exercises and Marches* (Cincinnati, Ohio: The John Church Co., 1891). See also E. B. Warman, *Warman's Physical Training, or, The Care of the Body* (Chicago: A. G. Spalding and Brothers, 1889; *Ladies' Home Calisthenics* (Boston: Educational Publishing Co., 1890).
27. Pamphlet for the Whitely Exerciser, ca. 1873, American Sporting Goods Co., St. Louis, Mo., Warshaw Collection of the Archives of the National Museum of American History, Washington, D.C.
28. See Mary Macfadden and Emile Gauvreau, *Dumbbells and Carrot Strips: The Story of Bernarr Macfadden* (New York: Henry Holt and Co., 1953), p. 16.
29. Robert Fielding, "What's Wrong with the Doctors?" *Physical Culture* 46 (July 1921): 24; Bernarr Macfadden, "Owning Our Bodies," *Physical Culture* 44, no. 1 (July 1920): 32.
30. Horace Fletcher to John Brennan, October 29, 1909, Fletcher Papers,

Harvard University, Cambridge, Mass.; Macfadden and Gauvreau, pp. 395–96.

31. *New York Times,* October 6, 1905, p. 9.
32. Ibid.
33. Ibid., October 7, 1905, pp. 8, 4.
34. Macfadden and Gauvreau, pp. 25–26, 28, 24–25.
35. Ibid., p. 182. For a listing of retailers, see, for example, *Physical Culture* 58, no. 6 (December 1927): 24.
36. Macfadden and Gauvreau, p. 65.
37. Ibid., pp. 100, 231.
38. Macfadden, *Macfadden's Encyclopedia of Physical Culture* (New York: Physical Culture Publishing Co., 1914), 1: 120.
39. See, for example, *Physical Culture* 46, no. 1 (July 1921): 99; 65, no. 4 (April 1931): 130; 44, no. 1 (July 1920): 4; 53, no. 6 (December 1924): 3. Any issue between 1920 and 1939 will do.
40. *Physical Culture* 44, no. 1 (July 1920): 1, 83, 97, 107, 118, 143, 145.
41. *Physical Culture* 44, no. 6 (December 1920): 1.
42. Ibid., pp. 1, 75.
43. *Physical Culture* 52, no. 6 (December 1924): 113, 21.
44. *Physical Culture* 58, no. 6 (December 1927): 106; "The Swoboda System," *Cosmopolitan* 31, no. 5 (September 1901): no page number; *Physical Culture* 65, no. 4 (April 1931): 101.
45. Albert E. Wiggam, "Should I Marry a Blond or Brunet?" *Physical Culture* 46, no. 1 (July 1921): 27, 29.
46. Ibid., pp. 80, 81.
47. Ibid., p. 84.
48. Macfadden, *Marriage a Life-Long Honeymoon* (New York: Physical Culture Publishing Co., 1903), pp. 213, 127, 124–25; Wiggam, "Can We Make Motherhood Fashionable?" *Physical Culture* 45, no. 5 (May 1921): 23, 93.
49. Wiggam, "Should I Marry a Blond or Brunet?" pp. 81–82.
50. *Physical Culture* 52, no. 6 (December 1924): 120.
51. *Physical Culture* 52, no. 4 (October 1924): 162; Macfadden, *The Power and Beauty of Superb Womanhood* (New York: Physical Culture Publishing Co., 1901).

CHAPTER TEN. OLD-TIME QUIET IN A BREATHLESS AGE

1. W. J. Burnett, M.D., to D. S. Sanford, esq., June 28, 1900, Bakken Library, Minneapolis.
2. Luther Gulick, *The Efficient Life* (New York: Doubleday, Page, and Co.,

1909), p. 107; William B. Forbush, *The Boy Problem: A Study in Social Pedagogy* (Philadelphia: Westminster Press, 1902), p. 145.

3. Horace Fletcher to James E. West, January 26, 1911, Fletcher Papers, Houghton Library, Harvard University, Cambridge, Mass.

4. T. J. Jackson Lears, *No Place of Grace: Antimodernism and the Transformation of American Culture, 1880–1920* (New York: Pantheon Books, 1982), p. 108.

5. Advertising brochure for the Sanitarian Equipment Company (Battle Creek, Mich., ca. 1927), Warshaw Collection of the Archives of the National Museum of American History, Washington, D.C.

6. Advertising brochure for the International Health Devices Corporation (New York, 1926).

7. Advertising card, Owen Belt and Appliance Co., Chicago, Illinois, ca. 1890–1900, Bakken Library, Minneapolis; advertisement excised from *Harper's Magazine* 84, no. 494 (December 1891), Bakken Library.

8. Advertisement from *Lippincott's Magazine*, ca. 1890–1900, Bakken Library, Minneapolis.

9. Riley Electric Company advertisement, *Munsey's Magazine* (January 1906): advertising section, Bakken Library, Minneapolis; catalog of the Chloride of Silver Dry Cell Battery Company, Baltimore, Md., 1898, Bakken Library, Minneapolis.

10. "Stop That Pain!" *Physical Culture* 58, no. 6 (December 1927): 119; *Physical Culture* 44, no. 1 (July 1920): 67; "Electric Health Brush," *Physical Culture* 44, no. 6 (December 1920): 89.

11. "Star Vibrator," *Physical Culture* 45, no. 6 (December 1920): 97; "Be a Credit to Your Sex," *Physical Culture* 45, no. 1 (January 1921): 67.

12. "Professor Chrystal's Electric Belts and Appliances," (Marshall, Mich.: ca. 1900), pp. 5, 11, 6; Bakken Library, Minneapolis.

13. C. A. Vander Beck, journal 1894–1897, pp. 265, 270, Strong Museum Library, Rochester, N.Y.

14. Professor Chrystal's Electric Belts and Appliances," pp. 14–16, 19.

15. Advertising pamphlet for O-P-C suspensories (Chicago, ca. 1910), unpaginated, Warshaw Collection of the National Museum of American History, Washington, D.C.

16. Ibid.

17. *Physical Culture* 44, no. 1 (July 1920): 100.

18. *Sixth Annual Report of the Boston Young Men's Christian Association* (Boston: Ticknor and Fields, 1857), p. 14; Mary Wood-Allen, *What Every Young Woman Ought to Know* (Philadelphia: The Vir Publishing Co., 1905), pp. 227–37; Emma F. Drake, *What a Young Wife Ought to Know* (Philadelphia: Vir Publishing Company, 1908), pp. 87–88.

19. Sylvanus Stall, *What a Young Man Ought to Know* (Philadelphia: The Vir Publishing Co., 1897), p. 241; Mary Wood-Allen, *Marriage, Its Duties and Privileges* (Chicago: F. H. Revell, 1901), p. 49; Bernarr Macfadden, *Marriage a Life-Long Honeymoon* (New York: Physical Culture Publishing Co., 1903), pp. 245–46, 82, 147–48.
20. Paul von Boeckmann, "Nervous Americans," *Physical Culture* 44, no. 1 (July 1920): 79. See also "The Force That Drives Us On—On and On," *Physical Culture* 44, no. 6 (December 1920): 77; "Nerves," *Physical Culture* 46, no. 6 (December 1921): 77; "Have You These Symptoms of Nerve Exhaustion?" *Physical Culture* 65, no. 4 (April 1931): 119; "Now You Can Master Your Jangled Nerves," *Physical Culture* 81, no. 5 (May 1939): 7.
21. *Vibration: Nature's Great Underlying Force for Health, Strength, and Beauty* (Detroit: Golden Manufacturing Co., 1914), pp. 2–3.
22. Frederick W. Coburn, "A Colonial Crafts Museum, *The Craftsman* 7, no. 2 (November 1904): 159.
23. Gustav Stickley, "From Ugliness to Beauty," *The Craftsman* 7, no. 3 (December, 1904): 315. See also Stickley, "How Boston Goes about Civic Improvement," *The Craftsman* 16, no. 4 (April 1909): 92–95.
24. Richardson Wright et al., "Williamsburg: What It Means to Architecture, to Gardening, to Decoration," *House and Garden* 72 (November 1937): 68–79. See also, "New Williamsburg Inn," *House Beautiful* 79 (July 1937): 24–25. Not everyone bowed reverently before Williamsburg; Frank Lloyd Wright called the style "codfish colonial."
25. Irene Sargent, "John Ruskin," *The Craftsman* 1 (November 1901), quoted in Lears, p. 71.
26. See Lears, pp. 84, 93.
27. Fletcher to "Fred," July 20, 1908, Fletcher Papers, Houghton Library, Harvard University, Cambridge, Mass.
28. Ibid.
29. See Lears, p. 101.
30. Stickley, "Some Pasadena Houses Showing Harmony Between Structure and Landscape," *The Craftsman* 16, no. 2 (May 1909): 216–21; Idem, "The Value of Permanent Architecture as a Truthful Expression of National Character," *The Craftsman* 16, no. 1 (April 1909): 80–91.
31. Fletcher to Paul Waddell, February 25, 1901, Fletcher Papers, Houghton Library, Harvard University, Cambridge, Mass.
32. Fletcher to West, January 18, 1914, Fletcher Papers, Houghton Library, Harvard University, Cambridge, Mass.
33. See, for example, Natalie Curtis, "A Bit of American Folk Music: Two Pueblo Indian Grinding Songs," *The Craftsman* 7, no. 1 (October 1904):

35–41; Irene Sargent, "Indian Basketry: Its Structure and Design," *The Craftsman* 7, no. 3 (December 1904): 321–34; Frederick Monsen, "Pueblos of the Painted Desert," *The Craftsman* 12, no. 1 (April 1907): 16–33; Frederick Burton, "Music from the Ojibway's Point of View," *The Craftsman* 12, no. 4 (July 1907): 375–81; Natalie Curtis, "The Creation Myth of the Cochans (Yuma Indians)," *The Craftsman* 16, no. 5 (August 1909): 559–62; Edward Curtis, *The North American Indian* (New York: Johnson Reprints, reprint of 1903–1930 edition).

34. Fletcher to West, July 30, 1912, Fletcher Papers, Houghton Library, Harvard University, Cambridge, Mass.

35. For detailed explanations of the continuing relationship between military ideas and sport, see Donald R. Mrozek, *Sport and American Mentality, 1880–1910* (Knoxville, Tenn.: University of Tennessee Press, 1983), pp. 28–66. For an intelligent discussion of militarism and themes of regeneration in turn-of-the-century America, see Lears, pp. 101, 112–13, and 116–17 especially.

36. Studs Terkel, *Hard Times* (New York: Pantheon Books, 1970); Warren Susman, *Culture and Commitment* (New York: George Braziller, 1973); Caroline Bird, *Invisible Scar* (New York: Longman, 1966).

CHAPTER ELEVEN. DIETETIC RIGHTEOUSNESS

1. Mary Wood-Allen, *What a Young Wife Ought to Know* (Philadelphia: The Vir Publishing Co., 1905), p. 48.

2. Horace Fletcher to John Harvey Kellogg, January 2, 1912, Fletcher Papers, Houghton Library, Harvard University, Cambridge, Mass.

3. Ibid.; Fletcher to Kellogg, ca. 1908—Fletcher Papers, Houghton Library, Harvard University, Cambridge, Mass.

4. Fletcher to Irving Fisher, July 26, 1914; Fletcher to Kellogg, December 14, 1910—Fletcher Papers, Houghton Library, Harvard University, Cambridge, Mass.

5. Wood-Allen, pp. 79–80; Kellogg, *Household Manual*, 51–59.

6. "Do Nine Out of Ten Persons Commit Suicide?" *Physical Culture* 45, no. 1 (January 1921): 103.

7. Ibid.

8. "Conquer Constipation," *Physical Culture* 46, no. 1 (July 1921): 87. See also "Are You Afraid of Constipation?" *Physical Culture* 58, no. 6 (December 1927): 118.

9. "You May Bathe Daily and Still Not Be Clean," *Physical Culture* 45, no. 5 (May 1921): 137.

10. Advertising card for Enno Sander Mineral Water Company, ca. 1905.

See also advertising pamphlet for Rubins Healing Springs Lithia Water, ca. 1910. Both in Warshaw Collection of the Archives of the National Museum of American History, Washington, D.C. Figures from James C. Whorton, *Crusaders for Fitness* (Princeton, N.J.: Princeton University Press, 1982), p. 258.

11. Advertisements for the "Health and Pleasure Resorts with Medicinal Springs" and "Health and Pleasure Resorts with Medicinal Wells," ca. 1910, Warshaw Collection of Archives of the National Museum of American History, Washington, D.C.; *Laurel Springs Courier* 4, no. 1 (May 1894): 1.
12. *Price List,* Morris and Schrader, Importers and Traders in Mineral Waters, New York, N.Y., ca. 1900–1910, Warshaw Collection of the Archives of the National Museum of American History, Washington, D.C.
13. On the insecurity and uncertainty of water and other facilities in cities at the turn of the century, see David Handlin, *The American Home, 1815–1915* (Boston: Little, Brown and Co., 1979), pp. 452–86.
14. *The Pasteur Germ-Proof Water Filter, 1894* (Dayton, Ohio: The Pasteur-Chamberland Filter Co., 1894), p. 2.
15. *Illustrated Catalog, 1894, McConnell Germ-Proof Water Filters* (Buffalo, N.Y.: 1894), pp. 8, 12–13.
16. Ibid., back cover.
17. Catalog for "The Ralston New Process Still" (New York: n.p., ca. 1900), pp. 17–21; catalog for "The Cuprigraph Sanitary Still" (Chicago: n.p., 1897), pp. 2, 7–8.
18. Fletcher's life is summarized in Whorton, pp. 168–69.
19. Fletcher to Paul Waddell, October 7, 1898, Fletcher Papers, Houghton Library, Harvard University, Cambridge, Mass.
20. Fletcher to Mary W. Waterman, October 31, 1909, Fletcher Papers, Houghton Library, Harvard University, Cambridge, Mass.
21. Handlin, pp. 193, 194.
22. Fletcher to Abby Fletcher, November 11, 1898, Fletcher Papers, Houghton Library, Harvard University, Cambridge, Mass.
23. W. G. Anderson to Russell H. Chittenden, June 25, 1908, Fletcher Papers, Houghton Library, Harvard University, Cambridge, Mass.
24. Ibid., pp. 2–4.
25. Ibid., pp. 5, 6.
26. Fletcher to Russell H. Chittenden, October 15, 1909; Fletcher to Gideon Wells, August 18, 1912—Horace Fletcher Papers, Houghton Library, Harvard University, Cambridge, Mass.

27. Fletcher to James P. Reilly, March 17, 1901, Horace Fletcher Papers, Houghton Library, Harvard University, Cambridge, Mass.
28. Fletcher to Robert M. Thompson, September 30, 1910, Horace Fletcher Papers; Fletcher to William James, November 7, 1905, William James Papers. Henry James to Horace Fletcher, January 5, 1906; Henry James to Horace Fletcher, September 21, 1905; Henry James to Horace Fletcher, July 22, 1908; Henry James to Horace Fletcher, December 4, 1907—Henry James Papers. All at Houghton Library, Harvard University, Cambridge, Mass.
29. Fletcher to William James, February 22, 1909; William James to Henry James (Fletcher's letter inscribed in William James's hand), ca. February 22–March, 1909—William James Papers. Fletcher to Kellogg, April 19, 1911, Fletcher Papers, April 19, 1911. Houghton Library, Harvard University, Cambridge, Mass.
30. Fletcher to Fisher, June 2, 1913; Fletcher to W. E. Berry, November 18, 1912—Fletcher Papers, Houghton Library, Harvard University, Cambridge, Mass.
31. Fletcher to General Leonard Wood, March 27, 1906, Fletcher Papers, Houghton Library, Harvard University, Cambridge, Mass.
32. Fletcher to Kellogg, July 29, 1911; Advertising Brochure for Fletcher, (n.p., n.d.) 10—Fletcher Papers, Houghton Library, Harvard University, Cambridge, Mass.
33. Fletcher to Kellogg, November 18, 1903, Fletcher Papers, Houghton Library, Harvard University, Cambridge, Mass.
34. Fletcher, *Optimism: A Real Remedy* (Chicago, 1908), pp. 15–16; Fletcher to William James, February 22, 1909; Fletcher to William James, September 27, 1908—William James Papers, Houghton Library, Harvard University, Cambridge, Mass.
35. *Horace Fletcher*, advertising brochure, ca. 1909, William James Papers, Houghton Library, Harvard University, Cambridge, Mass.
36. Fletcher to Berry, November 18, 1912; Fletcher to Kellogg, October 31, 1919—Fletcher Papers, Houghton Library, Harvard University, Cambridge, Mass.
37. Fletcher to Robert M. Thompson, October 1, 1910, Fletcher Papers, Houghton Library, Harvard University, Cambridge, Mass.
38. Horace Fletcher, *That Last Waif, or Social Quarantine* (Chicago: Kindergarten Literature Company, 1898).
39. Fletcher to Kellogg, August 2, 1910; Fletcher to Kellogg, August 6, 1910; Fletcher to Wood, May 20, 1903, Fletcher Papers, Houghton Library, Harvard University, Cambridge, Mass.
40. Biographical information on Atwater is in Whorton, pp. 141–42; Wilbur

O. Atwater and A. P. Bryant, *Dietary Studies of University Boat Crews*, U.S. Department of Agriculture, Office of Experiment Stations, Bulletin no. 25 (Washington, D.C.: U.S. Government Printing Office, 1900), pp. 66–72, quoted in Whorton, p. 228.

41. Woods Hutchinson, *Instinct and Health* (New York: Dodd, Mead and Co., 1908), pp. 18, 34, 46–47; "The Dangers of Undereating," *Cosmopolitan* 47 (1909): 388, quoted in Whorton, pp. 207–8.

42. Fletcher to Fisher, July 29, 1914, Fletcher Papers, Houghton Library, Harvard University, Cambridge, Mass.

43. Whorton, pp. 229–31.

44. Advertising cards for Ayer's Sarsaparilla, Lydia Pinkham's Vegetable Compound, and Magnetized Food, Strong Museum Library, Rochester, N.Y.

45. Whorton, p. 208.

46. Gerald Carson, *Cornflake Crusade* (New York: Rinehart and Company, 1957), pp. 93–94, 119–22.

47. Ibid., pp. 149, 151, 157.

48. Ibid., pp. 176–82.

49. Advertisement for Van Houten Cocoa, *The Ladies Home Journal* 10, no. 9 (August 1893): 15.

50. Advertisement, *The Ladies' Home Journal* 15, no. 1 (December 1897): 29.

51. "Driving the Brain," *Ladies Home Journal* 10, no. 3 (February 1893): 27; "Somatose," *Ladies Home Journal* 15, no. 1 (December 1897): 22; "Brains . . . ," *Cosmopolitan* 31, no. 5 (September 1901): back cover.

52. *Physical Culture* 44, no. 1 (July 1920): 89.

53. "Half a Man on a Whole Man's Job," *Physical Culture* 45, no. 5 (May 1921): 63; "Not All People Are Born Robust . . . Not All the Robust Live Long, *"Ladies Home Journal* 49, no. 11 (November 1927): 57; interview with Rudy Vallee, "Morning Edition," National Public Radio, April 17, 1985.

54. See, for example, *Physical Culture* 46, no. 1 (July 1921): 106, 107; 45, no. 5 (May 1921): 107; "An Advantage—Kellogg's All Bran," *Physical Culture* 52, no. 6 (December 1924): 102; "Ruts," *Physical Culture* 58, no. 6 (December 1927): 71.

55. "Pillsbury's Health Bran," *Physical Culture* 58, no. 6 (December 1927): back cover; "They'll Do You Good, Daddy," *Physical Culture* 52, no. 6 (December 1924): 75; "Mrs. Warren Writes to Mrs. Carr," *Physical Culture* 58, no. 6 (December 1927): 69; "Famous Women Say That Food Like This Is Essential to Health and Achievement," *Ladies Home Journal* 43, no. 8 (August 1926): 48.

56. "There's Strength in Every Shred," *Physical Culture* 65, no. 4 (April 1931): 79; "She *Could* Be Beautiful," *Ladies Home Journal* 43, no. 8 (August 1927): 54.
57. "Famous Doctor Eats Sauerkraut for Breakfast," *Physical Culture* 53, no. 6 (December 1924): 74; "Parkelp," *Physical Culture* 81, no. 5 (May 1939): 77, 81.
58. "Famous Women Say That Food Like This Is Essential to Health and Achievement," *Ladies Home Journal* 43, no. 8 (August 1926): 48.
59. Paul Starr, *The Social Transformation of American Medicine* (New York: Basic Books, 1982), pp. 113–17.
60. Ibid., pp. 136–37.
61. Interview with Dr. Winifred Curtis, Rochester, N.Y., November 14, 1984.

· PICTURE CREDITS ·

With the following exceptions, all illustrations appear courtesy of the Strong Museum, Rochester, N.Y.:

Illustrations on pp. 99, 110, 146, 156, 196, 197, 199, 200, 215, 240, 241, 278, 289, 292, and 293 courtesy Collection of Business Americana, Archives Center, National Museum of American History, Smithsonian Institution.

Photograph on p. 228 courtesy Division of Community Life, National Museum of American History, Smithsonian Institution, Hood College Collection.

Bottles and flasks illustrated on pp. 37, 126, and 304 are the gift of Dr. Burton Spiller to the Strong Museum, Rochester, N.Y.

Photograph on p. 209 below, courtesy Wyoming Historical and Geological Society, Wilkes-Barre, Pennsylvania, Erskine Solomon Collection.

Photographs on p. 244 courtesy Minnesota Historical Society Photographic Collection.

· INDEX ·

Neubauer, Ignatius, 250–52
neurasthenia (nervous prostration),
104, 136, 136–66, 231, 238,
271, 272, 273
causes of, 137–40, 165, 268, 321
definitions of, 259–60
treatments for, 140, 142, 145,
148, 149, 151, 158, 159, 166,
168, 174, 208, 260
New Guide to Health, A
(Thomson), 7
*New Gymnastics for Men, Women,
and Children* (Lewis), 138,
184, 188, 204
New Hydropathic Cook-Book
(Trall), 31, 45
New Nerves for Old (Blackstone),
268
New Theory of Disease, A (Wells),
168–69
Nichols, Mary Gove, 92

occupational hazards, 13, 21, 64,
74–75, 136
Olmsted, John C., 295–96
Olympic Games, 237–39, 242
opium, 40, 41, 43, 105
"Our Home on the Hillside," 65,
134, 247, 308
outdoor life, 87, 128–31, 139, 229,
237, 238, 261
overeating and overweight, 28,
30–35, 64, 95, 160, 179,
295–301
Owen, Calvin, 9, 12, 16, 59–60,
70

pace of life, 31, 62, 96, 137–39,
183, 268, 281
"Pangymnastikon," 188–89, 195,
204
Passing of the Great Race, The
(Grant), 253–54
patent medicines, 28, 39–40, 45,
126, 127, 138, 140, 149, 174,
286–87, 304–6
Patterson, John H., 295–96

perfectionism, 10, 13, 29, 44, 50,
54, 103, 182, 213, 249–50,
300, 320
Perkins, Elisha, 69
Perky, Henry D., 308
phrenology, 64, 75
Phrenology Known by Its Fruit
(Reese), 19–20
Physical Culture, 245, 249–52, 253,
255, 266, 267, 311, 312, 319
physical education, 12, 29, 52,
89–100, 181, 183, 213–14,
302–3
in college, 202–3, 204–5, 208,
227–28
evolution of American attitudes
toward, 95–100
instructors, 138, 184–91, 202–5,
210, 213–15, 321–22
mental education and, 23–24,
91–94, 183–84, 214, 249–50
nutritional research and, 302–4
*Physical Education and the
Preservation of Health*
(Warren), 91–92
physicians, 3–10
deference paid to, 28, 315–16
health-goods manufacturers and,
263
hostility towards, 10, 12–13, 59,
64, 103, 135–36, 166, 245
see also medical practice
Physiology and Calisthenics
(Beecher), 95
Pinkham, Lydia, 306
Pleasonton, Augustus James,
176–79
plumbing and drainage, 108, 125,
154, 156–57
Post, Charles W., 65, 294, 306,
308, 311, 312, 313, 314
Postum, 308, 309, 311
*Power and Beauty of Superb
Womanhood* (Macfadden),
257
*Practical Treatise on the Medical
and Surgical Uses of
Electricity, A* (Beard and
Rockwell), 171–72